THE
HOOD HEALTH
HANDBOOK

A PRACTICAL GUIDE to HEALTH and WELLNESS in the URBAN COMMUNITY

VOLUME ONE

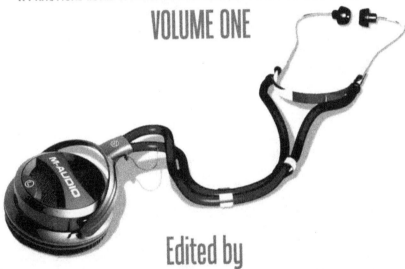

Edited by
SUPREME UNDERSTANDING and C'BS ALIFE ALLAH

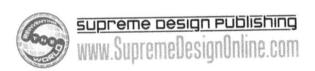

supreme Design Publishing
www.SupremeDesignOnline.com

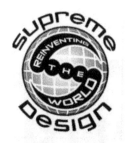

The Hood Health Handbook: A Practical Guide to Health and Wellness in the Urban Community. Copyright ©2010 by Supreme Design, LLC. All rights reserved. No part of this book may be reproduced in any form or by any electronic or mechanical means including information storage and retrieval systems without permission in writing from the publisher, except by a reviewer, who may quote brief passages in a review. Published by Supreme Design Publishing. PO Box 10887, Atlanta, GA 30310.

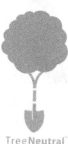

Supreme Design Publishing books are printed on long-lasting acid-free paper. When it is available, we choose paper that has been manufactured by environmentally responsible practices. These may include using trees grown in sustainable forests, incorporating recycled paper, minimizing chlorine in bleaching, or recycling the energy produced at the paper mill.

Supreme Design Publishing is also a member of the Tree Neutral™ initiative, which works to offset paper consumption through tree planting.

TreeNeutral

ISBN-13: 978-1-935721-32-1   LCCN: 2010934315

Wholesale Discounts. Special discounts (up to 55% off of retail) are available on quantity purchases. For details, visit our website, contact us by mail at the address above, Attention: Wholesale Orders, or email us at orders@supremedesignonline.com

Individual Sales. Supreme Design publications are available for retail purchase, or by request, at most bookstores. They can also be ordered directly from the Supreme Design Publishing website, at www.SupremeDesignOnline.com

Visit us on the web at

www.HoodHealthHandbook.com

FOREWORD

BY DICK GREGORY

I was born and raised knowing *nothing* about nutrition. For us growing up, if you got enough of whatever you liked when you were eating, and it didn't run out before you were full, I considered that "good nutrition." And if it ran out before you got enough of what you liked, I considered that "bad nutrition." There was so little information out there at the time. Even when I started searching for something better, I didn't know what that was. At that time, I was smoking four packs of cigarettes a day, drinking a fifth of Scotch every day, and my weight was on its way up to 365 pounds. For so many years, I didn't know the things I was eating or doing were bad for me, because the Ku Klux Klan didn't give it to me. My mother gave it to me. My father gave it to me. My church gave it to me. My school gave it to me. My friends gave it to me. Now, when I'd sit and go through my fifth of Scotch every day, none of my friends or anyone close to me called me a nut. When I would light cigarette after cigarette, no one called me a nut. When my weight was ballooning, nobody called me a nut.

Then one day, I went on a fast to protest the war in Vietnam, guided by one of the more brilliant minds that ever lived (pertaining to health and nutrition), a brilliant black woman by the name of Dr. Fulton. When I changed my lifestyle, no more smoking, no more drinking, no more weight problem, THAT'S when I was called a nut! All these things I was doing to destroy myself and not knowing what I was doing, and nobody ever called me a nut. But when I wanted to become healthy, then I was a nut. But the real nut is the one who's killing himself and he doesn't know or doesn't care. People ask me now, "You've been fasting for 40 years, what does your doctor think?" I tell em, "My doctor's been dead 30 years."

Before we can talk about health in "the hood," let me break something down for you: A "hood" is something you use to hide something. Think about the Ku Klux Klan. When they would raid at night, they would put on a hood. In America, when you get the electric chair, they don't want whoever's gonna do this to sit and look at you, so they put a hood on you. When people go before the firing squad, all around the world, they put a hood on you. So a "hood" is used to hide something. So when we refer to the ghetto as "the hood," there's something we're hiding. From racism, to sexism, to the way we been abused, to insanity, and we're not even aware that it's insanity we're hiding. We have to destroy what it is we're trying to hide, and we do that by purifying "the hood" and getting rid of all the things that make it so ugly you want to hide it. When we destroy this *hood*, it becomes a *community*. That's why white folks do not live in a hood. They live in a community, because in a community, you control your economy, you control your cops, you control finances, you control your educational system, you control your healthcare...and that we DON'T. But we can.

That is why this book is so important. In all my world travels, never have I picked up a book with the kind of love, concern, and information that I've seen put into this book. Money is not power. A degree is not power. Information is power. The power in this book is unimaginable. I thank the editors for taking the time and effort to teach the masses the truth about how important diet and nutrition are, in the mightiest nation in the world that has never done so for their people. I've never had something in my hand that has something useful, something important, something that's been "hidden" from us, on every page. On every page there's something you must know.

Some of you aren't even aware that you're eating bad or living unhealthy. You, especially, should read this book, and read it over and over. I can't help but think back to the great Elijah Muhammad, who talked about how diet is just as important as liberation. After all, what good is liberation if you're headed down the path to meet the Grim Reaper?

When my grandmother was alive, she didn't "analyze" much, because she dealt with *wisdom* and not intelligence. When you look at the Bible, it doesn't mention "intelligent" and "smart," it mentions *wisdom*. If I could put one label on this book and nothing else, I would call it *Great Wisdom*, and my grandmother would understand that. And because my grandmother trusted me, like millions of other people do today, I would relate to her by saying, "Put this book next the Bible." I wouldn't have to tell her anything else. She would know that this book was something *that* important for her to read.

When I was a little boy in Missouri, we would listen to the news on the radio and hear about forest fires burning in California. The governor would say, "If we don't get a shift in the wind, we won't be able to save it." I was born in 1932, and now it's 2010, and I have yet to read

4

where a state all the way burned down. Obviously, the winds changed. And this shift in the wind can only come from the universal God force. When I look at the state of health in America, particularly African Americans, I say, "My God, we need a shift in the wind." Now I can say to you that I believe this book is the shift in the wind we've been waiting for.

God Bless,

Dick Gregory

DICK GREGORY is a pioneer in both the worlds of comedy and social justice. He is one of the first performers to break the 'color barrier' in comedy, yet he never shied away from talking about race and poverty. Through the 1960s, Gregory spent more time on social issues and less time on performing. He has fasted in protest more than 60 times. He marched with MLK, ran for mayor of Chicago against Richard Daley, and ran for president against Nixon. In 1973, after developing an interest in vegetarianism, he became a health consultant and published *Dick Gregory's Natural Diet for Folks Who Eat: Cookin' with Mother Nature!* His social activism has continued into recent years, including a 1990 protest at CIA headquarters over their role in the crack-cocaine epidemic in Black communities. In 2001, Gregory announced to the world that he had been diagnosed with a rare form of cancer. He refused traditional medical treatment, and with the assistance of some of the finest minds in alternative medicine, put together a holistic regimen which ultimately resulted in his reversing the cancer. Today, he is 100% "cancer-free." He and his beloved wife, Lil, have raised ten children who have become highly respected members of the national community in a variety of fields.

TABLE OF CONTENTS

DISCLAIMER

Let's get one thing clear before we go anywhere. We're not doctors. Well, technically Supreme Understanding has a doctorate, but we're not medical doctors, bound to the rules and regulations of the Western medical establishment. Then again, some of the authors are medical doctors, but just pretend they aren't either. Just treat us all like people with opinions (opinions that some people disagree with very strongly), and we're simply providing our person opinions for informational purposes only. We don't hold ourselves to the code that binds many doctors to ineffective practices and corporate-sponsored madness. Yet we can't help but be bound to U.S. law, which some nut-job may try to use one day to ruin our lives. We don't want anybody suing us because they think we're prescribing medicine (we're not) or telling people to ignore their doctors and listen to us (we're not), so we've got to provide this sucky legal disclaimer.

Here goes: The information provided in this book should not be construed as personal medical advice or instruction. No action should be taken based solely on the contents of this book. Readers should consult appropriate health professionals on any matter relating to their health and wellbeing. The information and opinions provided here are believed to be accurate and sound, based on the best judgment available to the authors, but readers who fail to consult appropriate health authorities assume the risk of any injuries. This book is not responsible for errors or omissions.

Hip Hop's State of Emergency

Our Health Crisis

STATE OF THE UNION ADDRESS TO THE HIP-HOP GENERATION

BY SUPA NOVA SLOM, THE HIP HOP MEDICINE MAN

Dear Hip-Hop Generation,

This is a call to my fellow hip-hop artists, community, and generation at large:

WAKE UP!!! HIP-HOP IS DYING!!!! IT IS IN A STATE OF EMERGENCY AND WE ARE IN AN URGENT HEALTH CRISIS! HIP-HOP ARTISTS ARE DYING, OUR FAMILIES ARE DYING, AND THE HIP-HOP GENERATION IS THE FIRST GENERATION THAT MAY NOT OUTLIVE THEIR PARENTS!!!

As we mourn the passing of the Hip-Hop icon, Guru, I challenge all of his peers and fans to not let his death be in vain. There is no reason that Guru, and so many others under 45, should be passing away at the rate that they are. Every Hip-Hop head, sista in the club, college student, brutha on the corner, G, and hustler is personally (or knows someone who is), battling cancer, arthritis, diabetes, asthma, hypertension, obesity, or one of many other illnesses. These illnesses are mostly caused, or worsened, by the foods that we eat.

Don't think for one minute that your aunties, big Mamas, and parents are the only ones battling these sicknesses. African American and Latino communities lead the statistics for all of these crippling diseases, and people under 40 are being hit at younger and younger ages. (See "We The Illest").

You don't have to be old, poor, overweight, or live in the hood to be sick. Beyond being a Hip-Hop artist, I am a second-generation holistic health advocate. I have travelled on the road with Erykah Badu as her wellness consultant, and over the years I have encountered countless celebrities that are dealing with both minor and major ailments. (See "Hip Hop And Health?")

On the personal front, I am sick and tired of losing young people and reading outlandish statistics. At this point, NOBODY IS EXEMPT.

Everyone is vulnerable to these diseases, and unless you make some immediate, major changes, which incorporate healthier eating habits and lifestyle practices, you may not live to see 50.

If you are living on the American diet, YOU ARE A WALKING, TICKING TIME BOMB, ready to explode at any moment from the constant build-up of fast foods, fried foods, candies, sodas, sugar drinks, and chemical additives that you are constantly ingesting. I am talking to YOU in this letter. (See "The Wrong Foods")

People's number one excuse is that eating healthy costs too much, but most of these people are the same ones that spend hundreds of dollars on Jordans, Coach, Prada, car rims, and other material indulgences. When we tell these same people, who may buy two or three bottles in the club, to go buy a juicer, they say that that's too expensive. Our priorities are horribly messed up when it comes to spending money and taking care of ourselves.

It is easy to say, "Oh, we can't afford organic food," or to frown on the foods that we aren't familiar with, but we must look at the food situation in this country in the simplest and most straight-forward sense. Everyone has heard the terms, "only the strong survive," or "survival of the fittest." Well, the food war being waged on the poor people in this country is ensuring that we are not fit to survive. Compare the foods that are available in poorer areas to the food that is available in richer areas. Look at the menus of restaurants in well-to-do, trendy parts of town, and compare them to the menus at the fast food joints that are plentiful in the hood. Food has been transformed into a drug which kills off the poor people in this country. It's literally, modern-day, biological warfare and eugenics. Food is pumped up with chemicals and is force-fed to a very particular group of people, using colorful marketing, appealing smells, affordable prices, and a lack of options. (See "Spending Less To Feed More")

People in the hood are masters at knowing how to stretch what is available to them and making the most of it. This has long been the root of survival, and we must apply that same thinking to healthy living. In the past, African Americans have been directly targeted, restricted, and torn down with slavery, Jim Crow, a lack of voting rights, crack, unequal schooling, and the prison/"justice" system. We now can add FOOD to that list. We need to fight against their food attack in the same ways that we have organized and fought against their other racist attacks, but even harder. This fight is not just for equal access, or for just conditions. This fight is literally for our lives!

People have become accustomed to trying the new, green shake at McDonald's, or the new, glow-in-the-dark soda, and they never question what the ingredients are. But, the moment that these same people are offered a vegetable that they have never seen, or a healthy, green juice, they want to know exactly what it is, and everything that is in it. That is the type of mentality that has effectively been fed to us through advertising and marketing schemes. No one asks why chemicals are being added to foods and vegetables that were just fine without the sprays. Instead, our generation just thinks: price, taste, and packaging. Just as the Hip-Hop generation has become accustomed to defending its lives on the streets, so we must defend our lives with our food choices. We are always so quick to bang on each other, and so slow to bang for the things that matter, such as our own lives.

I recently wrote a book called, *The Remedy: The Five Week Power Plan to Detox Your System, Combat the Fat, and Rebuild Your Mind and Body.* It is the first, comprehensive wellness book written with the Hip-Hop generation in mind. It features testimonies from Melyssa Ford, Hype Williams, Tyson Beckford, Erykah Badu, Chuck D., and Jim Jones. They share with the reader the simple things that they do to maintain healthy and active lives. I provide the step-by-step plan to remedy your body, and work towards preventing future sickness through diet, exercise and positive thinking. Below is a list of tips that are easy to incorporate, and tools that can change your entire life:

- ❏ Commit to yourself and life. Decide that you want to live and feel good.
- ❏ Try to drink as close to a gallon of water a day, as you can.
- ❏ Eat something fresh and green in every meal.
- ❏ Substitute the bleached products with healthy alternatives, such as brown sugar, brown rice, wheat, spelt, or other whole grain flours.
- ❏ Cut out fried foods, or at least reduce your intake to once a week.
- ❏ Eat your heaviest meal between 12 noon and 6pm.
- ❏ Do some form of exercise each day.
- ❏ Start reading the labels on the foods that you are eating, and eat things that have the least amount of additives.

Big Pun passed. We didn't take heed. Nate Dogg had two strokes. Not much was said. When we lost J. Dilla, finally, people started to show some concern. When Phife Dawg exposed his battle with diabetes, people began to realize that there is an issue. But still, no one has effectively challenged our generation on a widespread scale, to reclaim our wellness, at every level. Today, I challenge every one of you to stand up, and take charge of your own health. We have just lost Guru, and Nate Dogg. The entire Hip-Hop community is in mourning. Let's take this opportunity to seize the time, before we find ourselves back here, again — with the next artist or family member dying too early and too soon. In the midst of the street beefs, egoism, misogyny, disunity, and materialism, I call for unity amongst us all on the issue of survival and health. It's about time that we get sick and tired of being sick and tired, and DO SOMETHING! In the memory of Guru, let's all get GANGSTARR for our health and wellness.

Salute!

Supa Nova Slom, the Hip-Hop Medicine Man

Originator of The Hip Hop meditation Ciphers, member of Bill Cosby's Hip-Hop project, The Cosnarati, and founder of "Unify the Hood, Heal the Hood," SUPA NOVA SLOM is a galvanizing force for today's youth and beyond. In early 2010 he released his first book entitled *The Remedy: The Five-Week Power Plan to Detox Your System, Combat the Fat, and Rebuild Your Mind and Body* and simultaneously released his album, also entitled *The Remedy*, which features Erykah Badu, Jadakiss, and The Game. Supa Nova is currently completing his second documentary, *Holistic Wellness for the Hip Hop Generation Part II*, and has recently launched his own wellness supplement line, Supa Foods. For more information on Supa Nova Slom and his work, visit www.supanovaslom.com and www.theremedybook.com

INTRODUCTION

HEALTH IS WEALTH

BY C'BS ALIFE ALLAH AND SUPREME UNDERSTANDING

State of Affairs in the Urban Community

We're sick. We're dying. And we need answers, insight, and practical solutions. We need ways that will work. And they exist. But we've got to start with what's kept us from finding these answers till now.

Let's be real. We can't talk about health in urban communities without coming to grips with a few basic things. First of all, "urban community" is just a nice way of saying "the hood." And by "the hood," we really mean poor Black and brown people. And when we talk about health among poor Black and brown people, we can't approach it the same way we would for another group of people...except maybe middle class Black and brown people, since they're just as sick. But the bottom line is that there's no way to separate race and health when you look at the outcomes. Blacks, Latinos, and Native Americans have the highest rates of cancer, diabetes, heart disease, high blood pressure, asthma, lead poisoning, reproductive damage, nutritional deficiency, food allergies, post-traumatic stress disorder, teen suicide, sleep paralysis, gonorrhea, syphilis, herpes, Alzheimer's disease...c'mon son! You name it![1]

So what makes you think that the CAUSES are different? And what do Blacks, Latinos, and Native Americans have in common, besides the fact that most of us live in the hood (or "barrio" or "reservation" but it's all, "the hood")?[2] Let's keep it simple. If white people

---

[1] Not an exaggeration. All the claims in this book are based on published studies and research.

[2] Don't get it twisted if you think you're not in this group. It's a well-documented fact that even so-called "middle class" Blacks and Latinos are not living the "American Dream" at ANY level even CLOSE to their white peers. Not to mention the fact, that – since our wealth is rarely generational – we're always a step away from being back in poverty... and in fact, many of our children end up poor, no matter how much money we thought we were making. Not to mention that an "I'm not ghetto" distinction makes no sense for THIS book, since middle class Blacks and Latinos are nearly just as sick as poor Blacks and

conquered your country, put you in slavery, and/or stripped you of your culture (religion, language, values, institutions, etc.), what makes you think they want you healthy and strong NOW? Go into the hood (or the barrio) and you are going to get bombarded with the same images. It's unmistakable. Everywhere you go, you will find Original people (otherwise known as "People of Color" or Indigenous people) [3] in their own "Great Depression." A "depression" isn't limited to the lack of economic opportunities. Depression is the condition describing all of those things that, together, cause our people to be unable to operate to the best of our ability. Health is wealth. And we're more than financially poor…we're afflicted with health poverty.

WHY THIS BOOK WAS WRITTEN

A bunch of us got together and decided that we needed to let people know that they don't need to be sick. You don't need to give up a chunk of your paycheck to doctors. You don't need a bunch of pills "just to get through the day." You don't need to be poor AND sick.

Let's keep this conversation one hundred percent authentic. Ever since white people have forced themselves into the societies of Original people (via colonialism, imperialism and slavery) they have been jacking up our health for the worst. The best example of this can be seen in the way we eat. The Standard American Diet is the culmination of white invasion. It is a diet that has you gobbling pork and beef like it was going out of fashion.

But it's bigger than food, It's not just our eating habits that have been devastated. An invasion implies that the whole landscape has been affected. We have become products of our environment, rather than the producers of our environment. Just open your eyes to EveryHood,

Latinos, thanks to similar diets, similar lifestyles, and similar lack of access to adequate healthcare. Never forget where you come from homey, because life has a hell of a way of reminding you.

[3] Throughout this book, "Original" will be used synonymously with Black or African-American, or as an umbrella term covering Black, Latino, Asian, Native American and other indigenous populations. While the use of the term "Original" to cover such a diverse population is not widely accepted, we argue that there is no other word that captures the deep commonality of people of color worldwide, without somehow being a subtle reference to a white or European standard. For example, "people of color" suggests that the norm is actually people without color, just as "minorities" suggests that Original people are somehow not in the majority worldwide. Similarly, "non-white" suggests that the standard is "white" and everything else is "other" and thus secondary. It is our argument that the world's first people, anthropologically known as indigenous people, may have been geographically separated and culturally distinct, but were never collectively oppressed, forceably marginalized, and systemically set at odds with each other (creating the present need for a collective identity) until Europeans distinguished themselves as "white" (and thus "different") and went to work throughout the world, completely changing our paradigms of identity and ideology.

USA and give us your honest opinion of the quality of the environment. There is a lack of basic resources like quality housing, affordable and healthy foods, access to community-based resources, and a quality education. (See "In the Ghetto")

"Every human being is the author of his own health or disease." – Buddha (563-483 B.C.)

This book was written because, in order for us to "make it" anywhere, we'll need a road map AND a blueprint. The road map will show us the way, and the blueprint will instruct us how to build a community, once we get there. Our goal is to take us from basically NOTHING to EVERYTHING. And until now, many of those who have tried to lead the people in the right direction have found the people reluctant, to say the least. "Getting healthy is too hard," they'd say. "Getting healthy is too expensive," is another common complaint. We understand all the complaints, and in many cases we agree. Getting healthy is certainly no "walk in the park" (although walks in the park can be part of getting healthy), but we've worked over-time to make this road map as easy to follow as possible. We've also worked to show where we came from, and how far we've come, to explain that we need only observe the meaning of the West African proverb *Sankofa*, which means to "go back (home) and fetch it." We're not going anywhere new. By living healthy, we're simply going back to being ourselves.

The simple beauty of this whole journey is that we have the answer. We've always had the answer. Your grandparents and great-grandparents were the answer. The traditions of your ancestors are the answer. Learning about your body and being able to listen to its messages is the answer. But you've got to start asking questions before you find your answers!

Resurrection

People are dying. More precisely, people simply aren't living. Our communities are in a state of depression and shock. Many of us are literally like zombies. We go through the motions, yet we rarely make much out of our lives. And what do zombies do? They stink. They look a hot mess. They sometimes lose body parts. And they can't keep up with people who are living. Sounds like a lot of us. As Marvin Gaye observed in "What's Going On," what most of us are doing ain't living.

"When a dying man cries, it is not because of where he is going which he knows nothing about, but because of what he wishes he would have done in the world he is leaving behind" – African Proverb

The destruction of our hoods has resulted in a fracturing of community. Without that unity, we keep spiraling down a hole where we all become self-centered predators, not caring about one another, much like the people who put us in these miserable conditions. This is also basically what a "dead people" will do. And when this happens, everybody suffers. Look at your own suffering right now, and imagine how it could be alleviated simply by adding one more person to your team to go through the struggle with you. Then you two add one more, and then one more, and so on. Think of everything that you could accomplish with a community of people, dedicated to a common cause. The way to develop a community is through the common language and culture of mental and physical health and well-being.

"Before healing others, heal yourself." – Gambian Proverb

Our personal health is just the beginning. Once we are on that road to healing (since you're never truly "done"), then we can begin to heal our communities. And if we keep it moving, guess what? We might just end up healing the world!

IS THIS BOOK FOR YOU?

If you can answer "Yes" to any of these questions, this book is for you:

☐ I had a parent die from a health condition that I don't want to die from.

☐ I want practical advice on how I can lose weight without a crazy diet.

☐ I need to know how to eat healthier, but on a budget.

☐ I want to improve myself, but I hate reading boring books that don't speak to me.

☐ I want to know about all the illnesses – from diabetes to gum disease – experienced by people in the hiphop industry.

☐ I've heard there are natural treatments and cures for cancer, heart disease, and other major illnesses and I want to know more.

☐ I want to know why Black and Latino people have more illnesses than anyone else.

☐ I've heard that pork is terrible for you, but I need some proof.

☐ I want to know if I can handle becoming a vegetarian.

☐ I want to know how to become healthy without become a vegetarian.

☐ I've heard you can use herbs for just about anything. I want to know how.

☐ I can't find any information on psychological health that speaks to me and my background.

☐ I want to know why I'm addicted to junk food.

☐ I've heard that they put chemicals in fast food and I want to know why.

- ☐ I need ideas on how to keep my home clean, but I don't have much time or money to spend.
- ☐ I need help on making sure my children grow up healthy.
- ☐ I don't want to be sick like so many other people in my family.

WHAT THIS BOOK IS NOT

This book is a lot of things, and it will definitely reach different people in different ways…but there are some things this book is certainly NOT. This book is not:

Only for people who are already healthy: There are a lot of "health" books (especially natural/holistic titles) that don't address the way most of us are living, right now. Instead, they preach to the choir, talking only to readers who are already on the right path. Not this book.

A guide on how to take your medicine: It's fairly easy to see that "more medicine" hasn't made our people "more healthy." Instead of promoting the Western medicine model (diagnosis of symptoms → prescription of chemicals), we're going to show you how to prevent sickness and how to heal without the chemicals (which actually make us sicker).

A diet/weight loss book: Our health problems are deeper than obesity. While it's good to be in shape, we're not going to teach you how to starve yourself to do so. We're also not going to promote the idea that a skinny person is healthy, just because they are skinny. "Holistic" health means "everything."

Super-holistic, super-natural, and super-difficult: Our books are written to address the needs of people who normally don't enjoy books about health, so we're not going to promote a lifestyle that is unrealistic for many of our readers. Our goal is to provide practical, sensible advice that almost anyone can use. Along the way, we'll throw in more challenging concepts here and there to keep things interesting.

Medical advice, replacing that of a professional, or meant to diagnose you: We're not trying to pass ourselves off as doctors giving you medical advice. We are simply providing information that you can take into consideration when you make your lifestyle decisions. If you have a condition requiring serious or immediate attention, then by all means, seek out a professional you trust.

Race-specific: The topics addressed in this book focus on Black and Latino people, but many of the health issues we talk about are relevant to just about anyone interested in improving their health. That means you don't need to be Black or Latino to benefit from this book.

Class-specific: Similarly, you don't need to live in the hood to benefit from this book.

A bunch of opinions: We are not "quacks" with crazy ideas. We have spent countless hours making sure that our information and recommendations are research-based. As often as possible, we've drawn on clinical studies and medical journals to develop our positions. When we came across an idea that "sounded good" but had no evidence to support it, we refused to publish it.

A scientific journal: At the same time, we have avoided including hundreds of footnotes and citations throughout the text. We have simplified the language to the point where everyone can read it without a dictionary on hand (though it wouldn't hurt). Our goal is to make this information accessible, not to sound smarter than everyone else.

A 'what you're doing wrong' lecture: We're not here to make you feel bad. While the hood is certainly very sick, nothing is hopeless. We're more interested in providing easy recommendation for change, than harassing readers about the mistakes they've made.

A 'change everything now or die' sermon: Revolutionary change is a process, not a one-time event. It made more sense to promote one step at a time than to tell you to change everything immediately.

A walk in the park: In spite of all of the above, this book will challenge you mentally and physically. It will challenge your pre-conceived notions and your current lifestyle choices. And, the truth might hurt occasionally. But without pain, there's no real growth. We promise it will be worth it.

WHAT'S UP WITH THE "WELLNESS" THING?

Oh yeah, that. We almost didn't put the word "wellness" in the subtitle of this book. Sounds kind'a "New Age," we thought. "People will think we're pushing something weird and expensive instead of something practical and affordable." But we kept the word because "wellness" has a meaning that's worth keeping. Wellness means more than just being in a state of good health. Wellness is being on the road to getting there. And wellness is things that the doctor often can't measure.

"As I see it, every day you do one of two things: build health or produce disease in yourself." – Adelle Davis

According to John Travis, author of *The Wellness Index*, "Wellness is not a static state. High-level wellness involves giving good care to your physical self, using your mind constructively, expressing your emotions effectively, being creatively involved with those around you, and being concerned about your physical, psychological, and spiritual environments." He goes on to explain that it doesn't matter what side of the "healthy-unhealthy" spectrum a person is on, but which direction they are facing.[4]

"To wish to be well is a part of becoming well." – Seneca, ancient Roman philosopher

So, how do we know where we're at – and where we're going – on the road to wellness (or the road away from it)? Simple. Take every test, quiz, and questionnaire in this book. Read every article and see where you fall in terms of your daily practices. This book is the first COMPREHENSIVE guide to health in the urban community because it covers nearly EVERY aspect of health AND wellness. When you're done with these two volumes, you'll know exactly where you stand, and where to go from there. Then, you can set your goals and move fast or slow. But the critical first step is KNOWLEDGE. And once you KNOW, wisdom – and wellness – follow.

"He who has health has hope; and he who has hope has everything." – Arabian Proverb

HOW TO READ THIS BOOK

❏ You can start from the beginning and work your way to the end, or you can find interesting headings in the Table of Contents and hop around from essay to essay. This book can be read in any order.

❏ When you come across a word you don't know, first see if you can figure out the meaning based on the rest of the sentence. If not, the word may be defined in the glossary in the Appendix of this book. If it's not there either, grab a dictionary or go to www.dictionary.com. You can also find basic definitions at http://medical-dictionary.thefreedictionary.com.

❏ The same thing goes for any person, place, event, or idea that's new to you. We don't want you to simply "believe" us. Look it up. If you don't feel like grabbing a book, you can start at www.wikipedia.org, www.webmd.com, health.about.com, or one of the many other websites we suggest in the book.

❏ Bring it with you wherever you go. Instead of smoking a cigarette or text messaging when you're bored or waiting for something, *read.*

---

[4] As holistic health writer Gretchen Goel writes: "If a person is currently suffering with cancer he or she can be moving forward or backward depending on their daily practices. They can decide to do chemotherapy and continue the same poor diet and health practices they had prior to diagnosis. The person may have decided in their mind that death is imminent. This would cause the person to continue to move backwards toward increased ill health and ultimately death. Whereas a person who decides they want to be well can move forward on the continuum. Their daily choices might look like this: eating a diet of mostly raw fruits and vegetables, exercising daily, practicing meditation and positive thinking, getting 8 or more hours of sound sleep daily."

- Find a partner or two who can get a copy of the book to read as well. When you meet, talk about what you're reading and what you think about it.

  "The best preservative to keep the mind on health is the faithful admonition of a friend." – Sir Francis Bacon

- Don't get overwhelmed. All this information can be difficult for someone who thinks they have to start changing everything all at once. As we said earlier, optimum health is a path, not a destination.
- Take notes. Highlight. Circle important sections. But only if this is *your* book. Otherwise the owner's gonna be pissed.
- Work to understand every idea that is discussed in this book. If you can do that, we guarantee that you'll know more than the average pre-med student.
- We didn't make everything easy. Some of this book is written in very simple language that anyone can understand, dealing with basic issues like weight loss. Other parts are more challenging, dealing with issues like herbal treatments for OCD. If this book didn't challenge every reader somehow, we wouldn't be proud to present it to the general public.
- Above all, the single most important thing you can do with this book is APPLY WHAT YOU LEARN. We cover everything from the low end to the high end, so EVERYONE can start using SOMETHING in this book to improve their lives. The key isn't to do it all at once, or even to do it all period, but to begin the process by doing something you haven't done before. That's all it takes. The journey of a thousand miles begins with one step.

Let me reiterate that last point. There are some parts of this book that will *totally* blow your day. You'll be feeling dusted and disgusted. You'll feel like you can't do *anything*, because *everything* out there is so unhealthy. Don't fall victim to that kind of thinking. The goal, again, is to simply **start doing better**, and to constantly be doing the best you currently can. Meaning, for example, you'll know that canned food ain't that good for you, but eating canned vegetables is better than NO vegetables.

HIP HOP AND HEALTH?

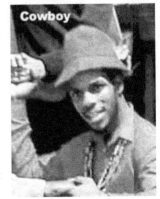
Cowboy

Why use Hip Hop as a reference point? Why not? Hip Hop is a reflection of the state of the urban (Black and brown) community in America. In fact, it's just as sick as we are; and in more ways than one. Beyond your personal tastes in music, the people who make up this industry are a diverse reflection of the people who make up our communities. They are not something other than us. As a result, they're sick like us. Using them as reference points makes it easier for us to show you that these issues aren't rare disorders you only see on TV. So, although it may not be obvious, Hip Hop and Health go hand-in-hand. While only a few big artists are brave enough to make songs addressing health issues (eg. KRS-One, dead prez, Prodigy, Wu-Tang Clan, etc.), that doesn't keep the rest of them from HAVING the health issues they don't rap about. Life-threatening health issues are everywhere in the Hip Hop community. And we've lost enough artists to know that the situation is serious. Just look at the following timeline of notable losses.

1989: On September 8, 1989, Cowboy (Grandmaster Flash and The Furious 5) died of complications from HIV/AIDS. He was two weeks shy of his 39th birthday.

1991: MC Trouble, the first female emcee ever signed to Motown Records, died of an epileptic seizure in 1991, on her 19th birthday.

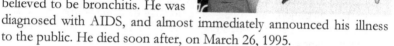

1995: In 1995, Eazy-E entered the hospital with what he believed to be bronchitis. He was diagnosed with AIDS, and almost immediately announced his illness to the public. He died soon after, on March 26, 1995.

1995: On December 10, 1995, Darren "Buffy, the Human Beatbox" Robinson (of the Fat Boys) died of a heart attack in Rosedale, New York. He was 28 years old and reportedly 450 lbs.

2000: After a long battle with morbid obesity, Big Pun suffered a fatal heart attack and respiratory failure on February 7, 2000. Pun, the first solo Latino rapper to go platinum, was only 28 years old and at least 450 lbs. He left behind a wife and three children.

2001: In April 1999, Grym Reaper (aka Too Poetic of the Gravediggaz) was diagnosed with a deadly colon cancer, and was given only three months to live. On July 15, 2001, Grym Reaper passed away, almost two years longer than the time he was given by the doctors.

2004: Ol Dirty Bastard collapsed at approximately 5:29pm on November 13, 2004 at Wu-Tang's recording studio. He was pronounced dead less than an hour later, only two days shy of his 36th birthday. He had a lethal mixture of cocaine and the prescription painkiller Tramadol in his system at the time of his death.

2006: On February 10, 2006, producer J-Dilla of Slum Village passed away from cardiac arrest, following a battle with thrombotic thrombocytopenic purpura, a rare blood disease, and lupus.

2007: Pimp C died on December 4, 2007, after suffering respiratory depression caused by the combined effects of him taking a large dose of promethazine and codeine (prescription cough syrup) coupled with a preexisting sleep apnea condition.

2008: Queens Bridge rapper KL of Screwball died of an asthma attack on March 28, 2008

2010: Queens Bridge rapper Killa Sha (aka Sha Lumi) died from diabetes complications on January 18, 2010.

2010: Flavor Unit emcee Apache, known best for his single "Gangsta Bitch," passed away January 22, 2010 after battling an undisclosed, protracted illness.

2010: On February 28, 2010, Guru went into cardiac arrest and, following surgery, fell into a coma. He died on April 19, 2010, at the age of 43, from multiple myeloma, a form of cancer.

THE 23 KEYS TO HEALTH AND WELLNESS

Your health is the most important thing you possess. These are 23 keys to health and wellness that one should keep in mind regardless of race, creed, class or environment. The articles in this book are written around these core principles, so you'll find yourself revisiting these ideas as you read.

1. The traditional lifestyles of Original people (otherwise known as "Indigenous people" or "People of Color") all over the planet were always in tune with their environment (even if they lived in cities).

2. Optimum physical health requires a nutritious diet, avoidance of toxins and other stressors that cause disease, and life's essentials: clean water, clean air, sunlight, exercise, and rest. Deficiency in any area causes most of the health problems we experience.

3. The eating practices of Original/Indigenous/People of Color, all over the planet, leaned towards diets that were focused on vegetables, fruits, grains, legumes, and other plant based foods. The consumption of meat has traditionally been a minor, if at all, part of the diets of Original people.

4. You can eat some meat and still be pretty healthy, but not if you're eating SAD (Standard American Diet) amounts of it, or eating the chemical and parasite-filled kind we find at most grocers.

5. Clean on the inside, clean on the outside. We should be free of nastiness and parasites inside our body, and this cleanliness should be reflected on our exterior as well. With healthy practices, we won't need to depend on artificial cosmetic processes and products to feel attractive. And because we live in a toxic environment, it's important to fast and cleanse our internal systems regularly, no matter what kind of diet we're on.

6. Western culture through White Supremacy (slavery, genocide, colonialism, terrorism) initiated the current downward spiral of sickness and disease amongst Original/Indigenous people all over the planet.

7. White Supremacy is anti-life. Through their doctrine of Manifest Destiny, they seek to be the ultimate consumers, devourers, users, conquerors with no thought as to how resources are to be renewed in the environment.

8. Original people don't need the help of white people to assist in the recovery of their health and wellness. The way that most "health-conscious," liberal white people approach our communities is patronizing at best. It's just another manifestation of colonization. Also, in actuality, their information and resources about a holistic way of life were taught to them by Original/Indigenous people.

9. We are not anti-Western medicine, yet we do reserve the right to critique it and take only the best part that benefits our communities.

10. Too much of anything is no good. Some things are more dangerous in their excess than their lack - others, vice versa. For example, too much salt is more dangerous than too little, but too little Vitamin A is more dangerous than too much.

11. At least 75% of disease is nutritional, either in terms of how disease is developed, or how it could have been prevented. Junk food, fried food, red meat, and other popular foods are killing you slowly.

12. Eating dead, burnt, toxic, chemically altered, genetically tampered, and/or inorganic matter leads to obvious consequences.

13. Everything that tastes good is not good for you. Yet, we eat these things because certain ingredients in our foods can be as addictive as hard drugs.

14. You can also overuse (abuse) parts of your body, particularly the organs that are in place to clean and filter your system. When you overload those organs with toxins, they eventually shut down and disease emerges.

15. Whenever a part of your body (such as a muscle) is not in use, it atrophies, meaning it dies. People who are not physically fit die sooner than those who are.

16. Losing weight is not about dieting, but about changing your habits. By eating right and exercising, it's easy to lose any amount of weight you desire.

17. Hospitals, doctors, drug companies, and the whole "industry" of Western medicine, is a big business. We understand that its goal is to maximize profits and that they may go against the goal of healing the people.

18. Healing and Wellness must be holistic. It is mental and physical. The individual and the environment.

19. Healing starts where you are at. It took you years, months, and days to get to your current state of dysfunction and will take an equal amount of time to rise out of it. Utilize the resources right around you, realizing that health and wellness is a journey not a destination.

20. One of the most powerful elements of health and wellness is preventative medicine.

21. Children are born with all the stress and toxins we put in our systems, even those from before they were conceived. Whatever they see us eating and doing, they will also want to eat and do. But children are more susceptible to toxins in the environment, as well as those in the foods we eat. In order to keep them healthy, we have to be healthy.

22. Get your mind right. Mental/emotional health is as important, if not more important, than physical health. Without a sound mind, it does us no good to have a sound body. But mind and body are interdependent, so living healthier can have us thinking and feeling healthier.

23. When you heal yourself, you'll, in effect, be healing the hood.

ARE YOU HEALTHY?

POP QUIZ: ARE YOU HEALTHY?

Before we jump into the content of this book, we've gotta be clear that this process won't work if you're not being honest with yourself – in terms of where you're at and where you need to be. But even the most honest of people don't necessarily know how "healthy" or "unhealthy" they are, because there's so much to that whole health thing. So we're gonna help you learn about yourself. Try the following quiz and see how you score. What have you got to lose? It's not like somebody's gonna see your score and laugh cause you're unhealthy. Unless you and your friends have this same book. Then, they might. Or you might get to laugh at them. Either way, it's cool because laughter is the best medicine. See, you're already on your first step to healing! Seriously though, knowledge is half the battle. The other half (more like 7/9ths) is putting in the work once you have the knowledge. You gotta start somewhere, start with this quiz!

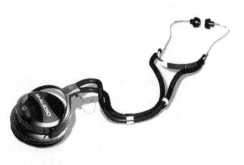

1. Do you eat fried foods?

a. Less than twice a week.

b. Occasionally, but I'm mindful of it.

c. Pretty regularly.

d. If it ain't fried, I probably don't want it.

2. How long would it take you to walk a mile?

a. Less than 10 minutes.

b. Between 10 and 20 minutes.

c. I'd have to take a few breaks, so I'm not sure.

d. Why would I walk a mile?

3. When seated with my legs straight in front, I can bend forward at the waist and reach...

a. Past my toes.

b. Near my toes.

c. My shins.

d. My knees.

4. I can balance on one foot, extend my arms, and stand still...
   a. More than 3 minutes.
   b. 1 or 2 minutes.
   c. About 30 seconds.
   d. I'm not even gonna try that and embarrass myself.

5. Do you drink sugary sodas and artificially flavored "juices"?
   a. Never. It's real fruit juice, tea, or water for me.
   b. Rarely. I go for days without having any sugary drinks.
   c. Sometimes. But I can manage a day without any.
   d. Often. It would be hard for me to go without them.

6. Do you exercise?
   a. I could be an athlete or a personal trainer (30 to 60 minutes most days)
   b. I'm in decent shape, but I'm not ready for the marathon. (About 30 to 45 minutes a few times per week)
   c. I can help you move out of your apartment, but not by myself! (About 30 minutes twice a week)
   d. Sometimes I have to walk across a big parking lot. (Very little, if ever)

7. Do you eat sweets or candy?
   a. What's a snickerdoodle? (Never)
   b. Where's the snickerdoodles? (Rarely)
   c. I need some snickerdoodles. (Sometimes)
   d. I *am* the snickerdoodle. (Often)

8. Do you eat red meat?

a. Never.
b. Not often.
c. At least once or twice a week (or "I eat beef but not pork")
d. They call me "Swinefeld"

9. Do you have breakfast in the morning?
   a. Yes, daily. And it's usually pretty healthy.
   b. Most days. And it's usually pretty healthy.
   c. Most days. But it's usually not that healthy.
   d. Does a cup of coffee count?

10. Do you smoke?
    a. No, and I never have.
    b. I used to smoke, but I quit.
    c. I don't smoke, but I live with or work around smokers who puff near me.
    d. All day. Nicorette ain't got a patch strong enough for me.

11. When was the last time you had your blood pressure and cholesterol checked?
    a. Within the past year.
    b. Within the past two years.
    c. Several years ago.
    d. I can't remember.

12. How much sleep do you get at night?
    a. 6 or 7 hours a night.
    b. 8 or more hours a night.
    c. Less than 6 hours a night.
    d. My sleep patterns are so irregular I couldn't even tell you.

13. Do you use any "recreational" drugs?
    a. Nope. I get high off my success.
    b. I might smoke a little weed on occasion, but that's it.

c. I might do a little bit more than weed.

d. I could be considered a junkie, if you were trying to be mean.

14. How is your dental health?

a. My dentist worships me.

b. I haven't seen the dentist in a while, but I brush and floss regularly and I don't have cavities.

c. I don't brush or floss like I should, and I probably have a few cavities I need to address.

d. I'm probably gonna lose some of these teeth.

15. How much sunlight do you get?

a. If I was white, I'd have an awesome tan.

b. I get at least an hour of sunlight daily.

c. I'm stuck indoors most weekdays, but I try to make up for it by getting some sun on the weekends.

d. I'm practically a vampire. I can remember the last time I spent a while in the sun.

16. How much water do you drink?

a. All I drink is water (More than 64 ounces).

b. 8 glasses a day, like the doctor say (48-64 ounces).

c. I don't drink as much as I should (16-48 ounces).

d. There are too many other things that taste better (0-16 ounces).

17. How do you deal with illnesses?

a. I know how to cure most things naturally and who to see when I don't.

b. I consult with a healthcare professional and develop a regimen that will combat the illness.

c. I see a doctor and hope he knows how to fix me.

d. I pop some pills, say a prayer, and hope for the best.

18. What kind of medicines do you take?

a. Mostly herbs, minerals, and whatever else Mother Nature provides.

b. Mostly natural stuff, but I use the synthetic stuff too.

c. Mostly the synthetic chemical stuff, but I've been trying natural remedies too.

d. Mostly pills, needles, and whatever else Medicaid provides.

19. Do you have mood swings or rapid emotional changes?

a. No way. That's crazy as hell.

b. It's rare, but it happens.

c. More than I'd like to admit.

d. All day. I'm crazy as hell.

20. When is the last time you fasted or did a cleanse?

a. Within the past month.

b. Within the past six months.

c. Within the past year.

d. The only detox I know about is the one you do for a urine test.

21. How often do you get headaches?

a. Rarely.

b. Sometimes, but I usually know what caused it.

c. Often, and they can get bad.

d. I got one right now, and I'll probably have another one soon.

22. How often do you eat fresh or steamed vegetables?

a. At every meal

b. At most meals

c. Not often...does rice and peas count?

d. Um...do the tomatoes in ketchup count?

23. When was the last time you had your stuff inspected? (Pap smear, STD test, breast exam, testicular exam, prostate exam)

a. Within the past two years.

b. Three or four years ago.

c. Five or more years ago.

d. I ain't doin none of that nasty stuff.

24. How often do you treat pains with an over-the-counter pain reliever?

a. I take one once or twice a year, or I used a natural remedy.

b. I use them occasionally.

c. I pop a pain reliever most days.

d. Over the counter? Please. Gimme that Vicodin baby.

25. How much alcohol do you drink?

a. I average one drink or fewer per day.

b. I drink once in a while, but then I'll often have four or more.

c. I have about two drinks daily.

d. I average more than two drinks a day; at times I can't remember how much I drank or what I did afterward.

26. What do you eat more of, pastries or fruit?

a. All fruit, no pastries or sweets.

b. More fruit than pastries and sweets.

c. More pastries than fruit.

d. Mostly pastries and sweets, almost no fruit.

27. What's your waist size?

a. Less than my hips

b. Bout the same as my hips

c. A little more than my hips

d. C'mon son! I'm FAT.

28. Do you have a family history of heart disease, diabetes, cancer, or other hereditary illnesses?

a. No parents or grandparents with any problems like that.

b. 1 or 2 of my parents or grandparents have 1 or 2 problems like that.

c. Most of us got something.

d. Everybody's got something, and some of us got everything. (or "I have no idea")

29. Which best describes your sexual practices?

30. I'm in a long-term, mutually monogamous relationship.

a. I'm not committed to one person; but I always use condoms when I have sex.

b. I'm not committed to one person; and I don't always use a condom.

c. I get it in, by any means necessary.

31. How do you typically cope with stress?

a. I regularly carve out time to recharge.

b. I vent about my crises to a friend or a family member.

c. I don't know what to do. Usually I just feel overwhelmed.

d. I depend on alcohol, food or another vice to help me make it through the day.

32. I experience fatigue...

a. Only after a strenuous workout or similar physical activity (ahem).

b. Usually after a long day of work

c. After climbing a set of stairs, taking a long walk, or carrying something heavy

d. Pretty much throughout the day, even when I haven't done anything

33. I experience back or muscle pain...

a. Never.

b. Sometimes.

c. Pretty often.

d. I stay with some kind of pain.

34. When I stand against the wall...

a. The back of my head, hips, feet, and shoulder blades touch the wall.

b. Only the back of my hips, feet and shoulder blades touch the wall. I have to change my posture for my head to touch the wall.

c. Only the back of my hips and feet touch the wall. I have to change my posture for my shoulder blades to touch the wall.

d. Only the back of my hips touches the wall. I don't want to talk about it

Scoring

Scoring Key	Items Marked		Points
A: 0 points	Number of As: ____	x 0 = ____	0
B: 1 point	Number of Bs: ____	x 1 = ____	
C: 2 points	Number of Cs: ____	x 2 = ____	
D: 3 points	Number of Ds: ____	x 3 = ____	
	TOTAL SCORE =		

Scoring Ranges and Explanation

0-10: OPTIMUM	You're either insanely healthy or just plain insane. Most people are nowhere near this level of optimum health, so we congratulate you (if you're telling the truth). If you lied, you may need to skip ahead and go straight to the section on psychological health, because that's just strange. Assuming that you were being truthful, you're a living example of the principles in this book. Because of how much information we've packed into the following pages, we're sure you'll still learn a lot. But you'll find this text most valuable if you use it as a teaching tool for the people you know who need it more than you.

11-25: EXCELLENT	A great score. You should be proud. You eat healthy, live healthy and probably even think healthy. Sure, there are some things you could work on, but with this book, you're definitely on the right track to optimum health and a long, satisfying life.
26-50: DECENT	Even with a score in this range, you're still doing better than most Americans. But if you think about it, that's not necessarily a high standard to measure yourself against. Perhaps you need to eat more fruits and vegetables and less junk. Perhaps you should be exercising more and spend less time indoors. Perhaps you should go see a doctor or a dentist soon. Whatever the case, you have plenty of room for improvement, and this book will make sure you cover it all.
51-75: UNHEALTHY	Don't be offended at being called "unhealthy." We're just being real with you. You knew you weren't too healthy when you took this quiz, so don't be mad at us for telling you what you already know. The question now is 'What am I going to do about it?' You can either continue on the downward spiral of unhealthy living, cut several years off your life, and finally end up dead before your time or sick and miserable in your old age...OR you can get on the upward spiral to better living. It's your choice. You have family members who chose not to address their health until it was too late. You've seen what happens. It's going to be some work, but this book will guide you through many of those changes, showing you both the big steps and the baby steps you can take. Aren't you tired of feeling the way you do? Make a decision. Your bad habits can still be changed!
76-90: SICK	You've got a LOT of unhealthy habits. You know you do. You've been treating your body like a rental car you don't plan on returning. But it's all gonna get billed to you in the end. You pay for all those habits, one day, some way. And it's never pretty. In your present condition, you're probably already sick. You may have diabetes, cancer, arthritis, heart disease...who knows? You may not even know what you have. But unless you're going to kill yourself now, you should consider this
91-100: DEAD	Seriously? How do you even get a score in this range? I know crackheads who would score higher. Either you were trying to be funny when you took this quiz, or you're an unhealthy crackhead. You can't even get 100 points on this quiz. It's mathematically impossible. Just like it's almost physically impossible to live much longer with the type of lifestyle you have, if you scored in this range. If you really scored between 91 and 99, this book could literally save your life.

The first step is knowing you can improve. Then you apply solutions.

You Know You're Unhealthy When...

You know you're unhealthy when...

- [ ] Your breath smells like sh*t.
- [ ] You can't take a sh*t.
- [ ] Your hair's comin out and you ain't 70.
- [ ] You get thirsty at work or school and drink a Mountain Dew...and it's 9:30 am.
- [ ] You can't run a single mile, even if someone's chasing you.
- [ ] You always feel tired, even when you wake up.
- [ ] You're seriously overweight.
- [ ] You're seriously underweight.
- [ ] Kool-aid is your idea of a fruit juice.
- [ ] You are a vegetarian, yet you never eat vegetables – just carbs and protein.
- [ ] You start discussing the fact that KFC should do delivery
- [ ] You're breathin hard and sweatin after only climbing a flight of stairs.
- [ ] You have a hard time breathing and you haven't done anything yet.
- [ ] You'd rather eat fast food because it "tastes better" than live foods.
- [ ] You don't even know what live foods are.
- [ ] You're addicted to junk food and don't know it.
- [ ] You think Miller Lite is healthy because it's "Lite"
- [ ] You have acne and you're an adult.
- [ ] You think sugar-free or low-carb means healthy.
- [ ] You sleep all day.
- [ ] You're addicted to something white (cocaine, heroin, Xanax, sugar).
- [ ] You can't sleep at all.
- [ ] Your parents are brown but your skin is pale.
- [ ] You think pork is the other white meat.
- [ ] Your mind is more toxic than your body.
- [ ] Your family has tried to do an "intervention" with you, and it didn't work.
- [ ] Your family has tried to put you on one of those weight loss Reality TV shows.
- [ ] You're an emotional wreck.
- [ ] Sh*t comes out your body that makes you say "What the f*ck?"
- [ ] Your feet stink even when you ain't been running.
- [ ] You make your eating decisions based off of TV commercials.
- [ ] You get sick, know why you are sick, and still do what makes you sick.
- [ ] You can't sleep without smoking a blunt.
- [ ] You live to eat instead of eating to live.
- [ ] You step over the backs of the people in front of you to get off the bus and take a smoke.
- [ ] You see vegetable fried rice, take the things that you don't like out and you just have rice.
- [ ] You're not interested in sex.
- [ ] You always have headaches.

- [ ] Your "annual checkup" makes you a nervous wreck for weeks before your appointment!
- [ ] Your urine is not clear enough to damn near see through!
- [ ] Your urine smells like stale movie theater popcorn.
- [ ] You can't do 20 pushups without a struggle (this goes for females too).
- [ ] Your "private parts" smell like "public sanitation."
- [ ] You put just about anything in (or on) your body.

Habits reflect just how healthy or unhealthy one is. Reevaluate how you live to improve your health.

THE LIES WE TELL OURSELVES

BY SUPREME UNDERSTANDING

Basic Useful Lies we Love to Spit to Help Ignore the Truth...
Also known as B.U.L.L.S.H.I.T. We tell ourselves a lot of lies to avoid change. We, meaning damn near all of us. It's a psychological principle called **"cognitive dissonance,"** which means that people normally respond to uncomfortable challenges by telling themselves the evidence is bullsh*t. In reality, we're the ones BSing. And most of the time, we know it. But we keep "self-medicating" with them lies so we don't have to feel bad about not changing. But you already know what happens to people who can't change. **Another principle called "survival of the fittest" takes effect, and whatever can't change DIES.** Let's examine some of the lies we tell ourselves about becoming healthy:

I already am healthy.

If you're like most of us, you're probably not. America is the sickest country in the world (it's a documented fact), and Black and brown people are its sickest citizens. We're the fattest, the most diseased, the most toxic, the most psychologically ill...basically, everything. Even those of us who aren't totally screwed are still residually affected somehow. So, we all have some growing to do. Why do you feel like you're the only one who has no room to improve? And isn't that a sign of being sick?

This[5] is my cultural heritage.

No, it's really not. These are the unnatural diets and lifestyles we developed living in an unnatural environment. Africans didn't eat most of the things we call "Black food" before slavery, and really didn't

---

[5] "This" refers to any unhealthy habit, from eating pork to smoking crack to drinking liquor when depressed. "That," on the other hand, refers to any healthy habit or lifestyle change.

even eat it DURING slavery. (See "The History of Soul Food")

You gotta die of SOMEthing, might as well do this and enjoy it.

In that case, everyone would smoke crack-cocaine. Crack's gotta be a more exciting rush for the senses than a pork chop, right? So, why not? Because we calculate our risks against the benefits we receive. So once you get past the taste (which is mostly chemicals and seasonings anyway), and realize there are almost NO health benefits to the crap we're defending, why are we still doing it? Easy. **It's addictive**. Just like crack. Don't believe me? Do what KRS-One said, and prove it ain't addictive by giving it up for a month. Watch the withdrawal symptoms you go through. If you're thinking "A little bit won't hurt me," again, you wouldn't say that about smoking crack or licking poop. **A "little bit" is the only true gateway drug.** (See "Junk Food is Crack")

My grandpa is 150 years old.

Or, more specifically, "My grandpa does this same bullsh*t every day and he's 150 years old." These kinds of stories are fun to listen to, but everybody knows you don't base your lifestyle off the "exception to the rule." Let's face it, out of 100 people with the same habits, only ONE lived this long. The rest of them died between 48 and 70. Beyond that, I've met some of these magical elders people talk about. Sure, they're alive, but they're in a wheelchair, missing a foot, and breathing with the help of an oxygen tank! I don't want to end up like that! The healthy ones are much rarer, but usually those are the ones who had a few unhealthy habits, but also worked 16 hour days of physical labor, never cheated on their wife, and only drank on Saturdays. Meaning their healthy habits outweighed the unhealthy. But how many pork-eatin', beer-chuggin', sleepin'-around, never-exercisin', barely-bathin' males or females do YOU know? (See "Elder Wisdom")

This was bad for you back in the day, but they fixed it.

No, you mean they made it worse. Sure, they've reduced the number of live parasites in a slab of beef from 300 to 250, but in the meanwhile, they also added 200 more chemicals, hormones, pesticides, and antibiotics. Same goes for damn near any other unhealthy habit we think science has improved.

I'm already on a diet.

That's why this book isn't about dieting. It's about living. Living healthier is a "holistic process," which means whole, not JUST what you eat, or how much you eat, but many other things, as well. You actually DIE from some of these stupid diets. The second thing is "process," which means it won't be over in 30 days. It's gonna continue for as long as you want to live.

I have medical coverage.

Despite all the evidence, people still believe that doctors and medicine can fix just about anything. But there are several problems with this pipe dream. **First, if you're Black or brown, you're gonna get worse treatment.** That's well-documented. **Second, if you're poor, you're REALLY gonna get worse treatment (or no treatment). Third, even if you DO get treatment, it's not gonna "fix" you. Western medicine doesn't cure. It covers up.** You'll get halfway patched up, or doped up to the point you don't feel yourself still dying. (Seen "Are All Doctors Mad Scientist?")

My cousin did that* and she's still unhealthy.

Again, this is an example of people using one person's experience as "all the proof they need." Chances are that she (a) did something that sounded healthy but really wasn't (b) did something healthy but only halfway, or (c) did something, but not the things she needed to do most to become healthy. **There are literally THOUSANDS of studies, involving hundreds of thousands of people, which show that the recommendations we make in this book WORK.** They'd even work for your cousin.

It's too late for me to change.

Totally untrue. Elderly people who have changed their lifestyles have been able to do everything from improving their memory to reversing their diabetes. And we're talking people aged 70+, so what's YOUR excuse?

That healthy stuff is too expensive, hard, weird, and nasty.

That stuff won't be half expensive as those medical or funeral bills, or as difficult as the death of a loved one. We're not telling you to eat garlic-curried spinach leafs or rock Jesus sandals and quartz crystals. What's weird about being that person everyone turns to for nutritional advice?

What's the point? Everything is bad for you.

Every time I talk about the chemicals in everything from our tap water to our air supply, people start using that as an excuse to keep their unhealthy habits. That's like me telling a woman that all men have some sort of issues (we do), so she uses that as an excuse to keep dating Bobby Brown. That's dumb! The smart thing to do is eliminate the worst things from your life first, and slowly work on the others! That way you minimize your risk, instead of maximizing it. But when people start talking all illogical like that, I already know it's the addiction speaking for em. And I've been addicted before, so I understand.

Don't fool yourself. Build an argument for what is healthy instead.

WHAT IS GOOD HEALTH?
BY SUPREME UNDERSTANDING

Your body's engine is in good running shape (Meaning your heart works.)	This means you don't have a weak heart, high blood pressure, low blood pressure, heart disease, heart attacks, strokes, or any of the other conditions related to your circulatory system.
Your body can produce the substances it needs to function.	These substances include insulin, antibodies, serotonin, white blood cells, Vitamin D, and thousands of other essential chemicals you need to function properly.
Your body is not in physical self-destruct mode.	Self-destruct mode can mean any number of auto-immune conditions, from Crohn's disease to cancer, where your cells are basically attacking each other.
You're able to produce healthy offspring.	This means you can make children or bear children without complications, such as impotence, infertility, miscarriage, and other reproductive issues.
Your body can eliminate toxins and waste.	This means your liver, kidneys, spleen, stomach, intestines, colon, and pores (yes, the pores in your skin!) work like they're supposed to.
You can escape a burning building...and save others.	This means you're in good enough physical shape to climb down a fire escape, jump out of a window, crawl through a smoke-filled hallway, and/or save people who are passed out.
Your body can defend and repair itself.	This means your immune system works and you heal naturally at a normal pace.
You're not in mental/emotional self-destruct mode.	This means you're in a state of good psychological/emotional health, and you're actually satisfied with living your life, not destroying it.
You can breathe without a problem.	This means your lungs work. Your respiratory health can be affected by asthma, bronchitis, pneumonia, and dozens of other conditions.
You don't look like crap.	This means you don't have problems affecting your skin, hair, nails, eyes, posture, weight, or

	other physical features that are causes by poor health.

Maintain all your bodily and mental functions. They decide the quality of your health.

WHAT YOUR BODY IS TELLING YOU

SIGNS AND SYMPTOMS NOT TO IGNORE

BY SUPREME UNDERSTANDING AND SCIHONOR DEVOTION

"A man too busy to take care of his health is like a mechanic too busy to take care of his tools." – Spanish Proverb

We regularly put up with many symptoms of early disease, and men do so for far longer than women, from obvious warnings, like a terrible fever that signals infection, to more subtle clues, like losing hair on your toes, which can be an early sign of vascular disease. Now, some signs that might scare the hell out of you may actually be harmless, but many things that seem minor can warn of a serious disorder.

Still others can be unclear: Does that growing gut mean you're just "letting yourself go," or is it sign of ovarian cancer? Only a professional can tell. But the problem is that most of us don't notice ANYTHING, even when the warning light is flashing and beeping at us to stop. For example, Miami rapper Trick Daddy just thought he had a bad case of "dry skin" until he got tested for Lupus (See "What Is Lupus?"). T-Boz of TLC just thought her painful headaches were another symptom of her Sickle Cell Disease – until an MRI showed that she had a brain tumor (See "Get A Second Opinion"). And Ghostface Killah thought he had the symptoms of a common STD until he found out he had diabetes (See "Diabetes"). All of these conditions are life-threatening! So why stay in the dark about what's going on in your body? Especially if it's trying its best to tell you what you need to know? Let's take the top to bottom approach, and analyze your body's "check engine lights." We also break down a lot of the following conditions, more specifically, later.

Hair

❒ Your hair may be dry and brittle because it's over-permed, you're applying to much heat, or just straight-up over-processed.

❒ Dry hair may also mean an under-active thyroid or nutritional deficiency.

❒ Thinning hair and baldness doesn't affect just the fellas. Female pattern baldness often runs in families, and can also be associated with aging, menopause, an over-active thyroid or an early warning sign of diabetes. Thinning hair can also be from over-processing.

❒ Metabolic and circulatory disorders can cause a loss of body hair.

Nails

☐ Ladies, make sure that your nail shop is up to code and uses sterile equipment. Otherwise, you may be paying top-dollar for a fungal infection with your mani/pedi.

☐ Besides being over-processed, thyroid disease can also cause your nails to become dry and brittle.

☐ Splinter hemorrhages are dark, horizontal (side to side) streaks under your fingernails or toenails. This can be a sign of trichinosis. Meaning, you're infested with parasites because you've been eating undercooked pork or wild game. However, splinter hemorrhages are also warning signs for psoriasis, peptic ulcers, kidney disease, lupus, rheumatoid arthritis, blood-clotting diseases, or endocarditis (an inflammation of the heart tissue).

☐ Beau's Lines are horizontal (side to side) and sometimes appear when your body experiences a period of significant stress or illness. Your body is busy, struggling to handle other priorities, so your nails take a little break, and then start growing again.

☐ If the skin underneath the nail (the nail bed) is white, this may mean that you're anemic. Nails that are white near the cuticle, and red or brown near the tip, can signal of kidney disease. Irregularly shaped brown or blue spots in the nail bed can be melanomas.

☐ Fingertips that are blue or clubbed are a sign of chronic lung disease.

Skin

☐ Rashes, or "break-outs," can be caused by allergies to various foods or detergents.

☐ That innocent spot on your skin, that you thought was just a mole or a scar, may turn out to be a sign of cancer. You can tell by using **the ABCDE self-evaluation method**: It may be malignant (cancer-causing) if it has an **A**symmetrical shape; a jagged or irregular **B**order; a suspicious **C**olor; a **D**iameter larger than a pencil eraser; and is **E**levated and uneven.

☐ Basal and squamous cell carcinomas tend to be red to pink, are

Normal Mole   Melanoma
Asymmetry
Border Irregularity
Color
Diameter

crusty, and bleed easily.

- [ ] If you have more than 50 moles on your body, you're at increased risk for melanoma, a deadly form of skin cancer.
- [ ] Lesions, or ulcers, on the skin that will not heal, are associated with diabetes. Diabetics have poor circulation, and as a result, heal very slowly when they suffer a skin injury. Large patches of dark skin on the neck and underarms are also indicators for diabetes.

Persistent Headaches

- [ ] **Headache that last for more than two to three days are a cause for concern.** If accompanied by vomiting or vision changes, it could mean something is wrong in the tissues surrounding the brain like a clot or a tumor.
- [ ] Headaches are also one of the first signs of dehydration especially if you're suffering from a hangover. So, drink lots of water or a fluid with electrolytes in it, like Gatorade or Pedialyte.

Eyes

- [ ] Seeing "floaters" (those spots or flecks that float across your field of vision) is pretty common. But, a sudden increase in floaters may mean that you have a retinal tear or even a retinal detachment, especially if flashing lights accompany the floaters. **This requires immediate medical attention.**
- [ ] Your eyes may feel dry all the time because of low humidity where you live. This can also be caused by drug side effects. If your eyes are dry all the time (chronically) this may also be a warning sign that you have an autoimmune disease, like rheumatoid arthritis, hyperthyroidism, or lupus.
- [ ] If your eyebrows no longer extend over the corners of the eyes, this may be an indication that you have an under-active thyroid.
- [ ] Dark circles around the eyes can mean that you have allergies, anemia, that your liver is overworked, or that you're just plain tired.
- [ ] Small yellow bumps on the eyelid may be fat deposits that signal high cholesterol. High cholesterol raises your risk for heart disease.
- [ ] Little bumps that look like cobblestones, on the inside of your lower eyelid, mean that you're probably allergic to something.
- [ ] The eyes motor (movement) responses can be used to diagnose many medical conditions, such as diabetes and schizophrenia.

Ears

- [ ] It's normal to hear your heart beating, especially when you're lying down. But, if you can only hear your heart beat in one ear, this may be a warning sign for a heart murmur, high blood pressure, or other vascular disorders.
- [ ] If normal noises seem louder than usual, you may be drinking too

many diet sodas that contain aspartame. **Super-sensitivity to sound may also be caused by a magnesium deficiency, or an autoimmune disease.**

❑ A diagonal crease in the earlobe may signal a greater risk for heart attack, but this isn't true for Native Americans and some other ethnic groups.

Nose

❑ Your sense of smell can be affected by any number of things. Cigarette smokers can't smell, or taste, as well as non-smokers. As you get older, your sense of smell also tends to fall off a little. Injuries to your nose, nasal polyps, or a deviated septum may also impact smell. Interestingly, zinc deficiencies, hypothyroidism (an under-active thyroid), diabetes, multiple sclerosis, Parkinson's, and Alzheimer's disease may also impact your sense of smell.

❑ An inflamed, red, and bulbous (round) nose is often a sign you've been hitting the alcohol, long and hard. This type of nose may also be caused by rosacea, which triggers, or worsens, this skin condition.

❑ Breathing thru the mouth may mean allergies, congestion, or you may be under serious stress. We're supposed to breathe through our noses because this stimulates our vagus nerve, slowing down our heart rate, relaxing our blood vessels, and reducing stress.

Mouth

❑ Suffer from "Yuck Mouth"? If you've got a terrible taste in your mouth, that won't wash away with mouthwash, this may be a side effect of a medication or vitamin supplement you're taking. But, **this may also be a sign of gum disease and cavities. Viral infections, gastrointestinal** (stomach) **disorders, Bell's palsy (facial paralysis), and "Burning Mouth Syndrome"** (a rare condition primarily affecting menopausal women) may also cause Yuck Mouth.

❑ Although gingivitis can cause your gums to become inflamed and bleed, diabetes and leukemia can also play a role.

❑ If your lips are cracked lips, you may have a vitamin deficiency.

❑ Missing teeth, or mad gaps in your grill, can be a sign of poor nutrition, advanced gum disease, or long-term drug use. Chronic Bulimia leaves tell-tale acid marks on the inside of the teeth.

❑ Say, "Aaaah..." A healthy tongue is covered in tiny bumps (papillae). If your tongue looks, or feels, very smooth and glassy, you may have a nutrient deficiency. It's time to take some folic acid, vitamin B12, or iron. **A smooth, red tongue may indicate pernicious anemia, or possibly mal-absorption syndrome** (your body can't absorb the necessary nutrients).

- ❏ You may also be breathing through your mouth because you're too fat, and breathing through your nose isn't allowing you to move enough oxygen, since you've got all that weight on your chest.

Breasts

- ❏ Now's your opportunity to cop a feel. Seriously! Lumps, beneath the arm, and in the breast, as well as dimples, swelling and discharge may signify breast cancer, and not just in females! Fellas, you can develop breast cancer too, with many of the same symptoms. Always seek medical attention if you find a lump.
- ❏ A condition which causes men to develop enlarged breasts is gynecomastia. This may be caused by an imbalance of estrogen (female hormones), and testosterone (male hormones). With all the hormones that dairy cows are fed to increase their milk supply, you may be drinking female hormones, without realizing it. **Gynecomastia also occurs during puberty, or with aging, and can also be a sign of kidney disease, or pituitary tumors.**

Stomach and Digestion

- ❏ A high body-mass index (BMI), or waistline measurement, is a red flag to clinicians. But, sudden, unexplained weight loss can be even worse, suggesting serious depression, a gastrointestinal illness, a mal-absorption syndrome, or even diabetes.
- ❏ If your stomach is rumbling a lot, this may only be because you're gassy from a diet that's too high in fiber, carbohydrates, or artificial sweeteners. Or, maybe, you're drinking too many carbonated drinks, (where do you think all those bubbles go?). Excess gas may also mean that you're lactose intolerant (can't digest milk products), or that you have other food or drug allergies.
- ❏ If your stomach is constantly aching, don't ignore it. You could be suffering from ulcers, a gall bladder condition, or pancreatic, appendix, or digestive issues. There's also a condition which usually occurs in children called, "abdominal migraine." This is similar to when adults get migraine headaches.
- ❏ If you haven't had a bowel movement, pooped, taken the Browns to the Super Bowl, or shat for 3 days, you are what we call "BACKED UP." We're supposed to be eliminating each time that we eat, but some of our bodies are so jacked up that we're happy to go once a day...some of us even settle for once, every other day! Drink lots of water and eat lots of fruits and vegetables to keep it movin'.
- ❏ And, if you've ever wondered why your kids are droppin' bigger turds than you, think about all the nasty stuff that's accumulating in

your system. Better out than in, right? If your stools are often small or thin, you may have a gang of blockage down there, which can be a warning sign for colon cancer, or its precursor, colon polyps.

☐ If you're eating smaller portions than usual, but feel full, and you are often nauseous, vomiting, bleeding, and experiencing fever or weight loss, you may have a bowel obstruction. This means that something is preventing you from pooping.

☐ Surprisingly, vomiting can sometimes be caused by stress.

☐ If you've had diarrhea for 2-3 days, you may have a bacterial or viral infection, parasites, or a colon problem, like cancer.

☐ Don't be afraid to look in the toilet after you go! **The color of your stool can tell you a lot.** Black, tar-like stools may be a result of taking too much iron, but can also be caused by bleeding in the stomach or the esophagus. Bright red stools may be caused by intestinal bleeding, but more often come from eating red foods, especially if they're artificially dyed. If your stool's very pale, this can be a result of too much calcium, or it may come from eating a lot of rice or potatoes. But if your stool is always pale, this may be a signal that your bile ducts are blocked by tumors, a pancreatic disorder, or liver disease (like hepatitis, cirrhosis, or liver cancer).

☐ **Stool with an extremely bad and unusual smell can indicate a more serious condition,** such as cystic fibrosis, Crohn's disease, ulcerative colitis, or chronic pancreatitis.

Urinary Tract

☐ The first time that you urinate in the morning, expect that your urine will be darker and smellier than it will be for the rest of the day. This is because, as you sleep, the minerals and toxins in the body accumulate. For the rest of the day, your urine should be light-colored and odorless. This is assuming that you have normal functioning kidneys, no bladder disease, and no infection.

☐ What you eat can also affect the odor and color of your urine. Asparagus causes your urine to smell strange and turmeric (a spice) can turn your urine bright yellow.

☐ Sweet-smelling urine is caused by the excretion of blood sugars and can be a warning sign for diabetes. This sweet smell is associated with ketonuria and may also occur as a result of excessive dieting.

☐ Red urine can indicate diabetic nephropathy (diabetic related kidney failure), papillary renal cell carcinoma (cancer), aloe poisoning, or simply eating too many beets or using certain prescription drugs.

☐ Frequent urination is also associated with diabetes.

☐ **Blood in urine can be a sign of a urinary tract infection or**

bladder cancer. Blood in the urine may also occur due to cysts, stones, infection or inflammation along the urinary tract.

☐ Very low urine output, known as oliguria, can be a symptom of renal failure, urinary blockage, or insufficient blood supply to the kidneys.

☐ Men with enlarged prostates, or prostate cancer, have difficulty with starting to urinate.

☐ Women who have difficulty controlling their bladder can practice Kegal exercises to strengthen their muscles and prevent leakage. A loss of bladder control is sometimes a result of multiple child-births.

☐ If you feel the need to urinate, but only a few drops trickle out and it hurts like hell, you could have a urinary tract infection, or you may be burning from an STD. Betta get that checked out homie.

Menstrual Cycle

☐ Normal menstrual cycles (if you have them) are timed anywhere from 21 to 35 days apart. More frequent, and they could indicate a gynecological condition like fibroids (benign uterine tumors), or endometriosis (a condition where the tissue that lines the uterus starts to migrate outside of it).

☐ Sometimes a woman has a really painful cycle and has no idea she's suffering from endometriosis. The endometrial tissue, which usually lines the uterus, attaches to other body parts and organs like the ovaries and bowels.

☐ If your menstrual cycles are erratic, you could have polycystic ovary syndrome (PCOS), a hormonal imbalance caused by an overproduction of male hormones – a condition thought to affect up to 10% of all American women.

☐ Abnormal bleeding can also be a sign of miscarriage, disease or pregnancy, and should also not be ignored.

☐ Some women in their 30s also start to notice heavier or more frequent bleeding, caused by hormonal changes. Either way, if you notice something out of the ordinary, it's a good idea to get checked out. And if you're a man, you definitely need to see someone.

While we're down here...the Reproductive Area

☐ Itching, burning, bumps, lumps, little bugs, sores, blisters, discharge, or anything else that's unusual around your genitals could be signs of sexually transmitted diseases (STDs).

☐ Painful, urination, pelvic pains and pain in the scrotum are signs of an STD.

☐ Go get checked out on the regular, so that you're not the one who is infecting and re-infecting others. That is *so* not a good look. Most STDs are treatable and curable.

Legs

❑ Swollen legs and feet are an indication that your body is not eliminating water properly. This is also called edema. Edema can be a sign of kidney or liver disease, or even heart failure. Congestive heart failure not only affects the lower extremities. It may also cause for your lungs to fill with fluid. This is called pulmonary edema.

❑ Pregnant women are also frequently affected by edema. But don't worry Sis, it's an excellent excuse to sit down and put your feet up.

Feet

❑ Numbness and tingling in the feet can be indicators of vascular disease and other circulatory problems. Nerve damage also often begins at the extremities (hands and feet). Numbness and tingling often occur as a result of nerve damage, and this condition is associated with uncontrolled diabetes. Since blood circulation is compromised for diabetics, even a minor scratch or sore on the feet can become infected easily. The lack of sensation can make it easy to ignore the wound. Gangrene can then set in, requiring amputation of the affected limb. People with diabetes are urged to check their feet every day for any kind of scratch or lesion.

❑ If you have pain, tenderness or limited motion in the joints of your feet, you may have arthritis. This is especially true if this pain worsens over time.

❑ If you are a male and over 30 with acute pain in the big toe or other joint, you may have gout. Gout results in hot, red, and swollen joints. "The Gout" is caused by high levels of uric acid in the blood, and is a chronic form of arthritis.

❑ If you have flat feet, you're at increased risk of exercise injuries.

❑ If your feet lose color and you notice increased or periodic swelling in the lower extremities, you may have hypertension.

❑ Pain in the ankles can be a sign of problems in your knee and hip joints.

Symptoms of all kinds are your body's way of communicating with you. Defined as a change from normal function or appearance, minor or serious, symptoms are warning signs! A diseased person can typically experience indicators over a long period of time before a diagnosis is made. As Peter McWilliams writes in *Life 101*:

> Pain (any pain, emotional, physical, mental) has a message. The information it has about our life can be remarkably specific, but it usually falls into one of two categories: We would be more alive if we did more of this, and, life would be more lovely if we did less of that.

Once we get the pain's message, and follow its advice, the pain goes away...The more severe the pain or illness, the more severe will be the necessary changes. These may involve breaking bad habits, or acquiring some new and better ones.

If we pay attention to these indicators early on, we might prevent the onset of disease altogether.

MORE SIGNS AND SYMPTOMS NOT TO IGNORE
BY SCIHONOR DEVOTION

Chest pain: Although chest pain may be caused by something as simple as heart burn, or indigestion, it can also be a warning sign for something much more serious! Your heart may not be getting enough blood. When your heart muscle doesn't receive enough blood, you'll experience an acute myocardial infarction (sudden heart muscle death)...or what we laymen like to call a "heart attack." Other symptoms of AMI are pain in the chest, pain in the jaw, and/or pain in the left arm. Difficulty breathing and profuse sweating are also associated with AMI. **We shouldn't have to tell you to call 9-11!**

Shortness of breath: Shortness of breath can be caused by many factors. **Because of the conditions that Original People often live in** (smog-filled cities, mold-filled housing, frequent exposure to tobacco smoke), **we suffer from asthma** (sometimes called reactive airway disease or RAD) **at higher rates than the general population.** Albuterol inhalers are prescribed as rescue inhalers for asthmatics. It's necessary to find out what your "triggers" are – what causes your asthma to "act up." Triggers can be anything from pet dander to pollen to exercise. Shortness of breath may also be caused by an exacerbation (worsening) of a chronic lung condition that tobacco smokers suffer from. This condition is called chronic obstructive pulmonary disease or COPD, and there is no cure for it. Do yourself a favor, and stop smoking before COPD or lung cancer sets in. Shortness of breath may also be caused by pneumonia or pulmonary edema. Both of these conditions limit how big a breath you can take. Whatever the case, if you're short of breath then find out why. The breath of life is important!

Coughing: Coughing may also occur as an allergic reaction. Any inhaled irritants will cause you to cough. These irritants may be tobacco or marijuana smoke, dust or smog.

Unintended weight loss: This could be a sign of an overactive thyroid. Sometimes unintended weight loss is the first sign of cancer or liver disease. Surprisingly, depression may cause you to lose weight as you may become less interested in eating.

Coordination: If you're so weak and unbalanced you can't walk straight without falling or bumping into something, you may be experiencing muscle or brain problems which are affecting your coordination. **Weakness and imbalance may also be signs of a stroke. Nowadays, people as young as in their early twenties are having strokes, so don't take this lightly.** If you're having coordination issues, weakness (especially on the left side), a loss of vision, and slurred speech...**put down this book and call 9-11!** These are definitely stroke symptoms. Headaches and loss of balance can be included.

Pain on right side of the body: This could be caused by gall stones. Gall stones are collections of calcium and cholesterol that accumulate in the gallbladder, which is a small sack beneath the liver. These stones can block the digestive tract. But don't worry! **Dandelion leaves from right outside.** Yes, the yellow flowers that we call "weeds" have medicinal properties. **Their leaves can help dissolve these stones.** Milk Thistle (another weed) can help, too. You'd be surprised what herbs you can find in the hood!

Body temperature: A rectal temperature reading is said to be the most accurate, but it isn't always that serious. A fever is a rise in internal body temperature to temperatures considered to be above normal. Normal body temperature is considered to be about 98.6°F or 37°C. You are considered to have a fever when your body's temperature is above 100.4°F or 38°C.

If you take your temperature when you wake up (when your body temperature is at its coolest), and it's below 98.6, this could indicate that you have a condition called hypothyroidism, or an under-active thyroid.

Fatigue: Fatigue may occur because you may not be getting enough quality, deep sleep, you may be stressed out, you may have just finished exercising or doing other strenuous activities, you may be jet-lagged, etc. Or, you may be experiencing chronic, or constant, fatigue because you have an iron deficiency, because you're "coming down with something" and your body is using its energy trying to fight off infection, or because you may be pregnant.

Get your mind right: Many of us suffer from mental illnesses and often overlook it. Sudden changes in the mental state can appear in many different forms: sudden confusion; erratic mood changes (like being really drained to severely agitated); extreme aggression; disorientation; sudden memory problems; delirium. Like Busta said, "This is serious!" And it is also "very dangerous!" The mind and body work closely together. **If your body is fighting an infection, or if you have low blood sugar, or are anemic, this can result in mental health issues.**

If you're normally interested in sex, but you're not anymore, sad after your baby is born, and you're even considering hurting the baby, or yourself, somethin' ain't right. Are you exhausted, even though you sleep all the time, suicidal, worried and always anxious? Do you hallucinate? Either seeing things that aren't real (visual hallucinations), or hearing the voices of people that aren't there (auditory hallucinations)? Something ain't right! Emotional problems are often over-looked in our communities and aren't considered to be very serious. Well, they are serious. Get some help. If you know someone else who is experiencing these symptoms, please be a friend and get them some help. In the society we live in, it is easy to fall into a slump. People are hungry, worked to the bone, overwhelmed, sad, and just sick and tired of being sick and tired. Don't beat yourself up. You have every right to be down. But, you can't allow yourself to stay down there. Make a move to pick yourself up. (See "Get Your Mind Right" in Volume Two.)

Most symptoms are curable with a change in lifestyle but don't dismiss medical attention. Hear the warnings.

IS IT ALL IN YOUR HEAD?
BY SUPREME UNDERSTANDING

What is Somatization?

Put simply, somatization is "a tendency to experience and communicate somatic distress in response to psychosocial stress and to seek medical help for it." In other words, it's when you feel like sh*t physically, but it's really because of something in your head. It's related to temporary "psychosomatic" conditions (those where your mind is affecting your body), as well as the full-fledged Somatization disorder, a psychiatric diagnosis applied to patients who persistently complain of varied physical symptoms that have no identifiable physical origin.

Now, this may sound crazy and rare to some of us, but it's really very common in our community. In fact, **studies suggest that somatization is more prevalent in Black and Latino communities than anywhere else. Some of this is tied to cultural beliefs** (I'm sick because she put a hex on me), **while in many other cases, it's tied directly to depression**...which we don't really talk about, so we just say we're in pain. The following test can help you see if any of this applies to you.

Pennebaker Inventory of Limbic Languidness

This 54-question self-test measures peoples' tendency to notice, and report, a broad array of physical symptoms and sensations. The questionnaire includes a list of 54 common physical symptoms and sensations. On each question, select the choice that reflects how frequent you've experienced that symptom or sensation. Please note: This test will only be scored correctly if you answer each one of the questions. The choices are coded in the following way:

NA:	L3:	EM:	EW:	M1:		
Never or almost never	Less than 3 or 4 times a year	Every month or so	Every week or so	More than once every week		

	NA	L3	EM	EW	M1		NA	L3	EM	EW	M1
Eyes water	NA	L3	EM	EW	M1	Itchy eyes or skin	NA	L3	EM	EW	M1
Ringing in ears	NA	L3	EM	EW	M1	Temporary deafness or hard of hearing	NA	L3	EM	EW	M1
Lump in throat	NA	L3	EM	EW	M1	Choking sensations	NA	L3	EM	EW	M1
Sneezing spells	NA	L3	EM	EW	M1	Runny nose	NA	L3	EM	EW	M1
Congested nose	NA	L3	EM	EW	M1	Bleeding nose	NA	L3	EM	EW	M1
Asthma or wheezing	NA	L3	EM	EW	M1	Coughing	NA	L3	EM	EW	M1
Out of breath	NA	L3	EM	EW	M1	Swollen ankles	NA	L3	EM	EW	M1
Chest pains	NA	L3	EM	EW	M1	Racing heart	NA	L3	EM	EW	M1
Cold hands or feet even in hot weather	NA	L3	EM	EW	M1	Leg cramps	NA	L3	EM	EW	M1
Insomnia or difficulty sleeping	NA	L3	EM	EW	M1	Toothaches	NA	L3	EM	EW	M1
Upset stomach	NA	L3	EM	EW	M1	Indigestion	NA	L3	EM	EW	M1
Heartburn or gas	NA	L3	EM	EW	M1	Abdominal pain	NA	L3	EM	EW	M1
Diarrhea	NA	L3	EM	EW	M1	Constipation	NA	L3	EM	EW	M1
Hemorrhoids	NA	L3	EM	EW	M1	Swollen joints	NA	L3	EM	EW	M1
Stiff muscles	NA	L3	EM	EW	M1	Back pains	NA	L3	EM	EW	M1

Sensitive or tender skin	N A	L 3	E M	E W	M 1	Face flushes	N A	L 3	E M	E W	M 1
Tightness in chest	N A	L 3	E M	E W	M 1	Skin breaks out in rash	N A	L 3	E M	E W	M 1
Acne or pimples on face	N A	L 3	E M	E W	M 1	Acne/pimples other than face	N A	L 3	E M	E W	M 1
Boils	N A	L 3	E M	E W	M 1	Sweat even in cold weather	N A	L 3	E M	E W	M 1
Strong reactions to insect bites	N A	L 3	E M	E W	M 1	Headaches	N A	L 3	E M	E W	M 1
Feeling pressure in head	N A	L 3	E M	E W	M 1	Hot flashes	N A	L 3	E M	E W	M 1
Chills	N A	L 3	E M	E W	M 1	Dizziness	N A	L 3	E M	E W	M 1
Feel faint	N A	L 3	E M	E W	M 1	Numbness or tingling in any part of body	N A	L 3	E M	E W	M 1
Twitching of eyelid	N A	L 3	E M	E W	M 1	Twitching other than eyelid	N A	L 3	E M	E W	M 1
Hands tremble or shake	N A	L 3	E M	E W	M 1	Stiff joints	N A	L 3	E M	E W	M 1
Sore muscles	N A	L 3	E M	E W	M 1	Sore throat	N A	L 3	E M	E W	M 1
Sunburn	N A	L 3	E M	E W	M 1	Nausea	N A	L 3	E M	E W	M 1
ITEMS MARKED						ITEMS MARKED					

Scoring

Scoring Key	Items Marked	Points
NA: Never or almost never: 0 points	NA: ___ x 0 =	0
L3: Less than 3 or 4 times a year: 1 point	L3: ___ x 1 =	
EM: Every month or so: 2 points	EM: ___ x 2 =	
EW: Every week or so: 3 points	EW: ___ x 3 =	
M1: More than once every week: 4 points	M1: ___ x 4 =	
	TOTAL SCORE =	

Scores on the PILL can range from 0 to 216, although most people generally score between about 34 to 84 (the average is 59).

Scoring Ranges and Explanation	
0 to 21: Below Normal Range	Your score is below the normal range. This could reflect the fact that you are exceptionally healthy, aren't under much stress, or you simply try not to pay too much attention to your body's signals. Some researchers or psychologists might question if you are actively avoiding paying attention to your body or even

	denying normal symptoms of fatigue and stress.
22 to 66: Well Within Normal Range	Your score is well within the normal range. You are attentive to normal variations in your body's symptoms and sensations but don't dwell on them too much. Keep up the good work.
67 to 84: Slightly Above Average, Within Normal Range	Your score is slightly above average but within the normal range. Your slightly elevated PILL score indicates that you tend to be somewhat introspective and notice subtle changes in your body when you are experiencing distress. It is also possible that you sometimes use your body's signals to figure out how you are feeling.
85 or Above: Top 25 Percent	Your total PILL score puts you in the top 25% of people who have taken this questionnaire. People who score high on the PILL tend to pay a great deal of attention to their bodily sensations. This preoccupation can reflect being under great stress, feelings of depression, or even periods of emotional conflict. If these feelings of stress are overwhelming, you might consider seeing a mental health professional.

The PILL has been used in a large number of medical and psychological studies to understand the nature of symptom reporting. People who report a large number of physical symptoms tend to go to physicians at higher rates suggesting that their health is worse. Many high symptom reporters, however, are objectively as healthy as low symptom reporters. Interestingly, high symptom reports tend to be more nervous, distressed, and unhappy. They are more likely to have had major upheavals in their childhoods and tend to keep these upheavals secret. Several studies have found that people who are asked to write about emotional upheavals in their lives tend to show drops in symptom reports in the weeks and months afterwards. Physical symptoms, then, reflect people's psychological states almost as much as they say something about their biological condition.[6]

Watch your thoughts. They can bring about an "imagined" ailment.

AM I FAT? PROLLY.

BY SUPREME UNDERSTANDING

Everyone knows that being fat (or "obese") is linked to damn near

---

[6] Important Note about Our Psychological Screening Tests: All tests in the book are meant to be used as a starting point, not as a diagnosis tool. The score is not intended as a mental disorder diagnosis, or as any type of healthcare recommendation.

every health problem you can think of, from diabetes to heart attacks. Yet some of us may be a little confused about what it means to be fat. Though many of us like to think we just have a "little gut" and are still healthy, that's not necessarily true. We think the risk factor is overall obesity, but it's actually more about your waistline than anything else. That's right, your gut. And we often think that having a little "gut" doesn't mean we're at risk for high blood pressure (because we are not "obese"), but this is wrong too. **Health experts agree that the bigger your belly, the bigger your risk for high blood pressure, heart attack, stroke, Type 2 Diabetes gallbladder disease, metabolic syndrome and numerous cancers.**

Waistline Measurement

The simplest indicator is a visual assessment of your waist-to-hip ratio:

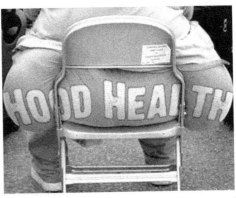

If you're a man and your waist is larger than your hips, or you're a woman and your waist is more than four-fifths of your hip circumference, that's a sign that dangerous visceral fat is surrounding an abdominal organ. That's where all the risk begins. Need an accurate assessment of how high your risk is? You can do a simple waistline measurement. All you need is a tape measure. Position it around your waist at the level of your bellybutton (You can also use the top of your hip bone as a guide). You might be surprised to find you've got "abdominal obesity" even though you aren't obese overall.

According to the International Diabetes Federation guidelines, the healthy normal waistline numbers by gender are as follows:

	Normal	Obese
Females	less than 32 inches (80 cm)	anything higher
Males	less than 38 inches (94 cm)	anything higher

WTR: Waist-to-Tallness Ratio

The BMI, or Body Mass Index, is how "obesity" is normally calculated. You can find your BMI in the chart provided in the appendix of this book. But the BMI isn't the best system. Waistline measurement is better, but there's an even better system to measure how much your weight is affecting your health. According to recent studies, your heart risk could be best shown by your waist-to-tallness ratio (WTR). **To figure out what your waistline should be for your height, take your height in inches and multiply it by 0.55 for men and 0.53 for women. That will give you a fairly good idea of the upper limit of a healthy waistline (in inches) for you.** Which means if you're a 5'8" tall male, you're 68 inches in height. 68 x 0.55 = 37.4, meaning if your waistline measures wider than that, you're at risk and fat.

Why is this better system? Keep in mind that for some people, like a huge football player who exercises as a way of life, the BMI index could show them as being obese when in fact they are in excellent physical condition.

> **Did You Know?**
> Recent studies have discovered that abdominal fat is even bad for your brain, as it's associated with the brain changes linked to Alzheimer's disease. Your waistline makes a big difference. The following is a set of ways you can tell if you're at risk.

Does a Big Butt Mean You're Fat?

Let me remind you that the idea of being "fat" is mostly in your head. That is, people who do NOT fit the description above (waistline bigger than hips) may think that are fat because they don't look like the European models on TV, but I don't even know if ANYONE wants to look like that anymore.

Still, women throughout the world continue to ask their mates, "Do I look fat?" But there's a difference between weight in the right places and weight in the wrong places.[7] **Research tells us that if most of your fat is in the belly area, your risk for a heart condition is greater than if the fat resides in your hips, thighs or rear (sometimes referred to as "pear shape" body type).** Meaning if you're a woman with big hips, big thighs, and a big booty...you're not fat, obese, or unhealthy...unless you have a belly to match. If you're a man with those features, you're not obese either, but you've got bigger problems. No, seriously. Those developments occur when a male's body is producing too much estrogen and not enough testosterone. (See "How to Boost Your Testosterone") Getting back to women, though, NPR recently published an article titled "Baby Got Back, and a Healthier Heart" that notes:

---

[7] Not to mention that mainstream models of "healthy" weight and size were based on European proportions, which are not always compatible with the otherwise healthy body shapes of many Original people. However, risk is risk, and unhealthy is unhealthy. Since straight-up obesity was not a typical feature of indigenous people, we shouldn't be using our ethnicity to justify not getting in shape. If you want to be culturally relevant, look at your ancestors and get in THAT shape.

It appears that "increased gluteofemoral fat mass"– science speak for "big butt and thighs"– may be healthy, concludes a review of the scientific literature just published by the International Journal of Obesity. The analysis by a team from Oxford University concluded that unlike people prone to belly-fat weight gain, those who tend to pad out around their bottoms are less likely to suffer from cardiovascular and metabolic diseases. They also pointed to recent findings suggesting that fat in the butt and thighs is more efficient at trapping and storing excess fatty-acids over the long haul, thus reducing weight gain elsewhere in the body. Dr. Konstantinos Manolopolous, the lead author, acknowledged in a statement that…the connection between belly fat and cardiovascular risk, for one, has been established. But, he noted that "it is only very recently that thigh fat and a larger hip circumference have been shown to promote health."

Yup. A big butt and thighs is good for a woman's health. And a big gut (or even a medium "paunch") is bad for everyone.

While we're on the subject, you can also learn to calculate your Body Fat Percentage, your Basic Metabolic Rate, and your Daily Calorie Needs using the tables in the Appendix of this book.

You should take all these things into consideration when you think about your weight and weight loss.

KNOWING YOUR FAMILY'S HEALTH HISTORY

BY SATORI ANANDA

Did You Know?
The "My Family Health Portrait" Web tool is a free and easy way to organize, save, and share your family history with your doctor and family members. Visit: www.hhs.gov/familyhistory

Living a loving, peaceful and happy life is what most people want for themselves and their families. Achieving this goal includes knowing as much as we can about the health and medical history of our close relatives. A record of health information about a person and his or her close relatives is called a medical health history. A complete record includes information from three generations of relatives, including children, brothers and sisters, parents, aunts and uncles, nieces and nephews, grandparents, and cousins. **We have many factors in common with our family including genes, lifestyle and environment. Together they provide a picture and give our doctors clues in our risk for developing particular conditions such as heart disease, high blood pressure, stroke, certain cancers, and diabetes.** Risks of rarer conditions caused by single cell mutations like cystic fibrosis and sickle cell anemia can be predetermined allowing more frequent and earlier screenings, changes in diet, and exercise.

Talking to our relatives about their health is the best and easiest way to get information about family medical history. Death certificates and obituaries are good resources as well. Keep records of the information, maintain it regularly and share it with as many other family members as possible.

Plan ahead. Take preventive measures.

---

13 Ways to Destroy Yourself

BY SUPREME UNDERSTANDING

ORIGINALLY PUBLISHED IN HOW TO HUSTLE AND WIN, PT. ONE

I know people think I'm playing when I say "kill yourself" throughout this book. Of course I don't want anybody to really commit suicide. But the truth is, most of us are killing ourselves ANYWAY. If you want some sure-fire ways to destroy yourself, just check out the following. Before you begin however, decide what age you want to live to. You'll need this number, so keep it in your head.

1. Stay Angry. A little anger here and there isn't all bad. It's actually better for you than other emotions, like fear and doubt. But like anything you can have too much of, is best in moderation. If you stay angry for long periods of time, you'll actually end up with health issues, like high blood pressure, sleep disorders and lung damage. As the Buddha said, "Holding on to anger is like grasping a hot coal with the intent of throwing it at someone else; you are the one who gets burned." (If this description applies to you in any way, take 10 years off the age you have in your head)

2. Sacrifice Sleep. Too little sleep (less than 6 or 7 hours a night) has been tied to many different health problems, including obesity, diabetes and cancer. Mental fatigue is also just as bad as alcohol when it comes to the worst risk factor for vehicular accidents. That's why you can get pulled over for driving drunk or just sleepy... and go to jail either way. (Take off 5 years)

3. Get into the Wrong Line of Work. Want to die for your country...way before you should? I don't only mean joining the army or the police force. There are plenty of jobs that will overwork and underpay you until you have nothing left to give. Oh, and let's not forget about all the illegal ways to make money, where most people never make it out successfully. (Take off 8 years)

4. Ignore the Doctor. It's almost impossible to get a man to take a physical exam. But if you want to find out anything before it's too late, you need to schedule an appointment. If you don't like doctors, see a holistic healer. If not, at least start reading books on health, like this one. If you don't want to listen to anybody, just kill yourself now. (Take off 12)

5. Dumb Down Your Brain. Reading, doing crosswords and problem-solving are good ways to prevent Alzheimer's, a degenerative brain disease that affects most people who live to be old enough. On the other hand, every 1% gain in your literacy increases your life expectancy by 2 years. Anyway, a dumb life is a life full of problems that never get solved. And those problems will kill you faster than losing sleep ever could. (Take off 14)

6. Have a Lot of Sex. Sex in itself isn't really bad. In fact, it's usually great. But depending on how you do it, you may be signing your death certificate. Keep avoiding those check-ups, checking out your partner's background, and forgetting to strap up. Watch what happens. Don't forget that 12 million Americans contract STDs every year, many of which can leave you unable to make or have children. (Take off 9)

7. Drink a Lot. The occasional drink of alcohol ain't so bad, as long as it ain't Thunderbird or Wild Irish Rose. Actually, a glass of red wine can be good for your heart. But more than two drinks per day, and you're looking at permanent liver damage or diabetes. Alcohol is also the root cause of nearly 100,000 deaths per year. Not to mention all the stupid, life-threatening problems created on "courage juice." (Take off 14)

8. Stress Out. Creating more stress in your life is a great way to invite all kinds of diseases to attack the body. When you're always stressed, your adrenal glands are forced to work overtime and will eventually wear themselves out, which seriously weakens your immune system. Next thing you know, you're stressed AND sick. Not to mention that

> **Did You Know?**
> According to a recent study published in the *Archives of Internal Medicine*, four bad habits can shorten your life by 12 years. The four bad habits are smoking, drinking too much, inactivity and a poor diet. The study examined 4886 adults over a 20 year span. In just 20 years, over 1,000 of the participants died – 431 from cardiovascular disease, 318 from cancer and 331 from other causes. The shortest lifespans were clearly associated with the above four risk factors. In fact, participants' risk of death increased with each additional bad habit. The healthiest participants were those who never smoked and those who had quit; women who had fewer than two drinks daily and men who had fewer than three; those who got at least two hours of physical activity weekly; and those who ate fruits and vegetables at least three times daily.

stressed-out people are more "ready to die" than regular folks. (Take off 20)

9. Watch TV. The average American spends a full 9 years of his life watching TV. Those are years that could be spent exercising, reading, or working for social change. Unless you only watch the science and history channels, you're on your way to being an overweight, lazy, TV-addicted couch potato. And that's a recipe for early death. (Take off 9)

10. Associate with the Wrong People. Whether it's a gang where people care more about whether you pay your dues than whether you live or die, or a relationship that drives you insane, there are a lot of people that will make your life shorter. If you want to live: Avoid people who don't care about their lives, because they won't care about yours, and avoid people who will suck the life out of you... even if she can suck the life out of you. (Take off 8)

11. Smoke. Tobacco-related illnesses are America's number two killer. They're also the most preventable. We all know that smoking leads to a dozen different cancers throughout the body. Smoking is also a major cause of heart disease, bronchitis, emphysema, stroke, and even contributes to the severity of pneumonia. Plus it causes asthma and cancer in the innocent people we smoke around. **Just one cigarette can immediately increase your blood pressure and decrease the circulation to your head and limbs. Imagine what a pack does to you.** (Take off 18)

12. Eat Junk. In 2006, at least 400,000 Americans managed to kill themselves based almost solely on what they ate. Heart disease is the country's number one killer and – although some of that comes from genetics – most of it's due to the crap we eat. Besides all the fat and cholesterol, the chemicals, hormones, and drugs they put in our food are killing us slowly no matter how you cut it. Not to mention all the worms and parasites already in your meat! (Take off 18)

13. Hate Yourself. Here's an easy way to die faster. Live a miserable life that you hate. Hate everything about it, including yourself. Before long, you'll either create the kind of problems that will eventually destroy you, or you'll just give up and kill yourself. (Take off 15)

Final Score

So...are you destroying yourself right now? What age did you end up with? I hope it's not a negative number! No matter what number you came up with, learn this lesson.

Live like you cherish life, not like you're anxious for death.

SETTING WELLNESS GOALS

BY KING DIVINE ALLAH

When setting goals, keep in mind certain factors can play a major role in your success. It can be useful to follow the S.M.A.R.T. (Specific, Measurable, Attainable, Realistic and Timely) Guidelines. Ask specific questions: What do I want to accomplish? Where will I do it? When will I do it? HOW will I do it? Do I need help with accomplishing my goals?

When setting goals, **it's important to think of the actions you need to change.** Everyone has room for improvement, so we all have things about ourselves that we can change. It's a great idea to take your family medical history into consideration (See "Knowing Your Family's Health History") know what has and hasn't worked for others, the same may apply to you. Use visualization techniques, visualize yourself being healthy, and see what you need to become that person. Create your own slogan, or vision statement, based on how you will look, feel, and behave. An example would be, "I will become a more balanced, less stressed, even-tempered person, who makes health a top priority."

Next, I recommend you set at least three goals based on your vision statement. Six month and one year goals can be set, but three month goals provide urgency, and encourage you to start today. It's also best to work on only three to five changes at a time. When we try to make too many changes at once, we can feel overwhelmed and defeated.

Determine your internal motivators for change and put them into writing, or say aloud to yourself daily what they are. When I decided to lose weight, my internal motivator was that a lot of females dissed me because I was overweight. I ended up losing over 100 pounds and created another internal motivator, I will never go back to being obese, again. You may develop some resentment from your friends and family because of this new lifestyle. They might clown you, or feel betrayed, and in ways discourage you but this is just another obstacle, like eliminating junk foods. **Don't turn them away, share what you know, get as much support as you can.** If auntie knows how to cook vegetables and primo exercises, get with them.

Figure out three things that you can do this week to achieve your short term goals. Make sure you can achieve at least 80% of this, if you can't you need to cut back and find something more achievable. Maybe start with getting a salad with your order instead of fries, or choose wheat or whole grain brad over white, one step at a time.

SO SICK: HOW IT ALL STARTED

WE WEREN'T ALWAYS THIS ILL

We weren't always this way. **Original people, in their native homelands, were typically disease-free, physically fit, mentally sharp, and emotionally sound.** That's not my opinion. That's based on historical accounts provided by both the European missionaries and the storytellers and griots (historians) of those indigenous communities. The missionaries might have said they were "pagan heathens" bound for hell, but they sure didn't say we were fat and sick. So what happened? Cause right now, we're fat as hell and sick as hell, so ain't nobody concerned about where we're going, because we're there already.

Well, once they decided we were bound for hell, the Pope cosigned us being physically "bound" as well. And Europeans told themselves they were saving us…by enslaving us. Then again, it was always more about profits than prophets, so let's not give anyone the benefit of the doubt. We were raped, robbed, and ruled for the benefit of those who got rich while we lost everything we knew. In the process of our exploitation and near extermination, there was also experimentation and examination. They cut us up, subjected us to infectious diseases, and tested all their methods on our vulnerable populations. Black and brown people throughout the world were introduced to European pork, European alcohol, European syphilis, and eventually the European diet.

You see, everywhere in the world where you find Black and brown people with some remembrance of their original way of life, we eat similarly. We eat a grain with a legume as our staple dish. In East Asia, it's rice and soybeans. In South Asia, it's rice and lentils. Among Native Americans, it's corn (or quinoa) and beans. In Africa, it's millet (or sorghum, tef, etc.) and lentils. We eat a ton of vegetables with our meals, and we eat fruit separately as a snack or a dessert. That kind of traditional diet is consistent everywhere, except among Europeans. What do they eat? Meat and potatoes, almost no vegetables. And what do we eat? Whatever our oppressors told us to eat. Although Africans and Native Americans had to teach the Pilgrims what to eat and grow to survive, (See "American Food Only Has A Dash Of White In It") the dinner tables have turned. As soon as Europeans were in a position of dominance over us, we started following their lead, sometimes by force, sometimes by influence, but never for the better. Before being dominated by Europeans, Original people throughout the world healed themselves using plants and herbs. We taught Europeans how to do this as well. And they found a way to reduce these natural methods to chemical processes (as they did with the food), and then mass-produce them cheaply, only to sell them back to us. Once we started patronizing them for our health and wellness, we soon forgot the old ways. And now here we are…

Our interactions with Europeans and the subsequent loss of our original culture coincides with our poor state of health.

IN THE GHETTO…

THE MAKING OF THE GHETTO

BY C'BS ALIFE ALLAH

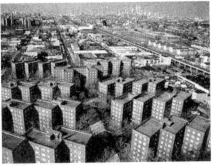

In white science fiction, you always have stories about UFOs that abduct people, take them away and perform godforsaken experiments on them. The reason why they tell these stories so well is because they sent their UFOs/slave ships to the coasts of West Africa and abducted Blacks. They then took them to the Americas and performed various psychological and biological experiments on them. These same "aliens from the planet Europe" had previously invaded the Americas, looking and sounding unlike anything that the Indigenous people had ever seen. In their wake, these white aliens left death and destruction.

The end result of this alien invasion is the creation of the ghettos, barrios and favelas, which, to Black and Indigenous peoples, are just like alien planets. The mental and physical health of Original people in the Americas is jacked up by design. The ghettos, barrios and favelas are all environments of limited resources that place stress on their inhabitants. This stress breaks down the physical and mental foundation of the community. For Original people, living in the hood is like living on another planet without a life support suit. Let's jump back in time and see what went down.

Maafa

The term, Maafa, refers to the Trans-Atlantic Slave Trade. It's important to understand many of the indigenous Africans had been living in metropolitan areas since the Middle Ages, highly civilized and advanced, performing medical procedures Europeans had no clue about (like eye surgery and cesarean births). They were taken from cities and sold to slave traders often as war captives. So, the first layer of mental illness was the psychological impact of war.

Secondly, the images of demons in much of African cosmology were white beings, and the sea symbolized the way to the after-world. These Black captives were psychologically terrorized with the fear of being

taken to a literal "Hell." And their journey into slavery was exactly that. They were packed below the decks of the slave ships amongst feces and rats. Many did not make it across the Atlantic due to these conditions. There are still areas in the Atlantic Ocean, along the route of the Trans-Atlantic Slave Trade, where sharks frequent, because 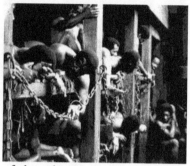 they carry a genetic memory of having fed on the masses of slaves who jumped or were thrown overboard.

Incidentally, there is some evidence that the Blacks that survived the Maafa, or the Middle Passage, carried a gene which allowed them to retain salt. They were not provided salt during the Middle Passage, but salt is necessary for such a long journey. **The theory is that this salt retention gene left the slaves' descendants vulnerable to high blood pressure, due to the high salt diet of modern-day Black Americans.**

The Invasion

As in Africa, the Indigenous Americans were highly civilized. The many city-states in South America dwarfed anything that existed in Europe, at the time. The Indigenous peoples had highly sophisticated metropolitan centers and technologies that were not understood by the white man. Some Indigenous societies were so highly organized that when it came time to draft the Constitution and other American documents, the Europeans modeled their documents and governments after the Indigenous designs.

Whites were not the only invaders to the Americas, and it was not just by "technological advancement" that the whites conquered. They carried with them many diseases. Many of these diseases wiped out whole civilizations. They brought along invasive plant and animal species. Not only did they spread diseases, their dirty asses brought rats to the "New World"! Rats congregate wherever waste and refuse are found. This has affected health up until the modern day because garbage litters the

landscape of any ghetto. Thus, the ghetto is set up to be a breeding ground for rats and roaches, which transmit various types of disease.

Breaking Grounds

Whites had to make sure that Blacks had their 'resistance' beat out of them. They had to transform them from free thinking men and women into chattel slaves. They would beat women in front of men. Slay babies in front of mothers. Utilize various torture devices rooted in the Inquisition. When a person is presented with a dangerous situation their body goes into fight or flight mode, flooding their body with various hormones like adrenaline and places the brain in a hyper-sensitive state. This state is necessary for fight or flight, yet when you are unable to do either and kept in this state, it becomes detrimental to your body and mind.

Talking 'bout the Ghetto

A ghetto is basically an ethnic enclave, meaning that it is racially segregated. In North America, the first ghettos were actually Irish, Italian, and Polish. In fact, during the early part of the 20th Century, Italians and Eastern Europeans were more segregated from the larger white community than Blacks were.

After slavery ended, and up until the Civil Rights laws of the 1960s, "ghettos" were formed. Many Northern, modern-day ghettos were established during the Great Migration in Detroit, Chicago, etc.[8] Blacks, especially, were forced to live in specific areas due to a lack of

---

[8] Though we are focusing on Black ghettos, Asian ghettos, like Chinatown, and Barrios for various Latino groups exist. There is an element of upward mobility in these ghettos due to a portion of the middle class and college educated being able to move out into some suburbs. Yet, these areas also have a constant influx of immigrants who are impacted by drugs, gangs, crime and other stress factors that affects the inhabitants of traditional Black ghettos.

post-slavery capital and sanctioned terrorism by the KKK, lynch mobs, and US government.

The Effects of Living in the Hood

❏ You have limited access to healthy food options.

❏ You have limited access to the economic growth opportunities that other parts of the US have, (banks, mortgages, etc), strictly because of location.

❏ The schools in your community receive less funding, have low-quality teachers and staff, and a poor curriculum. Your schools are also plagued with fewer high-achieving peers, many health and nutrition problems, residential instability, single-parent households, high exposure to crime and gangs, and other factors that negatively affect student performance levels.

❏ You will live with Environmental Racism. This determines how laws, policies, and practices impact low-income areas. In blunt terms, this is why garbage dumps are always in the poor part of town, why lead paint and asbestos are still in many buildings in the hood, and why there are so many rodents and pests in the hood.

❏ You have less access to exercise areas, and less information about the necessity of fitness.

❏ Your air and water quality are less than anywhere else.

❏ You are exposed to a higher rate of violent crime.

Have our history motivate you to improve. Learn from the positive and negative, and share your knowledge with the community.

THE HISTORY OF SOUL FOOD

BIG MAMA HAD A BIG HEART ATTACK AND YOU'RE STILL IGNORING WHY

BY C'BS ALIFE ALLAH

I know that everyone has their memories of the movie, *Soul Food*. Yet, all I can remember is the message that I got from it, which is that food kills! Big Mama is a symbolic person that is too often seen in the Black community. The woman who knows how to cook, and is feeding her whole family a slow (or fast) death. This death is brought on by food that is so-called, "good for the soul," yet, it screws up the body with high blood pressure or hypertension, diabetes, and a host of other PREVENTABLE diseases. **Because Africans in North America have lost many aspects of their varied cultures during enslavement, holding onto Soul Food is seen as retaining one's connection to Africa. The truth is that Soul Food, nowadays, has been warped and it ain't the same as it was during slavery.** Now that your internet-having and library-card-possessing ass has access to more information, you need to take ownership of Soul Food. You need to make this heritage cuisine work for you, instead of making your whole family diseased and sending them to an early grave.

What is Soul Food?

Like Jazz, Soul Food is a unique North American creation that is a direct result of the Maafa (See "In the Ghetto). Enslaved Africans in North America combined different foods, taking a little bit of this and a little bit of that, resulting in some good eating. The foods involved in Soul Food came from three main sources.

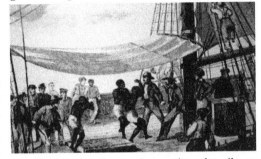

African Sources

Let's be clear. Whites didn't just steal *people* from Africa. In fact, in their brains, they weren't stealing *people*, but RESOURCES. A resource isn't only a person, they also stole precious minerals, oil, etc. Along with these resources, whites took food. Africans also brought over a lot of food on their own, as seeds that were braided in young girls' hair, or as seeds that were embedded in clothing. A lot of these foods could not grow in a European climate, so whites were completely unfamiliar with how to cultivate these crops. Even in the Americas, these crops were totally tended by enslaved Africans. One such crop was rice, which grows in a tropical environment that whites could not tolerate. Other crops that came straight from Africa were indigo, okra, sorghum, kola nut, sesame seed and various melons.

Indian (Native American) Sources

When enslaved Africans were brought to North America, many of them weren't down with being enslaved to white people. Some ran away. Others led all-out war and revolts against white slave owners. This brought Africans in contact with the various Indian Nations who were in the Southeast, such as the Cherokee, Chickasaw, Choctaw, Creek and Seminole. In many cases, formerly enslaved Africans were incorporated in Indian communities. Even those Africans that remained enslaved still interacted with various Indian peoples. This close connection allowed Africans and Indians a fruitful cultural exchange. One thing that happened is that Southern Indian foods and cooking techniques like boiling beans and curing meat over smoked hickory, found their way into modern Soul Food cooking. This became a way of preserving some of the cooking traditions found among Southern Indian Nations.

White Sources

Whites' primary contributions to Soul Food were the pig and the cow. In Europe, during colonial times, whites basically used every part of an animal. However, once it was found out that corn doubles as a key source of feed for livestock, white Americans increased their meat production to a degree that was substantially higher than the rest of the world. This led to greater consumption, and the current statistic, which is that Americans eat three to five times the amount of animal protein than the rest of the world. Because meat was in such abundance, wealthy whites in the Americas could choose to only eat certain, choice cuts of pork and beef. Only in the Americas did the notion of, "eating high on the hog" develop. So, while it is true that Blacks were given the scraps of the pig and cow, the reality is that poor whites were already eating pig intestines, head cheeses and jowls. Poor whites actually showed Blacks how to prepare pig and cow innards. While whites typically seasoned these dishes only with salt, Blacks also used various other seasonings, including onion, garlic, bay leaf and thyme.

> **Did You Know?**
> Soul Food classics like hominy, cornbread, grits and corn meal dumplings (hush puppies) are actually Indian dishes. Indians also shared the meats that they hunted and trapped with Africans. This is how the use of venison, rabbit, squirrel, and possum and raccoon meat found their way into the traditional Soul Food menu. Because Native Americans ate very little meat to begin with, they wasted no part of the animal and ate organ meats like liver, brain, and intestines. This same practice was applied by Africans in their dishes.

In terms of vegetables, whites forced Blacks to utilize "cast-off" greens like turnip, beet and dandelion leaves. Kale, cress, cabbage and mustard were also introduced to Soul Food by whites. However, ironically, many of these fruits and vegetables didn't have a European origin. These foods had found their way into Europe via the Silk Road, (the trade route that stretches from Europe to the civilized world: Africa, India, Arabia and the Far East), during Grecian and Roman times. So, although many consider turnips and beets "white" foods, they actually came from Morocco, North Africa.

Health

There is an emotional connection to Soul Food that links into part of our own romanticism of slavery. Along with the Christian religion, Soul Food is seen as one of those ways that helped Blacks make it through slavery. So, when one speaks out against Soul Food, they are seen as attacking, (what many people see as), a fundamental part of being a Black American. Let's look now, at three major points:

1. You aren't working like a slave.

When a runner is getting ready for a marathon, he or she will eat a heavy meal, the night before, of pasta. This is because pasta releases its sugar/energy slowly. So, when the runner is getting tired down the line, their body can use the pasta's energy as fuel. The marathon runner eats in order to be successful at his or her profession. During slavery, work was from sun up to sun down, often in humidity and heat. **The foods that Africans ate were heavy in fat and calories to aid them with this heavy labor. Nearly no one nowadays is working like a slave, so eating like they did isn't beneficial.** In fact, it does nothing but push us into obesity and disease.

2. Slaves didn't eat three big meals a day.

They generally had one big meal a day that they had towards the closing of their day. They wouldn't have been able to work if they ate huge meals at breakfast and lunch. This is because the body automatically goes into digestion mode, taking energy from the rest of the body to aid in digestion in the stomach and intestines.

3. They didn't eat a whole bunch of deep fried meat every day.

Anyone who cooks knows how much time that it takes to prepare meals. Frying and barbecuing meat takes a lot of time. This is time that slave masters did not give slaves. Seeing that the slaves were only getting scraps of meat from the slave master, slaves didn't have a surplus of meat to go wasting every day. The majority of meat scraps were utilized to season pots of greens, beans and other vegetables. **There is evidence that the historical "slave diet" was heavy on vegetables. Definitely heavier in vegetables than the current American diet. What we also know, for sure, is that slaves generally at large portions of meat only once a week.** Holidays were another time when slaves ate large portions of meat because the slave masters were having feasts, leaving the slaves with the left-overs.

How to Make Soul Food Healthy

We are not telling you to throw the baby out with the bathwater. What we are saying though, is that you can change the game and get your health up. Start off by taking out pork (See "The Other Worm - Er, White – Meat") and replacing it with an organic, high quality meat, if you're not turning vegetarian anytime soon. You can season those greens or beans with smoked turkey neck bones or with Wiley's Southern Classic Seasoning, which has no meat or fat. The vegetable base of Soul Food is extremely healthy. Everything from the greens to the spices is invaluable so get plenty of that! (See "The Healing Power of Vegetables" and "Herbs=Medicine"). Also, It' important to leave the lard alone (See "What Is Lard?") and experiment with baking/broiling (See "Basic Cooking Techniques") to cut back on deep frying. All oils aren't created equal, some can be heated, some can't, others have no business on your food, and none should be recycled! (See "Oils Are Not Health Foods")

If you're eating like a slave maybe you're thinking like on too. Dig deeper in history and know the true foundation.

ARE ALL DOCTORS MAD SCIENTISTS?
WHY BLACK FOLK DON'T TRUST DOCTORS
BY C'BS ALIFE ALLAH

"The fear of medicine is based on real events. And real events go way beyond – way before and way after – Tuskegee. There are things that are happening now that will keep [Blacks] from going to the hospital." – Medical Ethicist Harriet A. Washington

Though lack of money, education, and access to medical resources are all factors in the state of health throughout the Original community, **Original People often avoid the doctor because, deep down inside, they don't trust the same people who lynched them, sent dogs after them, and turned water hoses on them.** At first it seems like a collection of badly written conspiracy theories. "Tropical Fantasy soda causes low sperm count in Black males." "The KKK owns Churches Chicken and is putting extra salt and fat in the chicken." Though things like this seem 'too crazy to be true,' when you dig into the books, you will see a REAL pattern of experimentation and intentional harm done to people of color.

The Hypocrite Oath

You know that famous oath that doctors take, where they pledge to help those in need and not do any harm? It's called the Hippocratic Oath. Its origins are in ancient Greek medicine (and was evidently inspired by the Egyptians). The fact is that no one takes the original oath anymore. It has been changed many times and there are several versions hanging around. In the original you weren't allowed to do abortions or euthanasia (helping a person commit suicide), you were supposed to give the children of your teacher free medical training, and you weren't supposed to have sex or relationships with your

Did You Know?
Female slaves were used to start a well-known medical field today, gynecology. J. Marion Sims, the father of gynecology, did experiments on slave women whose vaginas were damaged during violent child births. The common belief at the time was that Black women did not feel pain, so even though anesthesia was available, it wasn't used on the slave women when he experimented. Dr. Joy Leary goes into painful debt on what was done to these women in her book, *Post Traumatic Slave Syndrome*. And it continued, as women from Puerto Rico were used as guinea pigs in the development of "the pill."

66

patients or any member of their family. As you can see, a lot of that is moot today. The larger picture, though, is this: You know how the Army interrogates prisoners? All of the time, a doctor is present. In fact, many times, it is the doctor who is torturing, oops, I mean "interrogating" the prisoner.

They Treated Us like Animals

The slavery that happened in the Americas is referred to as chattel slavery. That means basically denying the humanity of the slave viewing them literally as livestock. Once you view a person as an animal it is easy to do anything to them. For instance, in the white world from Europe to the Americas there was a tradition of what is called a human zoo. **Look into people like Ota Benga, Saartjie Baartman, and Ishi. These were all Original people who were kept in zoos or exhibitions to be gawked at by white people.** Ota Benga was kept in the Bronx zoo in a cage right next to animals (as "evidence" of the popular "Blacks = monkeys" theme). Saartjie Baartman, called the "Hottentot Venus," had her body violated in many ways, even after death. Ishi was placed in an exhibit to be entertainment for white people. This was all part of viewing Original people as animals. This isn't just in reference to African-Americans. To varying extents, Native Americans, Asians, and other groups were viewed as savages or exhibited as "oddities" and "curious wonders" also. But there is no denying that people from Africa received "special attention." Often, whites paid to poke, prod, and probe the flesh of these vulnerable captives. This went hand in hand with the practices of slavery, particularly the "exhibitions" and "inspections" at slave auctions. Naturally, people who were treated like animals would eventually be used as guinea pigs.

Jack your Body

The historical record of human experimentation by the medical and scientific community in the West is extensive. They try to make it seem like only the Nazis dealt with human experimentation. In chattel slavery, a slave master would breed his slaves like cattle, trying to make slaves of superior 'stock.' Since slaves were treated as property, a slave master couldn't be held liable for anything that he did to his slaves. As a result, every gruesome and inhumane thing imaginable was tested on slaves. Even now fertility drugs and birth control devices are often tested on third world countries. Also defective formula, recalled prescription medicine, defective condoms which don't pass the safety regulations of the U.S., and even tainted blood plasma are often sold and dumped in third world countries.

Blacks, Indians, American Eugenics, and Nazi Germany

In America, during the late 1800's and early 1900's, there were communities that were referred to as "tri-racial isolates." These were basically groups that were combinations of Blacks, Indians and poor whites. Through intermarriage over a period of time, they understood themselves to be different. They basically became communities of people of color that were hard to tie down as specifically Indian or Black. Whites felt threatened by them because they couldn't classify them. As a result, there was a huge eugenics campaign ("eugenics" meaning the science of changing a population by controlling who people can sleep with and reproduce with) against these groups. States started to pass eugenics laws in the late 19th century. These laws allowed them to 'mercifully' kill those who they labeled as mentally ill (or the open-to-interpretation label 'feeble minded') and to perform forced sterilization and forced abortions. This was always tied to race. In fact, one of the earliest groups advocating eugenics was the Immigration Restriction League in 1894. They wanted to limit immigration from 'select' countries because they didn't want the (white) stock of the Americas to be diluted. So eugenics became a tool against the poor and people of color. Oh yeah, by the way, in 1916, Margaret Sanger, one of the founders of Planned Parenthood, was a huge advocate for eugenics and strategically placed clinics in Black neighborhoods. She wanted to purify her race (though people nowadays like to soften the reality by claiming she was only trying to improve America as a whole, ignoring the fact that her work was clearly focused on eliminating undesirables which, again, were predominantly Blacks and the mentally ill). **And though people focus on what Hitler did to the Jews, they leave out part of the story: Hitler was inspired by the Eugenics movement in the Americas.** Another little-known fact: Even though there weren't many Blacks in Germany at the time, Hitler was so concerned about their presence that he vowed, in *Mein Kampf*, to eliminate all children born of African-German descent. The Nazis set up a secret group, Commission Number 3, to organize the sterilization of these "Rhineland Bastards" to maintain the purity of the Aryan race. In 1937, all local authorities in Germany were to submit a list of all the mulattos. Then, these children were taken from their homes or schools without parental permission and put before the commission. Once a child was decided to be of Black descent, the child was taken immediately to a hospital and sterilized. In addition, Raffael Scheck's book, *Hitler's African Victims*, tells of thousands of Blacks killed during Hitler's regime.

The Tuskeegee Syphilis Experiment

One of the most famous experiments on the Black body is the Tuskegee Syphilis Experiment. **This is one of the main foundations in the Black community for the aversion to doctors.** The U.S. Public Health service gathered up 399 Black men who had syphilis. The men were never told they had syphilis nor were they treated for it. They were told they had 'bad blood'. The experiment wanted to observe the progression of the disease. They were given free medical exams, free meals and free burial insurance. What made this test so horrible is that there was already a cure for syphilis in penicillin, yet none of these men were given it. The experiments went on from 1932 to 1972. The cure was found in 1940. By the end of the study, only 74 of the test subjects were still alive. Twenty-eight of the men had died directly of syphilis, 100 were dead of related complications, 40 of their wives had been infected, and 19 of their children had been born with congenital syphilis.

The Guatemalan Version of Tuskeegee

Between 1946 and 1948, U.S. government medical researchers intentionally infected hundreds of people in Guatemala, including institutionalized mental patients, with gonorrhea and syphilis without their knowledge or permission. **Many of those infected were encouraged to pass the infection onto others as part of the study.** Like what was happening at the same time in the U.S. in Tuskeegee, many (if not most) of those infected never received treatment. In September 2010, Secretary of State Hillary Clinton made an apology. Of course, they didn't admit to the hundreds of other similar incidents the U.S. was involved in, nor did they say they'd stopped doing such "reprehensible research" Of course not, because they didn't.

Project 4.1

In the 1950s, Project 4.1 was a medical study done on the residents of the Marshal Islands, who were exposed to radioactive fallout from tests at Bikini Atoll. The U.S. did many nuclear experiments in the Pacific after World War II to keep up with Russia during the Cold War. The first five years after the tests, the indigenous Rongelap women saw their rates of miscarriages and stillbirths double. Within ten years, there were developmental difficulties in their children along with elevated rates of cancer. All the "doctors" did was watch and take notes.

Can't Even Rest In Peace

Did you know that between the 1600's all the way into the early 1900's in North America, grave robbing wasn't a felony? In fact, police would see it happening yet wouldn't do anything to stop it. Even Lincoln's body had to be moved several time due to grave robbers. Though many robbed graves to steal buried valuables, others stole the actual bodies to sell to doctors. Why? When medical universities such as Harvard and Yale were founded in 1636 and 1701, they had a problem. Where were they going to get all those cadavers to use in their training and anatomy classes? They immediately turned to the Black market, literally. They started jacking bodies from the grave. And dead people, just like the living at the time, were kept segregated. So it was easiest to steal bodies from the graves of poor people of color.

And to keep things simple, they'd hire Blacks to do the dirt. **If you've seen the movie Candyman, that "Black boogeyman" figure wasn't created for the film.** In fact, that character is a staple in the mythology of many Black communities. **He is based off of the Black men who would grave rob and sometimes even kidnap children to sell to white medical schools.** In fact, one of the rumors during the time of the Atlanta child murders was that Black boys were being kidnapped to harvest a hormone found in their genitals that would help with AIDS. As we can see, that fear was rooted in a historical reality.

The fear of the Western medical profession is rooted in the treatment of Original People by white people. It's hard to extol the virtues of Western medicine when there is a legacy of debasement, torture, and experimentation.

Let your doctor know that you're in charge of your health and you know your history. Control your interactions with the medical industry.

DESTRUCTION OF THE TRADITIONAL AFRICAN DIET

BY EBONI JOY ASIATIC

Before slavery, the traditional African diet was much healthier than the Standard African American Diet of today. But what was the "traditional" African diet? This is a tough question for a number of reasons. For one, Africa - contrary to popular belief - is not a country. Africa is a massive continent with incredible cultural diversity and an unbelievably long history. What we may now consider "traditional" African cuisine may not necessarily be so. Let me explain.

A thousand years before Europeans stepped foot on the African continent, African peoples were trading herbs and spices, rice, banana and sugarcane with Asians. When Europeans arrived in Africa, they carried with them foods from the Americas, including maize (corn), cassava (yucca), peanut, tomato, chili pepper and pumpkin. Before the Asian and American introduction of foreign foods, a traditional African diet consisted of edible "leaves, roots, tubers, corms, rhizomes, bulbs, seeds, buds, shoots, stems, pods, or flowers." Also, various African peoples had distinct methods of cooking and food preparation. As stated in *The Lost Crops of Africa*:

> During the colonial era the process of discarding indigenous crops gained further momentum, as the official focus shifted to those familiar crops of mercantile interest, such as cane, chocolate, coffee, cotton, and other durable, transportable, and valuable crops of that sort. Indeed, during those times subsistence crops were almost entirely neglected in organized agriculture, while valuable exportable cash crops were cultured, harvested, graded, and protected against rodents, insects, and decay with exceptional efficiency and dispatch. And an end result of these historical trends was that most of Africa's food these days comes from a mere 20 or so species, almost all of foreign extraction.

Did You Know?
Of the continent's 100 highest yielding crops, only cowpea, yam and okra are indigenous to Africa. Although the "traditional" African diet has been altered by the introduction of various foreign food staples, indigenous African crops are still grown and have a variety of health benefits. Among these native crops are amaranth (greens), Bambara beans, baobab, celosia, dika, eggplant (garden egg), egusi, enset, lablab, locust bean, long bean, marama, native potatoes, yambean, and Shea. Shea butter is often used as a skin care product throughout the world, however in Africa it is also used as a cooking butter.

Health Deficiencies Due to Diet

Many illnesses that peoples of African descent suffer from are due to the Western Standard American Diet, (SAD). This diet either provides too few or too many, vitamins, minerals and nutrients. A lack of or overabundance of certain elements in the diet can conflict with the melanin-based biochemistry of African people. We eat SAD foods that have been

71

created to support the needs and desires of a melanin-deficient people, and this diet is incompatible with the Africans body chemistry. This is why Africans in America have higher cholesterol than the general population, resulting in a variety of circulatory issues, including arteriosclerosis (hardening of the arteries), heart attack, stroke and hypertension (high blood pressure).

The West Africans' original diet was comprised of vegetation – cassava, yam, sorghum and millet – which produced nitriloside and thiocyanate. Nitriloside is a chemical which inhibits blood clotting. Blood clotting commonly occurs among individuals with Sickle Cell Anemia (See "Sickle Cell Anemia"). A deficiency in nitriloside and cyanate may be responsible for the greater damage that occurs among Africans in America that have been diagnosed with this condition. Barbara Dixon states in her book, *Good Health for African Americans.*

> In Africa, an estimated 25% of the population carry the sickle cell trait [a natural developing immunity to malaria], yet the incidence of sickle cell disease itself is rare. In fact, from 1925 to 1950, it was estimated that fewer than one hundred cases of sickle cell anemia were reported throughout the continent.

Eat what your body is designed to live off.

HEALTH Y HISPANIDAD
BY DENIZ LOPEZ

When thinking about Hispanics and health, the first thing that must be spoken on is the diverse identities that the word 'Hispanic' encompasses. 'Hispanic' is used to describe people with origins in Mexico, Central and South America, and the Caribbean. So, for the purpose of this piece, I want to be clear that I'm writing as a *Xicana* about the Hispanic as she/he came to be in the wilderness of the United States – with acknowledgement of the ethnic and socioeconomic things that could make some of what I say not applicable to all 'Hispanics.'

Folk meets Modern

It's definitely true that due to the history of our migration into the US, most Hispanics have acculturated into Americanism – that is, taken some American customs, habits, and values, and adopted them into

> **Did You Know?**
> Depression, caused by joblessness or a lack of interpersonal relationships with other people, was minimal in traditional society. Every individual was given a purpose and a network within their communities. In modern times, our men and women are taught to write resumes, coordinate a good interview outfit, hope for a "good job," and remain individualistic. As a result, we are now prescribed chemicals to cope with the anxiety that all of this entails.

our lives, without losing the ones we already culturally exhibit. Yet, how true this statement is depends entirely on what generation of Hispanic you are discussing, and on how much that individual desired to take on Modern/European/Western habits. **Part of assimilation and colonization was to "help" us unlearn our own remedies and ways of taking care of ourselves.** Our grandparents and great grandparents had a recipe for every ailment known to man, and relied on the advice and guidance of their community in dealing with ailments. **Food was our medicine. We had the knowledge of its purpose and prepared it with this in mind.** The more we been forced to adopt Modern/European/Western thinking and living, the further away we've gotten from these understandings and practices. We've come to rely on the treatments and medicines that have been created by the same people who robbed us of our own knowledge, for help with pain, obesity, depression, and the like. This has created an interesting paradox for Hispanics, and for all people of color, who are trying to navigate between so-called "folk medicine" and modern medicine.

Health maintenance through folk practices, incorporated massages, *platicas* (open communication, discussion, and counseling talks), *limpias* (cleansings using herbal bath soaks, rubs, and scents), meditation and exercise, productive work within the community, and a diet incorporating mostly fruits and vegetables. While this may sound very basic and practical, think about the practices we are taught to incorporate in modern medicine. Instead of a massage, or activity, or medicinal herbs and foods, we allow doctors to cut us, prod our bodies where they hurt, and/or prescribe us chemicals to dull the pain – not cure the pain – but, *dull* the pain. This, of course, leads to even more dependence on the doctor, the drug, and the entire modern health care system. Another example of dependence on the "system" is that instead of us relying on traditional diet and productive activity to stay healthy and slim, we are taught that we must count calories, purchase a gym membership, become a Jenny Craig member, and take more pills to lose weight.

I must note that not all modern health practices are "bad," but, we have to consider what brought us to the point of being sliced by strangers, and living drug induced, idle life-styles.

While Hispanics still incorporate folk practices when dealing with health, we (and generations to come) will have to deal with the paradox of finding ourselves existing somewhere between a traditional and a modern health lifestyle, and all that that brings.

The Healthcare System Experience

In speaking on Mexican-Americans, comedian George Lopez hit the nail on the head when he said that we will not go to the doctor, no matter what. While a lot of the reason why is rooted in the folk practices that I

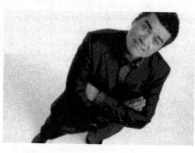

touched on, this also has to do with our experience when we do go to a health care provider for help. It's usually cold in the doctor's office, and I'm not just talking about the temperature. Doctors hardly make eye contact, while touching you in a very personal manner. And for Hispanics, there's also the language barrier, the physician's bias, and a lack of insurance.

Communication is already difficult when you share the same language, customs and ideas with the person you're speaking to. Imagine trying to explain something about your body – something very private to Hispanics – when the persons listening don't share the same culture, and have a minimal understanding of what you are trying to describe. Now imagine that there is no one there to translate for you. Now you're anxious and the attending doctor and nurse are frustrated. I worked in a scheduling department for a well-known Ophthalmologist Center in Houston, and when a Spanish speaker called, if I couldn't talk to them, they were either left on hold until I could attend to them (which was sometimes up to 20 minutes), or transferred to someone who was annoyed by the fact that they had to translate outside of their department, or they were hung up on. Imagine being a literate and respected person in your own community, but being stripped of all dignity, and shown no courtesy, when you walk into a doctor's office for help – help that you didn't even want to resort to them for in the first place!

Miscommunication and mistreatment often go unaddressed in the health care setting due to the doctor's prejudices, and the *respecto* (respect) and *machismo* (power-play) factors of the Hispanic identity. Tack on the inherent segregation of health care access, bias related to your insurance carrier, and you may wind up feeling even sicker than you were when you first decided to go to the doctor. So, we are left wondering what the alternative is when we've unlearned the Original methods of treating ourselves.

It has to be taken into account that in our history, we've dealt with the conquest of our people, and shifts from our traditional way of life to one of modernism. That conquest continues today and is exhibited by the fact that we continue to let go of ownership of our land, medicine, and our own Selves, based on habits and standards that we are forced to adopt. This is a vicious, fear-driven cycle.

Our struggle with health, as Hispanics, has come from internal and external influences, and can vary greatly based on our acculturation and place of origin. We have to decide what traditional practices we will keep, and which modern things we will adopt. We have to be aware of what we put inside of our bodies and learn how these things affect us. We have to take back ownership of our own thoughts and actions, and make our own decisions again, based on our history, knowledge, facts, and our incredible ability to survive, despite constant oppression.

If grandma or dad don't speak English, go with them to the doctor. Ask your elders what traditional folk practices you can try.

"AMERICAN FOOD" ONLY HAS A DASH OF WHITE IN IT
NATIVE AMERICAN FOUNDATIONS OF AMERICAN COOKING
BY C'BS ALIFE ALLAH

The pilgrims, and other whites, who were a part of the first wave of the European invasion into the Americas, were poor people. They came, generally, from the lowest rungs of European society and didn't plan out how they were going to survive in the new world.

Most of the food they brought from Europe wouldn't grow. **They had no knowledge of native fruits or vegetables, and lacked hunting skills.** A sport reserved for the upper class, illegal and considered poaching to hunt on land one did not own. **But they survived because the indigenous peoples showed the invaders which foods they could eat, and how to hunt.**

So, when you see Billy Bob on the Country Network hunting in his camouflage, remember that his ancestors were taught these skills. Europeans were taught the skills of camouflaging, trapping, grease-painting, and the use of decoys to hunt deer, rabbits, ducks, geese, pigeons, turkeys, alligators, caribou and bison. As well as new methods such as down South barbecue, which comes from the Taino word, *barbicu*, referring to the method of applying a dry rub of spices to meat, and slow-grilling it over a fire pit. Add blueberries, sunflower seeds, various squashes, pecans and nuts to this new diet. Four special crops native to the Americas are Tomatoes ("xitomatl," from the Aztec language of Nahuatl), Coco/chocolate ("cacao"), corn ("maize"), and potatoes (from the Taino word "batata" and the Quechua word "papa"). See "The History of Soul Food") for information on the impact of indigenous traditions and food on American cuisine.

NATIVE AMERICAN HEALTH – THEN
BY WILL STOLLER

Many of us have a stereotypical view of who the Natives were, picturing leather moccasin-wearing, buffalo hunters, who lived in animal-skin teepees, and ate a meat-based diet. However, this type of lifestyle was not commonplace and was almost exclusive to the Apache Indians. Most of the other Nations lived very differently, and only changed their way of life as a direct result of European expansion. When the Europeans arrived, they undermined the sensibility of the Native lifestyle, calling them "savages" and "heathens" – all the while "borrowing" everything they could use from Native culture. These Europeans did not possess half of the extensive medical knowledge they observed, or even know how to grow food. It was the "noble savages" who taught them. While the Natives had everything from toothpaste to shampoo, the Europeans were the real "dirty heathens," outlawing bathing, which caused their diseases to spread rapidly.

The Sweat Lodge and Tempering

Today, medical experts have no problem telling you that they don't have a cure for the common cold. However, the Natives had the answer to the common cold, arthritis, headaches, and many other ailments. This answer is the Sweat Lodge, and it may be the most beneficial activity towards improving ones' health. Why? Because sitting in a Sweat Lodge creates fever-like symptoms that force each of your internal organs to expel impurities, which results in detoxification. In fact, heavy sweating greatly improves your health and your physical appearance, affecting everything from body fat to acne. Just think about it. Without the proper amount of perspiration, the pores in your skin clog. No amount of face wash can open your pores. Only sweating causes them to open and be purified.

On the polar end, there's tempering. Until the advent of heated water, most people, who didn't live near a hot spring, would bathe in cold water. During the winter, they might have had to use ice water. While this might sound unpleasant, like sweating, this is also very good for you. Tempering improves your blood circulation, which is probably getting worse by the minute. In fact, by the age of 30, most people show signs of organ eutrophication (wasting away), which is caused by poor circulation to the capillaries. The capillaries are the smallest veins, and they are thinner even, than a strand of hair. The circulatory system transports your blood, anywhere from 60,000 to 100,000 miles, running throughout your entire body. We can only imagine how difficult it is for our blood to make it to every end of every capillary. This is where tempering helps blood circulation to take place. You can apply this technique to your lifestyle simply by adding ice to a cold bath. **Sweating and tempering go hand and hand, stimulating the body to find and destroy diseased cells, resulting in a reverse of degenerative diseases of the liver, heart, kidneys, and, in some cases, the mind.**

Native American Healing with Plants

Native Americans lived in a constant exchange with the Earth. While being careful not to take too much, they would use all that nature had to offer. When sick (and usually before it got bad enough to be called "sick") they relied on plants as their medicine. In fact, the American pharmaceutical industry grew out of the voluminous body of Native American (and enslaved African) medicinal knowledge. Over 200 medical drugs and their sources (including aspirin) can be linked back to Native Americans.

"The Great Spirit is our father, but the earth is our mother. She nourishes us: that which we put into the ground she returns to us, and healing plants she gives to us likewise. If we are wounded, we go to or mother and seek to lay the wounded part against her, to be healed. Animals too, do thus, they lay their wounds to the earth." – Big Thunder (Bedagi) of the Wabanaki Algonquin

Sometimes ailing animals were followed and observed to see what plants they would eat to heal and get well. The bear, revered for its intelligence, was considered a reliable source of herbal remedies. Thus, you have Native Americans who recall "legends" where they say, "It was the bear who taught us how to do this." And indeed the bear did!

"…Everything on the earth has a purpose, every disease an herb to cure it, and every person a mission. This is the Indian theory of existence." – Mourning Dove-Salish (1888-1936)

The healing practices can vary from individual spiritual tradition, prayers, and rituals because there are about 500 Native American Nations. Each having their own unique knowledge and understanding on the value of healing plants that "Mother Earth" gives us. See ("Herbs = Medicine")

Most of the ailments these plants would treat are the kinds of things you'd experience if you were living a natural, healthy life…not like us, nowadays, needing medicine for man-made diseases like diabetes and cancer. Why do I say "man-made"? Because man has made himself sick with unhealthy habits and a toxic environment. And if you REALLY want to get deep with it, it was the "made man" (them) who made Man (us) as sick as we are today.

Try a sauna or a cold shower. Matter fact, break a sweat and get your blood circulating with a run. Detox and strengthen that body.

NATIVE AMERICAN HEALTH - NOW
BY DENIZ LOPEZ

This piece is based on my conversation with the writer, mother, wife, and activist, Diana Joe.[9] From the onset, I expected her to tell me about the lack of healthcare options in Native American communities. She corrected this misconception, right away. She said that in the reservation she lives on, health care is provided and accessible. The problem with this, though, is that the 'care' is not so 'care-ful' of the history of her people.

The term, "Native American," is used to refer to the Indigenous people of North America, who are living within the boundaries of the United States. Prior to European exploration, and their eventual genocide of the Indigenous 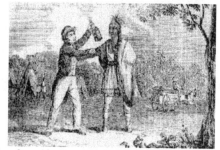 peoples, the Native lifestyle and culture had roots that extended from Chile to Alaska. These people had extensive knowledge regarding medicinal plants due to their lengthy study of the land and nature. (See "Healthy Hispanidad")

Diabetes/Hypertension – The more that Native Americans have been contained on reservations, and forced to adopt Western ways of eating and living, the unhealthier they've become. **The real after effects of the colonization and genocide is evident in the 68% increase in diabetes from 1994 to 2004 in American Indian and Alaska Native youths ages 15-19, and the 95% of the Native American population afflicted with type 2 Diabetes.** Hypertension caused by poor diet, lack of exercise, obesity, and alcoholism, is present in 1 in 5 Native Americans.

Alcoholism – Alcohol was introduced to the Indigenous people

---

[9] Diana Joe lives with her husband on a Navajo Reservation in Lukachukai, AZ – located near the Chusca Mountains where she educates through storytelling. She has raised 6 children and now has 13 grandchildren. She writes for rights.

during their early contact with European settlers, traders and explorers. Traders, who sought to gain the upper hand in their dealings, gave the Natives alcohol because of its effects on thought and reasoning. **Think, opium in China, or crack cocaine in the Hood.** It wasn't long before Native Americans lost their hold on their lands, goods, and their age-old knowledge.

It's been estimated that 80% of Native American youth have experimented with alcohol, compared to 50% of U.S. youth in the general population. Internal conflicts between traditional and modern culture, as well as post-traumatic stress and low self-esteem related to their subjugated role in dominant society, have resulted in disproportionately high cases of alcohol use, abuse, and addiction among Native American youth. Diana Joe shared that today, alcohol is illegal on the reservation, but because of dependency and addiction, as well as profiteering, bootlegging is a common practice.

Mental Illness –Few studies have been done regarding mental illness among the Natives. One small study, which had a 20-year follow-up, found that the lifetime prevalence of mental disorders among Natives can be as high as 70%. This same study found that males, ages 15-24, account for two thirds of all Native suicides.

Diana shared that she personally went through depression and stress. For several years she was on Zoloft, which was supposed to balance her, and soon found that it 'messed up her naturalness.' She was being numbed, not cured, and had to deal with new effects that affected her well-being to a whole other degree. She got off the Zoloft, and turned fully to Native ways to deal. (See "Traditional Medicine Vs. They Medicine")

Further Assimilation – In discussing the shift from traditional to modern living, Diana noted that the Elders continue to be highly regarded, and that the community still seeks their advice and healing. Yet, as time passes, more and more youth are turning away from their Indigenous ways. She said this begins with formal education. Children in the reservation are sent away to boarding school, once it's time for their formal education to begin. They are taken away from their homes and indoctrinated with a Western world-view and thought pattern. Adding insult to injury, many of the schools that they attend are unhygienic, and the education that they provide is sub-par. Some families have opted out of sending their children to school for these reasons.

In the past, children were brought into the world by the hands of their loved ones, with traditional medicine and good energy. Now, more and more Native women are going the modern route in regards to child-birth. Diana said that, now, a child is brought into the world with a knife…and if I might add, with drugs. And we all know that once you have given birth in a hospital, everyone entering your room afterwards will offer you birth control!

The Cure – So, how does the Native person come full circle in a society that has designated where and how they can eat, sleep, live and create? Diana says that we should ease ourselves and our youth back onto our cultural base, focus on building a warrior mentality, and teach our youth to listen to the Elders, and be open to re-learning the old ways. We need to re-gain the wisdom of our direct connection to all that is around us – from the food that we eat, to the people that we surround ourselves with. Be more aware of our words, and how they affect us. And, in closing, she humbly noted:

> Thank you in advance. Blessings to you. I feel as people of these Americas, we have to make an effort on a common level to educate the youth about the truth. Let's use the things the Earth has granted us in education, and we can avoid disaster.

I want to thank Diana Joe for sharing with me, while she spent time with her grandchild. After our conversation, things have become clearer for me, and I know that she has helped me to re-claim some of my own genetic memories. She reconnected me with my own struggle as an Indigenous *hermana*, and affirmed that the road to true health is one that we already have the knowledge to navigate.

There is no substitution for our original way of life, only consequences. See the commonalities? We're all suffering.

FAKE VS. REAL CHINESE FOOD
BY SINCERE JUSTICE ALLAH

Because I'm Chinese, people often come up to me, telling me how much they love Chow Mein and Orange Chicken. That's offensive on a few levels. But, it's also funny, because it's like cats are braggin' about rockin' a bootleg. C'mon now. Chop Suey? Beef and Broccoli? General Tso's Chicken? Sound familiar? All of these dishes were made to serve Americans, specifically, white people. The real Chinese traditional diet is much different. Let me explain.

Chop Suey. This, literally, means "odds and ends" (or leftovers) in Chinese. This dish was originally developed in the late 1880s, when Chinese immigrants with limited resources used vegetable scraps and animal entrails to create Chop Suey. The popularity of Chop Suey started in the 1900s in New York City, when it became sophisticated to go to a Chinese restaurant and order some Chop Suey to impress a date. This is called "slumming" and whites also went slumming when they visited Harlem to drink and dance.

Beef and Broccoli. What do Americans like more than beef? Beef and Broccoli. C'mon! Chinese don't mess with this! Most Chinese were farmers, so cows were often used for farming, meaning they were rarely eaten. Also, the type of broccoli used in Beef and Broccoli actually originates in Italy. However, the Chinese do have their own broccoli, known as *gai-lan* (or Chinese Broccoli in many supermarkets here).

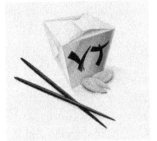

General Tso's Chicken. Sweet, Fried, and Chicken is just what Americans love. This dish has nothing to do with General Tso or the Taipeng Rebellion of the 1850s. Even General Tso's relatives in Changsha, China, don't recognize this dish. For all you Orange Chicken fanatics, this is similar to General Tso's Chicken. In fact, the creation of McDonalds' Chicken McNuggets borrows much of its influence from General Tso's Chicken. The two original sauces that were served with Chicken McNuggets were Sweet and Sour Sauce and Hot Mustard – both of which are used in Chinese cuisine.

Why does any of this matter? Because this is another example of how authentic cultures get co-opted (stolen), processed, repackaged, and sold back to the people in a form that is no longer Original. Instead, the remake is a weak, less nutritious, imitation of a people's traditional ways. This is popular among white people, who like "going ethnic" but not "going too far."

So what's real Chinese food? What do Chinese people eat in their homes?

Generally speaking, Chinese have a diet that consists of mostly leafy greens (such as bok choy or other vegetables), and a small serving of fresh meat or seafood. China's cuisines are divided into 8 distinct regions. The four most popular cuisines are the Cantonese in the South, the Szechuan in the West, the Shangdong in the North, and the Huaiyang in the East. Keep in mind that there are regional distinctions, such as the fact that Northerners are known to eat steamed buns and use more wheat based foods than rice. Also, traditionally in the North, soups often accompany meals as a first course.

Remember, there's no way in hell that real Chinese food would be as greasy, fried, and MSG-laden as what's found in the West, because many Chinese are influenced by the principles of Taoism, Confucianism, and Buddhism. **Many Chinese based what they eat on the Taoist Five Element Theory, which advocates an alkaline diet – meaning a lot of fruits and vegetables.** (See "Traditional Chinese Medicine")

If you really want to get down and try the real deal, find yourself a Chinese friend that will either invite you to their house for dinner or take you to a restaurant that they frequent. Strive to go during a Lunch Special hour for a cheaper meal, or order a specialty item. Often, the authentic dishes are listed in Chinese on flags that line the walls. Oh, and use some chopsticks, homie!

Here are some dishes for starters: Kung Pao Chicken, Mapo Tofu, Ong Choy with Chili & Garlic, Winter Melon Soup, Snow Fungus Soup, Soy Sauce Chicken. And if you're feeling brave, try you some Stinky Tofu.

Further Reading

The Fortune Cookie Chronicles: Adventures in the World of Chinese Food by Jennifer Lee, and The China Study by Colin T. Campbell.

Try some authentic food from different cultures. Think homemade not fast-food. Better yet, look up and prepare an authentic dish.

FAT AND DRUNK IN EAST ASIA
BY SUPREME UNDERSTANDING

When people think about East Asian countries like Japan, China, and Korea, they don't think about obesity and poor health. We conjure up images of monks doing Tai Chi, people eating tofu with every meal, doctors using traditional herbal medicine instead of Western drugs, and ridiculously petite women everywhere you look. But I've spent a decent amount of time in both Thailand and Japan, and perception is not reality. While people in the East certainly are healthier than people in the West, it's not like everyone out there is healthy. In fact, you'll find people drinking heavily, chain-smoking, and eating fast food every day in many of those countries. Of course, we know that most of that started when Europeans came over (study the Opium Wars), but it's getting worse every day. That's why you've probably seen that video of the 2-year old Indonesian boy smoking cigarettes like a pro, or heard about the wild drunkenness that is common among Japanese business executives. Sure, the traditional Chinese diet is healthier than our diet, but people don't really eat like that anymore unless they live in small towns and villages. Since the first McDonald's in China opened in 1990, China has become the #1 growth market for McDonalds (outside of the US), with 960 restaurants and over 60,000 employees. KFC, which opened there in 1987, now has around 2,200 stores dotted around China's 465 cities. That tells you, it's not long until the rest of the world ends up sick like the people here.

While American-style fatness is still pretty rare, the rates of obesity are steadily rising throughout East Asia. And the large number of cancer patients (6.2 million, compared with 1.6 million in North America and 3.4 million in Europe) could be traced to excess body weight, according to a recent study.

The most obese countries in Asia are Japan and South Korea, where 3.2% of the population has a BMI over 30. Not bad compared to America, where over 33% are obese! But it's a sign of a growing trend. And not only are the Japanese and Koreans the most obese Asians, they also have the worst drinking habits. Studies show that Koreans and Japanese drink the most alcohol and do the most binge drinking out of all Asians.

Why them? Think about what those two countries have in common. Both were "conquered" by the U.S. military. After the Korean War and World War II (where the U.S. dropped a nuclear bomb on Japan), both countries were "rebuilt" by the U.S. And in the process (of course), they were taught to love America and Western culture (kinda like "Reconstruction" for Blacks in American following slavery, if you know the real history).

Before WWII, sumo wrestling was the national sport of Japan. After WWII, it was baseball. Soon enough, other aspects of Western culture found a home where it had been previously rejected. **At one point, East Asians identified with the Black struggle in America** (Read *How to Hustle and Win* for details). **But now, they've got American-style racism there! Back in the day, East Asia rejected everything European, whether political or cultural** (since they're all related). That's why it took so long for McDonalds and KFC to get in the door. But now, as McDonalds' CEO Jim Skinner explains, things are different:

> We do extensive focus group studies of Chinese consumers, and one of the things that Chinese consumers say over and over again is that "we come to you because you are a Western brand, if we want to eat rice or congee we can eat at home or in Chinese restaurants, we want to sample the Western brand."

In fact, some mental illnesses ONLY found among Western (white) people, like anorexia, are now emerging in places like Korea as well. So what's the cause behind the poor health that's developing among Japanese and Koreans? The same cause behind the poor health that's nearly destroyed the rest of us here in America. And to drive the point home, Asians who were born in America have much poorer health (more obesity, more mental health problems, and worse drinking habits) than Asians who were not born here. That should tell you something about this "land of opportunity" you live in!

Don't accept what's forced upon you. If the people around you are a negative influence, teach or leave them. Use this book!

WHAT'S NEW? 12 MODERN DIETARY CHANGES
BY SUPREME UNDERSTANDING

In *The Macrobiotic Diet*, Michio Kushi writes:

> We are what we eat. Change of what we eat changes our physical, psychological, and spiritual conditions. Change of body, mind and spirit results in the change of social and cultural expression as well as personal health and development.

Kushi notes 12 major dietary changes in modern times:

Loss of principal food. The consumption of whole grains, the principal food of all previous civilizations, has declined sharply. And grains are now mostly eaten refined, not whole. (See "An Essential Guide to Grains")

Increased consumption of animal food. Meat, poultry, eggs, dairy products and fish have replaced grains and beans at the center of the modern meal. (See "How to Eat Like Fred Flintstone")

Increased consumption of sugar. Many foods today contain sugar, honey and other sweeteners, including artificial ones. (See "Is Sugar Bad for You?")

Change in vegetable consumption. People today eat only a few vegetables, like tomatoes, potatoes, lettuce and cucumber. These are mass produced with chemical fertilizers. Often, they are canned or frozen, not fresh. (See "The Healing Power of Vegetables")

Change in fruit consumption. Wild and naturally cultivated fruits have been replaced by uniform, hybrid species. People eat more canned, frozen and sugar-treated fruit, fruit juice and fruit from different climatic zones than fresh or naturally dried native fruit. (See "The Healing Power of Fruits").

Change in legume use. Beans and lentils used to be the principal source of protein. Today, they are fed mainly to animals. (See "A Simple Guide to Legumes").

Emergence of non-essential foods. Candy bars, soft drinks, ice-cream sandwiches, and other non-essential snack foods are being consumed in vast quantities. These are usually packed with sugar, fats, salt and chemicals. (See "Junk Food is Crack").

Change in farming quality. Natural, farming has been replaced by modern methods which rely heavily on chemical fertilizers, pesticides and other chemical sprays. (See "Food, Inc")

Change in salt quality. Natural, un-refined sea salt has been replaced with refined salt. This salt lacks other minerals that are essential for health. (See "Is Salt Bad for You?")

Rise in vitamin consumption. Natural vitamins have been removed from modern foods and a few are replaced by synthetic vitamins that often wash off or can't be processed by our bodies properly. Many people take vitamin pills and supplements instead of getting nutrients naturally. (See "Take Your Vitamins?" and "The Essential Vitamin Guide")

Rise of artificial foods and cooking methods. Thousands of synthetic chemicals, most of which have not been tested for their safety, have been added to modern foods. Microwaves and deep fryers have replaced cooking with natural fire. (See "Fried and Died")

Rise of biogenetically engineered food. These include foods that combine the genes of animals and plants, such as tomatoes that contain fish genes to give them a longer shelf life. Foods are also being irradiated to make them last longer. (See "Processed Foods" and "Genetically Modified Foods").

Use this knowledge to evaluate and gradually make changes to your diet. Take the "Are You Healthy Quiz?" again and compare scores.

WE STARTED THIS CAPTAIN PLANET THING

THE ORIGINAL FOUNDATION FOR VEGETARIANISM AND ENVIRONMENTALISM
BY C'BS ALIFE ALLAH

The self-righteous granola eating hippie comes into your hood. They have lettuce sandwich stuck in between their teeth, all the while going on about saving the rabbits. They go into a long sermon about how you aren't supposed to eat meat, and how you should be saving Mother Nature. If you break down their speech, it will basically sound like this:

☐ Y'all Original/Indigenous People are f*cked up
☐ We white folk know what is best for y'all because y'all are too stupid to realize this

- ☐ Our way/solution/idea is the best, and the most appropriate approach to ANY situation
- ☐ We got "some" of this information from Original/Indigenous people yet that doesn't matter because we're the owners of this information now

Not Eating Meat

Let's start with vegetarians, specifically vegans – those who don't eat any type of animal or animal byproduct for health and ethical reasons. The way that the majority of mainstream white vegans operate is no different than Christian missionaries during the age of European Imperialism. They work to impose their diet and views on people using guilt, shame, and in many cases force. **Because the vegan terminology is loaded with much of the baggage from white supremacy, many Original/Indigenous/People of Color have adopted different terminologies to refer to their eating habits. Some of these terms are, "decolonized diet," "pure vegetarianism," "plant-centric diet," "green gangsta," "right foods," and "eating to live."** Regardless of the term, what everyone must realize is that white people didn't start this "vegan" stuff.

If you look at Europe, ancient and modern, they have THE most meat saturated diet in the world. This has ALWAYS been true. The only time that there has been any tradition of vegetarianism, anywhere in Europe, was amongst small groups of Greek philosophers, who were influenced by their studies in Egypt. Europeans do not have any vegetarian traditions to build a modern day tradition of vegetarianism on. In fact, once they colonized the Americas, they began to export their surplus meat back to Europe. This is that foundation on which the American, Meat and Potatoes Diet has been built. This is also the beginning of that lie that vegetarians are going to suffer from protein and calcium, (due to a lack of meat and dairy products).

Now, when you flip it, and start looking at Original/Indigenous/People of Color all over the world, you will find diets that are not meat-centric. Meat is served as a side dish, if at all. This practice is found embedded in many religions outside of Europe (that naturally grew out of cultural practices). In East Asia, you will find vegetarianism in the traditions of Hinduism (especially the Vaishnavas sects that worship Vishnu), Jainism, Buddhism – about half of all Buddhists worldwide practice vegetarianism – and among some sects of Sikhism. Christian traditions outside of Europe (like many of the monastic traditions in North Africa) have traditionally practiced a vegetarian diet. In fact, a lot of the Eastern Christianity traditions (such as the Coptic Orthodox Church of Alexandria, the Oriental

Orthodox Churches, and the Ethioptic Coptic Orthodox Church) practice vegan fasting during Lent. They also fast during other periods, as many as 210 days out of the year. Taoists, some members of the Bahai faith, and some Sufi orders of Islam all practice forms of vegetarianism. And let's not forget the Rastafarian tradition of Ital, which forbids the eating of flesh, artificially preserved foods, and foods that have been salted, artificially flavored, or chemically altered in any way.

The above examples are rooted in the religions of Original/Indigenous/People of Color, yet even if you put religion aside, and examine only the cultures, you will not find eating traditions that "worship meat." For instance, in pre-Columbus America, there were no animals that were domesticated purely for food stock, unlike Europe's domestication of chickens, cattle and pigs. Meat in early America was an incidental part of the diet. Though the image of the Plains Indians has become part of Americana lore, these were, generally speaking, the only Native peoples whose culture revolved around a single animal (the bison). The Plains Indians' bond with the bison is not the same as post-Industrial America's obsession with pseudo-meats. The Plains Indians revered the bison, and didn't waste any part of the animal.

By looking at the religious and cultural traditions of non-white people, you can tell one thing. We have vegetarian traditions that go far beyond them sticking their nose in our business.

Killing Meat

In the world, outside of Europe, people have always had a close connection with their food source. A disconnect occurred in Europe, early on, for two reasons. For one, only the wealthy were allowed to hunt. Secondly, American colonists began to ship their meat surplus to Europe. Outside of Europe, religious traditions were always concerned that compassion be shown towards one's source of nourishment. Orthodox Jews have a tradition of *shechita*, by which the trachea, esophagus, carotid arteries and jugular veins of an animal are cut, using a super-sharp blade (*chalef*), killing the animal instantly and painlessly. This also allows the animal's blood to drain out, almost immediately.

Aside from this, there are no European traditions which promote the compassionate killing of animals.

Now, when you check into the rest of the world, you have the *jhatka* tradition of Hinduism (by which an animal is slain by a single sword or ax stroke, which passes through the spine, killing the animal instantly), the *dhabihah* tradition of Islam (a quick incision into the neck which slices the jugular veins and carotid arteries), and even the *ike-jime* tradition in Japan (a method of paralyzing and bleeding fish by inserting a spike quickly into the hind brain which causes an immediate and painless death and maintains quality). Even the Native Nations in the Americas realized that you shouldn't scare the animals that you are hunting. **When an animal knows that it is about to be killed, it floods its body with adrenaline and other hormones that saturate the meat, making it tough and causing it's flesh to be a repository for hormones, which aren't good for humans to digest.**

PETA-Punks

For those who don't know, PETA, or People for the Ethical Treatment of Animals, is an organization that is devoted to the protection of animals. **This organization is racist to the core.** As you can see in the preceding paragraphs, Original People have always had a peaceful relationship with animals. A peaceful relationship with animals does not translate into an abnormal relationship with animals that borders on, or crosses the line into, bestiality. People that know me know that I ain't no PETA-pet. I rarely use the term "vegan" because it has been co-opted by white, anorexic women in recovery (or on the down-low). And frankly, PETA be slipping too close into bestiality for me to really be feeling them. All-in-all, I see that PETA overemphasizes the welfare of animals, as opposed to showing an interest in the effects of post-colonialism, racism, genocide and slavery that continue to plague Original peoples. So, rolling with PETA-pets oftentimes makes me nauseous. **For example, in order to get their point across, at one point PETA decided to compare animal cruelty to the slavery of African-Americans, without even thinking, or not caring, that they were comparing African-Americans to animals.** They also tend to have a racist focus when it comes to choosing their battles. This is why PETA organized to vilify Michael Vick, or Latino cock-fights, but don't expend as much effort to shut down white politicians that hunt animals for sport or chicken farms.

Rooted in white culture is an unnatural relationship with animals. This is fully exposed and projected in their vegan and anti-animal cruelty movements. It is not enough for them to 'save' animals. They have to welcome them as full members of their families. And I really don't even have to mention how often you see those toy dogs being kissed by white females. Pets in the white household are exalted above the other human races. How many animal rescue commercials do you in the

United States, versus commercials encouraging child adoption?

We Don't Kill Cats, (Like Future-Serial Killers)

I hate that damned term, "animal abuse." No, I ain't for starving dogs, kicking cats, etc. Yet, since that term exists, in a legal sense, raising animals to be slaughtered should be termed "animal abuse." Oh wait…you treat it "good," and then you eat it, so it's "OK." Dumbass.

This is the same double-standard that exists, making it wrong for Santeria practitioners to practice animal sacrifice, but allowing Jewish people to slaughter goats on their holy days. Also, dammit…the farmers are just one slaughtering away from animal abuse. There is something that needs to be said. The PETA types are one end of the spectrum. They are, in some cases, literally, animal LOVERS. On the other end of the spectrum, you can see the manner in which this post-Industrial, Western culture applies their standard of white supremacy and racism. **There are some animals that are "good"** (basically pets like cats, dogs, and exotic birds), **and then there the lower animals** (cattle, chicken, pigs, etc.) **that you eat because they aren't fully 'feeling' or 'emotive'.** This makes it okay for them to be killed brutally. **It should come as no surprise that the notion of chattel slavery started amongst those Europeans who traded in livestock.**

The horrible treatment of animals during the production of food and goods (such as leather) is often the duty of poor, Original people, who are forced to labor in this inhumane industry. This impacts the individual workers, as well as the community, because these factories often leak toxic materials into the surrounding areas. Farms, processing plants, textile factories, etc. are always located on the poor side of town, which is inhabited by poor people of color.

During the Age of Imperialism, when whites entered Africa, Asia and the Americas, they brought along a narrow focus on "cash crops," (tobacco, cotton, corn, sugar), which were produced and exported for profit, while the Indigenous people were forced to stop growing local, sustainable food crops (See "Destruction of the Traditional African Diet"). Needless to say, this messed up the ecology and economics of the Indigenous people in all of these regions. Now, after having bled these agricultural areas dry, European and American corporations maintain economic power over their many former colonies, or "Banana Republics"[10], who can't even produce enough food to feed their people. Thus, these former colonies became dependent on Western non-foods, and were forced to give up their traditional diets.

The above reasons are solid reasons to "treat animals with compassion." However, one need not go to either extreme. When you look at Indigenous methods of animal slaughter, you can see that the Indigenous people understood that this is to be done with compassion. Indigenous people also understood that the depletion of natural resources is not an appropriate use of what nature has provided.

Indigenous Environmentalism

The biggest joke is when white people come into Original communities and try to preach to the Original people about the environment. White people have been the number one poisoners of the Earth's environment, hands down. Often, they prefer to attack non-white people's "destruction of the environment," instead of dealing with their own historical destruction of the environment. White people also ignore, as a whole, the current devastation of the planet's various ecosystems by white institutions and corporations. The hardest-hit countries are those in the "Third World." **Oftentimes, all that Original People need from white environmentalist is that they be left alone, and that the environmentalists take the rest of the white colonizers home with them.**

When the Spaniards arrived in the Americas, they brought pigs with them, that they then let loose in the forests of America. These pigs reproduced at such a rate that the subsequent European explorers had a ready-made food supply. These pigs, however, ate the seeds and shoots of the Native American gardens, destroying large tracts of their agriculture. These domesticated pigs also went feral, growing tusks, and becoming aggressive.

Whites have stolen, and continue to steal gold, ivory, oil, diamonds, uranium, coltan (an element used to make cell phones), and various other commodities from Africa. They steal food, vegetation, and even genes (by taking the blood of certain Native Nations and patenting the

---

[10] "Banana Republic" is a derogatory term for a nation, always a former European colony, whose entire economy is based on a single, cash crop. This is why the clothing store which shares this name, originally marketed European, safari-styled clothing.

gene sequence) from South America. The Gold Rush, which occurred in the Western United States during the late 1800s, flooded the local environment with mercury and sulphur – this after the Native Nations had been forced westward. There is a current rush on gold and uranium which is currently flooding the same environment with cyanide.

In 1991, the government of the East African nation of Somalia (which is located on the Horn of Africa) collapsed. Its nine million people have been teetering on the brink of starvation ever since. Many of the ugliest forces in the Western world have since used this instability as an opportunity to steal the country's food supply and dump nuclear waste in their seas. **The Somalian fishermen and sailors who lived off of the fish in these waters have known about this for years. When they finally decided to** 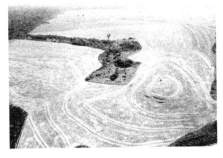 fight back (with the support of the people) **the world labeled them as pirates!**

I can also mention the atomic waste that has been left in various Pacific Islands and Japan as a result of nuclear weapons testing and use of atomic weapons, or the destruction of the rain forest by Western fast food cattle magnates, or the huge flotillas of trash in the ocean. I could go on and on. The common theme is that white people need to clean up their own stiff before preaching to other people about environmentalism.

Original People have always taken care of the Earth. Most Indigenous traditions embraced the stewardship of the planet vs. the European's doctrine of Manifest Destiny, the goal being to subdue and conquer the American West, and every other corner of the planet, for that matter. This philosophy is rooted in the Bible's Book of Genesis, 1:28.

> God blessed them and said to them, "Be fruitful and increase in number; fill the earth and subdue it. Rule over the fish in the sea and the birds in the sky and over every living creature that moves on the ground."

To get in tune with Environmentalism from a People of Color Perspective, check out the National Black Environmental Justice Network at www.nbejn.org, as well as the Indigenous Environmental Network at www.ienearth.org.

Take the above steps to push for environment justice in your community.

I'LL BE YOUR PUSHER: THE FDA

BY PHYLIS IQBAL

"If people let government decide what foods they eat and what medicines they take, their bodies will soon be in as sorry a state as are the souls of those who live under tyranny." – Thomas Jefferson

Everyone who is concerned with their health should get familiar with the Food and Drug Administration, or the FDA. This is a federally run organization which was created to protect citizens from the adverse effects of pharmaceutical drugs, food, tobacco, vaccines and even veterinary products, amongst other things. However, these days it seems that the FDA has gone from being our protector, to a drug pusher and peddler.

The regulation of products, drugs, and food can be a good thing. However, when government-run programs, which are there to serve us, become the pushers for wealthy drug companies, this is bound to take a toll on our collective health, well-being, and lifestyle. Most people in the general public tend to believe that if they see an FDA approval symbol on the product that they're buying, they're safe. But, what does it really mean to have a product approved by the FDA, versus a product that is not?

The only real difference is that one is backed by, not only a huge government program, but also a big medical drug company. The other product may be good for you, but it does not have the backing of the FDA. For a long time, the FDA has set up safety offices around the world to protect our food. However, the products that need the most protection, our pharmaceutical drugs, are not truly tested by the FDA.

This is because the FDA relies on a number of individual, privately owned, pharmaceutical companies to tell them whether their own product is safe or not. The FDA expects these companies to do their own testing and tell the truth about their results. That means that if a drug company has, say, an anti-depressant that they want to release, they "test" the drug and simply tell the FDA that it's safe, whether it is or not. From there, the FDA will put their stamp of approval on it, and allow it to be manufactured and sold to the public. Seems like the Big Pharma and the FDA are just drug pushers, right? That's because they are.

Because our medical field today is littered with doctors, scientists, and pharmaceutical companies who believe in chemical medicine versus healing, the population has been made into lab rats that are used to test the latest inorganic compound. How many times a day do you see drug commercials, starring famous celebrities? And then at the end of the commercial, a fast-talking announcer barrages you with the many side effects, that only a truly sick, disease-ridden individual would have. And yet, we still run to the pharmacy to fill our prescriptions.

This all really begins when a student is in medical school. Perhaps a big drug company approaches them, offering to pay for their education with the added stipulation that the medical student must push the company's drugs to their future patients. That student is then in the drug companies, and when they become a doctor, they will hold up their end of the bargain, prescribing unnecessary drugs to their patients.

This big drug company simultaneously approaches the FDA, whose commissioners and chair members are former pharmaceutical reps themselves, and offers them funding in exchange for their stamp of approval. Of course the FDA, like the doctor and the pharmacist, ends up working with the giant drug conglomerate. Meanwhile, you're still sick, and no matter what drugs you try, the results are always the same!

There have been studies done proving that doctors don't really "treat" their patients. Instead, if a patient walks into a doctor's office requesting a name brand drug, chances are that whether or not they actually need it, the patient will get the prescription. Thanks to the drug pushing FDA and pharmaceutical companies, the doctors, too, have become drug pushers.

In the past, people in the know relied on herbal remedies, vitamins, supplements, a healthy diet and exercise to heal their selves. Now, the FDA has a new partner, called the Codex Alimentarius Commission. This Commission has been around since the 1960s, but never before has it regulated our use of herbal medication as it does today, under the FDA.

This Commission is made up of approximately 146 nations and it regulates the dosage levels on vitamins and what mineral and herbs can be used for. All supplements have to undergo the Codex's approval process. The Codex Alimentarius (Latin for "Food Book") was put into effect in 2009, and has already created substantial difficulties in the holistic health community.

Recently, the FDA investigated Kombucha as an alcoholic beverage. Anyone who is familiar with Kombucha, (a fermented tea), in particular the raw bottled kind which is available everywhere, knows that there isn't enough alcohol in one bottle to get worried about. While, drugs, like Accutane, which causes Irritable Bowel Syndrome and Crohn's Disease, and which are frequently made of inorganic chemical compounds, are not usually under investigation. And yet, an all-natural herbal tea, that's actually good for you, is under governmental scrutiny? Seems kind of fishy, doesn't it?

The FDA could be an entity that actually works for the people, and providing us with accurate information and real results. Unfortunately, the reality is that it has become an organization which is controlled by the very pharmaceutical companies that it is supposed to regulate.

The meat, corn, and dairy industries also exert control over the FDA, many of its board members are former CEOs and chairmen of the meat, corn, and dairy industries. This dangerous liaison means that much of our food is unsafe, and certain products, which are not necessarily a part of a rounded diet, are promoted through government programs and subsidies. Think WIC.

It is up to us to try and figure out what's best for our bodies. You can be fooled to take things on face value, so do your research.

Notes:

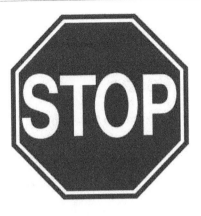

Take a break.
Put this book down for a minute.

Do NOT go back to reading this book until you do one (or more) of the following things:

- ❏ Call somebody who is going through some rough sh*t and make sure they are okay.
- ❏ Eat something that your body is telling you it needs, or drink some water.
- ❏ Wrestle, spar, or slapbox someone to make sure you "still got it."
- ❏ Take a walk through your neighborhood and see if somebody needs help with something.
- ❏ Clean up a part of your house, or organize some f*cked up part of your life.
- ❏ Tell somebody about this book and what you're learning. Invite them to come read it.
- ❏ Give this book away to somebody who needs it and get another copy for yourself.
- ❏ Cook something good, and make enough to share. Invite people.
- ❏ Check yourself out in the mirror and pick something to improve.
- ❏ Identify ten positive things about your life and stop forgetting them when you're stressed.
- ❏ Tell somebody you love them, cause it might be your last chance.

This has been a PSA from 360 and SDP.
Once you're done, carry on.

THE WRONG FOODS

PROCESSED FOODS

BY SUPREME UNDERSTANDING

What do we mean when we say "processed" foods? Basically, if it was grown in the soil under the sun, it's natural. If it was made in a factory or a lab, it was processed. To keep it simple, think "grown" or "made." Natural foods come from whatever you find in nature, like an innocent child who society hasn't touched yet. By this analogy, a processed food would be a 54-year-old prostitute with 12 kids and 8 STDs. Basically, it's been through a lot before it got in your mouth.

Eat Sh*t and Die

It is our body's job to process food once we eat it. That's how we extract the nutrients and energy from it. Once our body is done processing, we're left with crap...literally. This waste – which scientific people call "sh*t" – then leaves our body, because – nutritionally – we have no need for it. If it DIDN'T leave our body, it would make us sick, causing anything from infections to colon cancer. Now, if you're eating foods that have ALREADY been processed (which strips them of most nutrients), you're basically eating sh*t.

Let's talk about what you typically find in most processed foods:

Enriched Bleached Flour: It's what most breads, cereals, and granola bars are made from. The 54-year-old prostitute is perfect example here. They take some brown wheat and strip it down, bleach its skin white, make it lose all of its healthy qualities and then dress it up with some synthetic vitamin makeup so you'll be fooled into thinking it's healthy.

> **Did You Know?**
> The "bleaching" of food also has a connection to the phenomenon of skin bleaching that "dark" people practice, all the world over. This is all due to the fact that white people thought (and still think) that people of color were (and are) "evil," "dirty," and "filthy." This false perception has been pushed onto the rest of the world, just as their religion, languages and foods.

Sugar: Same thing. Start with tasty sugarcane. End up with a white powdery drug, with no nutritional value beyond the calories. And put it in damn near everything. **The**

average American child consumes 5 pounds of sugar a week! Sugar can be found in everything from canned soups to salad dressings. And if you can't find sugar, you'll find High Fructose Corn Syrup.

Partially Hydrogenated Oils: The unhealthiest (and cheapest) oils you can put in food, full of Trans Fat, one gram of which increases your risk for heart disease by 20% for that day. The Most Americans get 5 or more grams, even when selecting "Trans Fat Free" products. (See "Butter Vs. Margarine")

Artificial Food Dyes and Flavorings: These contribute to ADHD, cancer, and even brain damage. Eighty percent of so-called ADHD children who are taken off processed foods are cured of ADHD in two weeks. Sadly, this is what most kids are eating on a daily basis at home, at school, and when they visit the corner store and candy lady. (See "What Are Carcinogens?")

Salt: And we're not talking sea salt. Tons of processed foods are made with refined salt, which is another unhealthy form of a natural product that wasn't so bad for you to begin with. Salt, like sugar, and a number of chemical preservatives, is used to make processed food last longer. Know what else makes the processed food last so long on store shelves? The fact that all the living food qualities are DEAD. Just keep reading.

But if the food is so bad, why is it at the top of every shelf?

If you didn't know, food manufacturers actually "buy" shelf space and positions at grocery stores. That's why the most profitable foods (the ones with the cheapest and lowest quality ingredients) are the most visible. It's not because they're the "best" products. Also, most grocery products that make loud health claims on their packaging are usually nutritionally worthless, since the standards for making those claims are so easy to dance around. **The most nutritious foods are actually those the FDA doesn't allow to make any health claims whatsoever: fresh fruits and vegetables.** (See "I'll Be Your Pusher").

What the Hell is Irradiation?

Irradiation is a common process, where foods are blasted with radiation to eliminate bacteria, mold, and viruses. But, if you've ever seen the Incredible Hulk, you know that getting blasted just makes them mad and strong. Seriously, it makes the bugs become more resistant and, therefore, stronger. It also helps the surviving bacteria, who will no longer have natural enemies. For example, when radiation destroys salmonella bacteria (the bacteria that cause botulism) another form of food poisoning will flourish.

Anywhere from 20 to 80% of a food's vitamins are lost or damaged by irradiation. Among irradiated foods, fruit juices lose more vitamins than fruit, which lose more than vegetables and grains, which, in turn, lose more than meat. Vitamin E, in particular, is so badly damaged that even if it is put back as an additive later on, it will still get destroyed.

> Did You Know?
> While irradiation destroys bacteria, it does not destroy the toxic chemicals produced by bacteria. Irradiation increases the level of aflatoxin, a toxin associated with liver cancer. These increases ranged from 31% for corn, to 84% for onions. Irradiation also creates "free radicals," which are unstable molecules than can contribute to cancer and other bad things you'd associate with radicals running free.

Oh, and how could we forget hormones?

If you eat meat, you're eating a "processed" food also, because you're damn sure not eating it raw. By the time you get it, it's either TOTALLY different from its original state (such as a hot dog or chicken nugget), or just several steps away, full of antibiotics and hormones. **If it comes from an animal in any form, and the packaging doesn't say "no hormones," then, trust me, it's got hormones in it.** And that stuff is not good for the animals, or for you. See "The Dangers of Eating Meat."

What about Halal and Kosher food?

Ahh…the "labels." Okay, neither of those words means healthy. Those two words only mean that the food was processed in a way that adheres to the rules of traditional Islam or Judaism. **In the case of the "Kosher" label** (where you'll see a "K" or "U" on the box) **it typically means the food has no pork in it, but the way you get those labels is by paying a specific "Kosher certification agency"** (which is why the symbols look different), **and some agencies are more "lenient" than others.** Meaning "kosher gelatin" is still made from pig, but a certain group of Rabbis said it was cool. Similarly, in case you're under the impression that Halal meat is better, that's not necessarily true. While SOME Halal meat producers are also organic, pasture-fed, antibiotic-free and so on, **75% of Halal meat in America produced in the year 2000 came from pork fed cows, according to Dr. Stephen Emanuel, from Agway Feed Company.** According to Mazhar Hussaini, president of the North American Halal Foundation:

> In the United States the cows are being fed pork based protein, like pork meat byproducts, pork bone meal. It is also the same with chicken. Muslims are directed in the Quran to eat food that is Halal and Tayyib. Halal is defined as food that is permissible according to Islamic law.

Tayyib means wholesome, pure, nutritious and safe. Traditionally, Muslims in North America have emphasized the Halal over the Tayyib when it comes to meat consumption...For instance, great emphasis is placed on ensuring that animals slaughtered for consumption are done so in the Islamic manner (the practice known as Zabiha). However, little to no attention is given to whether or not the animal itself is healthy, free of disease, hormones, antibiotics, and chemicals at the time of slaughter.

Don't matter if your Muslim or Christian, Jew or Gentile, meat-eater or vegan, you're probably eating some crap. You too can improve.

BEEF (WITH PINK SLIME), IT'S WHAT'S FOR DINNER
BY DIERDRA BAPTISTE

Because cattle are now warehoused instead of farmed, they are corn-fed, and not grass-fed as nature intended. Their stomachs are not equipped to break down the corn properly. This means that the digestive process is slowed down, creating an ideal environment for bacteria to grow rapidly. One such bacterial strain is Escherichia coli, commonly referred to as E. coli. While many strains are harmless, some can cause food poisoning. Instead of forcing meat producers to allow cattle to graze naturally, the FDA decided to remedy the E. coli issue by allowing meat producers to chemically "wash" the meat.

Ground beef is processed by sweeping up scraps of cow flesh from slaughterhouse floors, and then pulverizing the scraps into a paste. This paste is then sent through a maze of tubing, where it's "washed" in ammonia hydroxide, which kills the E. coli. **Ammonia hydroxide is now found in 70% of all ground beef in the US, and the meat industry proudly claims that it will be in 100% within five years.** That means NO CHOICES!!

Even an FDA microbiologist, Gerald Zirstein, has called this ingredient, "nasty pink slime." As reported in *Grist*:

> It's the cheapest, least desirable beef on offer – fatty sweepings from the slaughterhouse floor, which are notoriously rife with pathogens like E. coli 0157 and antibiotic-resistant salmonella. [Beef Products, Inc. or BPI] sends the scraps through a series of machines, grinds them into a paste, separates out the fat, and laces the substance with ammonia to kill pathogens.

After the ground beef is washed in ammonia, it's sent out to our grocery stores, fast food chains and restaurants. Next time you bite into that Whopper, think household cleaner. Mmmm...tasty.

And this "pink slime" isn't just in U.S. ground beef. Beef Products, Inc. deals with other food products and other countries as well, boasting:

> [Our] ultimate goal is to have our products incorporated in all ground beef and other further processed meats produced in the United States. Our products can also be found in Canada, Mexico, and Japan with expansion plans for Central America, Europe, and Pacific Rim countries.

That's ON TOP of the fact that some of the cows ain't even "real" cows. They're more like resurrected, zombie clones. **According to Brady Hicks of JR Simplot** (a US-based cloning company) **some of the cattle that are cloned to boost food production in the US have been created from the cells of dead animals.** Hicks said that his organization was among many that had tried out the technique successfully. In August of 2010, he told *BBC News*:

> The animals are hanging on a rail ready to go to the meat counter…We identify carcasses that have certain carcass characteristics that we want, but it's too late to reproduce the genetics of the animal. But through cloning we can resurrect that animal.

If "zombie cows" don't seem appetizing, eat more fresh fruits and vegetables. If you can't quit the beef, look into veggie burgers.

THE DANGERS OF EATING MEAT
BY MENTAL SUN

"And hear it first-hand from the intelligent brown man/ A vegetarian: No goat or ham/ or chicken or turkey or hamburger/ 'cause to me that's suicide, self-murder" – KRS-One, "My Philosophy"

Too often we come across evidence of how we've been mis-educated. Since public school we've been taught about the basic food groups. We've been told that things like chicken, beef, pork, eggs and milk are natural parts of the human diet. Unfortunately, that kind of misinformation has had many harmful effects on our health, and these effects only have gotten worse with time. Every year, more and more people die from meat-related illnesses, such as heart disease, cancer, diabetes, small bowel obstructions, and many other sicknesses associated with obesity.

Have you ever wondered who was responsible for the food pyramid charts that we used to see hanging in our classrooms and all over the schools' cafeterias? Most people (including myself) believed that these charts were an unbiased, scientifically backed project that had the health of the people in mind. Instead, they have been shown to be a recipe for sickness and obesity, which are manipulated and controlled by big food corporations. Intense lobbying from the food industry has already questioned the validity of the food pyramid and dietary guidelines that are being taught to our young children all throughout the public school system, where school lunches are typically shipped out by the same companies that supply the food for prisons.

The next time that you see one of those pyramid posters, check the fine print and see who is responsible for it. You will see that it is usually the National Dairy Council, or some other industry trying to push their product.

Meat and Heart Disease

Consuming animals and animal bi-products has been one of the major contributors to the growing epidemic of heart disease in America, and more specifically, in the Black community. High cholesterol diets are the main contributors to these self-inflicted diseases and deaths. Cholesterol plays a very important part in the everyday functions of our cells, but excessive amounts contribute to the heart disease epidemic. **Cholesterol is a compound that is only found in animals, making it easy to assume that we need to consume animals to have cholesterol. However, the human liver produces enough cholesterol to satisfy the needs of the entire of the body.** The human body contains a feedback mechanism that keeps the serum concentration of cholesterol almost constant. The liver, itself, manufactures about 600 mg of cholesterol a day, but that amount varies on the intake of cholesterol in the daily diet. (See "Heart Health").

Meat and Cancer

The most common types of cancer affecting Americans today are breast cancer (among women), colon/rectum cancer, prostate cancer (among men) and lung cancer. All of these different forms of cancer can be fatal. However, when a person chooses a plant based diet, instead of a meat based diet, the occurrences of these diseases are rare. **According to the World Health Organization, 30% of all cancers in Western countries are diet-related.** Many studies have been advanced to figure out the link between eating meat and the risk of getting cancer.[11]

The most obvious factor is that meat contains absolutely no fiber, and lacks other nutrients that provide similar benefits. Meat, however, does contain animal proteins, saturated fats, and other carcinogenic (cancer-causing) compounds that increase the risk of cancer. (See "What Are Carcinogens?")

---

[11] However, it's legally dangerous for any of these scientists to tell you that eating meat can contribute to cancer. Just ask the ones who've been sued for even HINTING at it. This is why the "experts" will always say you can reduce your cancer (or heart disease) risk by eating more vegetables, but will never tell you to eat less meat. The meat industry and FDA (who are in cahoots) would have their heads, as they've done on several occasions.

Consuming high fat foods, such as meats, dairy products, eggs, fried foods and even vegetable oils, can cause a woman's body to produce an excess amount of estrogen that encourages the growth of cancerous cells in the breasts, and other organs. **This means that if a woman avoided high fat foods throughout her life, the risk of developing hormone related cancer decreases significantly.** Men suffer a similar risk, the difference being fatty acids increase the production of testosterone, which increases the possibilities of developing prostate cancer.

No matter what form of cancer or heart disease, it seems impossible to find a doctor or a holistic healer that won't advise a patient to reduce their meat and fat intake, or eliminate it completely, after being diagnosed, and increase the intake of plant-based foods. On the other hand, it's always suggested to increase the intake of plant-based foods such as fruits and leafy greens, along with eliminating other important factors, like tobacco, alcohol, and stress.

Aside from the inherent dangers of eating meat, the risks involved are even greater now, considering the way that modern factory-farming and corporate food giants operate. (See "Beef –With Pink Slime – It's what's For Dinner") Nevertheless, we need to study our bodies more, study what we are putting into our mouths, and study the ingredients listed in the foods that we eat. (See "Reading – And Understanding-Food Labels")

By decreasing your intake of meat you decrease your risk of disease. Save yourself the unnecessary complications.

GET OFF THE COW TITTY

WHY PEOPLE OF COLOR DON'T NEED NO DAIRY
BY C'BS ALIFE ALLAH

I had a conversation with one of my friends about the use of cheese throughout many European dishes. Yo, their food really has no flavor! Indians got curry, Jamaicans got jerk, and African Americans got hot sauce (yes, I do spritz it on my garden salads). Europe's got nuthin'. This is why, on those Silk Road adventures, whites brought back MAD SPICES. So, in the absence of spices, what does a dairy-rich, spice-poor culture do? They use cheese to cover up EVERYTHING. This practice has found its way into American cuisine.

Let's deal with some basic geography, weather climates and historical facts. Historically, white people drink a lot of milk and eat a lot of dairy by-products, like cheese, mayonnaise, and ice cream. The reason that they do this is due to several, simple reasons:

- Europeans inhabit colder climates, where milk doesn't spoil
- The domesticated cow has long been a part of European culture
- The gene which allows adults to digest milk, causing them to be lactose tolerant, appeared in Europe, approximately 6,000 years ago
- Most people in the world, other than Europeans, some degree of lactose intolerance

Now, how stupid are all of these "Got Milk?" commercials? Milk has been promoted as the primary source of calcium for "strong teeth and bones," but most of the world's population can't even physically tolerate it!

The U.S. Dietary Guidelines provide a perfect example of institutionalized, dietary racism. These guidelines push the consumption of milk and dairy products, even though 100% of Native Americans, 70% of African Americans, 90% of East Asians, 89% of West Africans, and 53% of Mexican Americans are lactose intolerant[12]. The same "suggestions" for meat consumption exist as a blanket statement, despite the fact that disproportionately high rates of meat-related cancers and heart disease affect Original people.

Now, if the school lunch program (which a high percentage of children of color depend on) is based on these institutionalized standards of dietary racism, is it any surprise that the stomach aches, the bloating, and the many other side effects of dairy consumption have had an effect on our children's academic performance?

So where are we supposed to get calcium from?

Where do we get our calcium from? Well, where does the cow, whose milk we drink, get its calcium from? The cow gets its calcium from the same place that we used to get ours. From bok choy, broccoli, collards, Chinese cabbage, kale, turnip greens, watercress, mustard greens, and okra. Not to mention from grains, beans, fruits, and vegetables. It's interesting that other mammals and primates have no problem meeting their requirements for daily calcium consumption, without drinking milk boxes and eating American cheese.

> **Did You Know?**
> No other animal on the planet drinks another animal's milk or past infancy, but there are clear historical reasons for why diary is a major part of the diet of Original People who, as a whole, are lactose intolerant... It's called slavery, colonialism, and imperialism.

Milk Substitutes

---

[12] Among adults. Typically, lactose intolerance worsens with age. So while only 45% of African American children show clear symptoms, this intolerance emerges fully by adulthood, raising the rate to 70% having total intolerance and 90% having some degree of intolerance.

There are now many milk and dairy substitutes that can be found, just about everywhere. Many of us are familiar with soy milk, yet other milk substitutes are just as available, and generally better for your health. There are many varieties of rice milks, almond milks, hemp milks, etc. You can find these alternatives in most large supermarkets, including Target and Wal-Mart. If they're not in the dairy section, they'll be in the health foods section. It's also easier than you may think to make your own milks. Basic recipes can be found in the Appendix section of this book.

A Few More Facts about Dairy Foods

It's well known that dairy proteins contribute to allergies, asthma, and sinus problems. Antigens in dairy may also contribute to rheumatoid arthritis and osteoarthritis. The galactose in dairy products may even contribute to ovarian cancer, as cancer rates worldwide parallel dairy consumption.

Other conditions that can be attributed to dairy consumption include acne, arthrosclerosis, bellyaches, a bloated abdomen from excess gas production, bronchitis, pulmonary (lung) infections, cramps, diarrhea, eczema, gastrointestinal disturbances, hay fever, hemorrhage, high blood pressure, hives, Juvenile Rheumatoid Arthritis, Multiple Sclerosis, nasal congestion, kidney disease, pyoderma (skin rash producing bumps and pus), and even sneezing. Furthermore, toxic pesticides and antibiotic residues are frequently found in dairy products, despite limited government efforts at screening.

Although you've probably heard that you need to drink milk for strong bones, that's not true. Weight-bearing exercises and eating greens are more likely to help your bones develop than dairy. In fact, consuming dairy is linked to osteoporosis (See "pH A Matter of Minerals"). **Countries that DO NOT consume dairy often have lower osteoporosis rates than the U.S.!**

Am I Lactose Intolerant?

You mean that you can't tell that your stomach is bubbling? Hippocrates reported negative to cow's milk, such as gastrointestinal problems including indigestion and flatulence (or farting) as early as 370 B.C. Ghostface Killah reported his own observations in 2009:

> Be careful. I mean, you know, whatever whatever, to each his own, though, but...that milk? That coffee? Y'nahmean? Hot chocolate and sh*t? Milkshakes? Son, you f*ck around, you'll be sh*ttin on yourself

and you got somewhere to go that's mad important, man, y'nahmean? I'm tellin you, G. Don't just get up and act like you drinkin some milk, nigga, and you bout to bounce. 'Cause you gonna f*ck around and sh*t on yourself. If you stuck in traffic, nigga, you gonna sh*t on yourself. Y'nahmean? I'm tellin you, so just take it...take it from me and sh*t. Y'nahmean? It's like, yo. I'm your man.

If you are Original/Indigenous/a Person of Color, you don't need to be sucking on a cow's titty. Make a fruit smoothie instead!

GENETICALLY MODIFIED FOODS
BY SUPREME UNDERSTANDING AND MIN. MUTWASZE

You might have heard people talking about "No GMOs." You might also know that GMO stands for "Genetically Modified Organism." But what exactly are Genetically Modified Organisms, and why are they such a bad thing? "Supreme healthologist" Minister Mutwasze explains it quite simply:

> "Genetically Modified" means that companies like Monsanto and big banks like Wachovia (who financed genocide thru slavery back in the day) are creating seeds in the laboratory consisting of 2 species, also known as "transgenic hybrids" of say, a fish gene and a tomato gene. They mix them in a dish and let them express themselves!
>
> Here is why they do this: A fish has a gene that allows it to not get frostbite. A tomato does not. However, if we cross (splice) the fish gene into the tomato gene – we will get a tomato that can withstand frostbite!

Sounds like some "weird science," doesn't it? Like a new Frankenstein story? In fact, it's exactly that...which is why people call these foods "Frankenfoods." And it doesn't stop at fish genes in your tomatoes. Scientists are genetically modifying damn near everything we eat. They do this to make it cheaper to produce, easier to grow, and less likely to be "reproduced." What does that mean? That means most GMO crops don't have seeds so they can't be planted in your backyard somewhere. Meaning you've gotta keep comin to THEM to get your food supply, which is getting further and further away from even being "food" in the first place. Min. Mutwasze's stance is that GMO foods – stripped of their natural ability to produce seeds – are unable to produce life and are basically dead as well.

So not only are scientists turning everything GMO, they're using crazier and crazier combinations. If you thought fish in your tomatoes was bad...you'll really freak out about human in your rice. **In 2007, the US government granted permission to Ventria, a biotech company, to produce rice that contains human genes.** Yes, human genes in your rice. And they said WE were the cannibals? **Ventria plans to harvest the human-rice proteins and use them in**

Did You Know?
Now, GMO crops like Canola are turning up in the wild as well! That means that even nature is being replaced by plant-life that is entirely unnatural. Researchers believe that the reason GMO Canola crops are turning up everywhere is because the seeds are transported on flatbed trucks, and they fly off and end up everywhere. It's just something about the past 200 years of world history that tells me it's not as "accidental" as they're making it seem.

drinks, desserts, yogurts and cereal bars. Ever seen the movie *Soylent Green?* Guess it's coming true.

What's ironic is that we were the originators of this science, as well. **The first genetically modified foods were hybrid crops bred by US in ancient times.** Min. Mutwasze continues:

Some of our most ancient foods are hybrids. How do we know this? I give you the 1,000 – 2,000 year old lemon or orange…both ancient and healing. And both hybrids! Yup, sho' is.

You've been eating hybrids all along, which were first developed in Afrika and Asia. So again, don't trip on what are essentially "first generation hybrids" because first generation hybrids have seeds (as we know for oranges and lemons). The science of hybrid engineering was necessary to extend the life of food crops so that a people could be fed all year round. Also you must remember that foods were seen just as much as medicine as food a few thousand years ago. (See "The Healing Power of Fruits")

For example, fruits were highly prized for their abilities to cure via creating an electrical charge inside the body, without which we would die. It takes Vitamin C for this – the sourer, the better. Thus, [we made] lemons! One of the most acidic fruits has the ability in simple experiments, for example, to light up a bulb! Many citric fruits do.

And that's the point. Fermentation is important, not only in fruits, but in our bodies, because it assists in generating electricity and generating Adenosine Triphosphate, aka ATP, which is the nuclear explosion khemical of the cell! If you do not have this khemical reaction being produced inside your cells, you can have chronic fatigue, for instance. You are eating, but not enough ATP production is happening at the ceullular level…that's Vitamin C you are deficient in (other things considered).

This makes sense then, that medically speaking, Vitamin C is also vital for the heart (electrical motor of the body) because the heart basically runs off an electrical charge going through/around it…and you can get this from those famous hybrids – lemons and oranges! This tells us that certain genetically modified foods (such as these first generation hybrids) are not all bad.

But once Western scientists got a hold of this idea, they went in a very different direction. Min. Mutwasze continues:

The problem with all this gene modification is that the evil Frankenmeds/Dr. Jekylls of the world never know when to stop! Again, his-story shows us that they always take what they learn from mucking with plants and try it out on people. In fact, it was the study of plants that led to genetics in the first place!!! A German monk named Gregor Mendel, who was a botanist, is credited with the discovery of genetics. Thanks to him we have Mendelian Genetics (and Eugenics)...All this goes right back to genetically modified foods. F–ing around with plants and animals to see what they can do on people, and calling it medical research for the sake of humanity. Sure. That's the way it has always gone with the diabolical ones.

Thus, an ancient, life-giving strategy became a modern, life-threatening industry. Am I exaggerating? Do you think all that "weird science" isn't gonna affect your health? C'mon son!

One of the main features of Genetically Modified Organisms, or GMOs, is that they can resist pests better than "organic" (meaning "normal") plants. But it's not that the bugs just "stay away" from the GMO. **The GMO plant actually "resists" the bugs with its own built-in pesticide.** Yes, pesticide. Inside. When a bug eats a GMO plant, the toxin splits open their stomach and kills them. Now what happens when people consume the same GMO? **Studies have found that rats fed genetically modified potatoes had an increased thickening in the lining of their stomach and intestine and a weakening of their immune system.** But most of the scientific community says there's no evidence that GMOs pose a threat to humans. That's only because there have been no long-term studies on humans. I wonder why? Perhaps because most of America's biggest cash crops (like soy, corn, and canola) are based on the success of GMOs. Either way, smaller studies have linked GMOs to food allergies, low fertility and birth weight, increase in autoimmune diseases, heart disease, respiratory illness, anemia, and cancer.

Read food labels, cut back on processed foods, buy organic when possible, try community farms and markets...or grow your own food.

F.T.P. AND DON'T SHELL-OUT
F.ORGET T.HE P.I.G. AND OTHER SCAVENGERS
BY C'BS ALIFE ALLAH

People call the police "pigs" as an insult...yet, go on to eat like pigs. People complain about us acting like "crabs in a barrel," and then go eat some crabs out of a barrel. One's words should always line up with one's actions, and one's actions should always line up with one's diet.

When you read the dietary laws of various religions, such as Judaism, Islam and Christianity (yes, Christians have dietary laws – these laws just aren't observed in the West), they all share something in common. They all prohibit the eating of animals that are scavengers. What's a scavenger? A scavenger is an animal that will eat anything. It's a living garbage disposal. Society's got y'all eating scavengers and has you believing that it's the nutritional truth. (See "The Other Worm –Er, White – Meat")

Now, shellfish are just as dangerous as pork. Many people don't know this because pork gets all the headlines. Lobsters, shrimp, oysters, clams, crabs, crawfish, scallops, and mussels are all shellfish. Lobsters, shrimp, crawfish and crabs are the roaches of the sea. If you crack open a roach, it has the same internal "meat" as those four. Why don't you just collect up a few roaches from around the way, crack them open, and enjoy them with some butter? Disgusted? What about oysters and clams? They're snot. And you know this because of how they look and feel.

All of the above are bottom feeders. They live at the bottom of the ocean and eat anything that falls to the bottom. This means that they munch on all of the waste that is produced by every organism in the ocean. Plus, like the pig, their internal "meat" is fat-based. That "meat" stores toxins in their bodies, just like with pigs. If you've noticed, a lot of shellfish only have that one vein to get rid of waste – think about the one vein that runs down a shrimp's back. So, shellfish eat crap, but their bodies aren't equipped to get rid of that crap – just like a damn pig. That's the reason why, **out of 145 sites that were recently sampled for the presence of mercury in shellfish, mercury was found at every single site.**

At the ocean's bottom, shellfish are also eating all the toxins dumped into the ocean. Now, only about 0.1% of shellfish are eaten raw, yet that tiny portion is responsible for a huge amount of the food-borne illnesses that are reported. This is because shellfish harbor bacteria, viruses, and heat-stable toxins, which are industrial contaminants, including heavy metals.

Along with shellfish, you can add fish that are over a foot long and that weigh over 50 pounds, to your list of what not to mess with. These large fish are scavengers, also. The smaller fish tend to be vegetarian, and therefore, don't scavenge. For the record, catfish ain't no good for you, either. Catfish don't have scales (no way to excrete toxins from their bodies), have a huge toxin retention rate, and damn…come on…you know they look weird!

___

Scavengers are never healthy for you…If you eat fish, ask where the fish came from and check the mercury levels of that area online.

___

THE OTHER WORM – ER, WHITE – MEAT

BY SUPREME UNDERSTANDING

ORIGINALLY PUBLISHED IN HOW TO HUSTLE AND WIN, PT. ONE

The following is an excerpt from an April 2001 *ABC News* article entitled, "Woman Contracts Parasitic Worm in Her Brain from Pork Taco":

> What sounds like science fiction was all too real for Dawn Becerra, who found a parasitic worm lodged in her brain after eating a pork taco while vacationing in Mexico. Doctors at Arizona's Mayo Clinic in Scottsdale believe the taco contained Taenia solium, a parasite that is surprisingly common in Latin American countries, and is often transmitted by eating undercooked pork. Becerra said the snack made her ill for three weeks. And soon after, she began suffering seizures…Doctors at the Mayo Clinic discovered Becerra had neurocysticercosis – a lesion in her brain, caused by the parasitic worm. Last November, she was told that if she wanted to live a normal, seizure-free life, she would need surgery…As an egg, the worm attached itself to the intestinal wall, and eventually moved into her blood stream and to her brain, said Dr. Joseph Sirven, who operated on Becerra…"All of a sudden, I realized they were going to cut open my brain, and take a worm out of my brain" she said…"The fascinating part about this is that it's much more common than people think," notes Sirven…The World Health Organization says neurocysticercosis is a common cause of epilepsy in Africa, Asia, and Latin America.

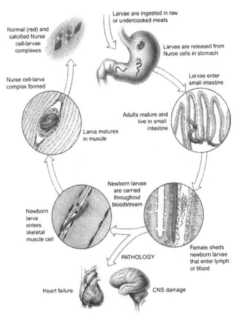

Larvae are ingested in raw or undercooked meats

Normal (red) and calcified Nurse cell-larvae complexes

Larvae are released from Nurse cells in stomach

Nurse cell-larva complex formed

Larvae enter small intestine

Adults mature and live in small intestine

Larva matures in muscle

Newborn larvae are carried throughout bloodstream

Newborn larva enters skeletal muscle cell

Female sheds newborn larvae that enter lymph or blood

PATHOLOGY

Heart failure

CNS damage

So uh...people STILL eat pork?

Of course, there are a lot bigger problems for us to deal with, but pork is a good one to talk about, because it not only makes us sick, but it says a lot about the way we still think. Here's the way most people who still eat pork think about those nasty chunks of disease:

☐ It tastes good.

☐ It hasn't killed me yet.

☐ It can't be THAT bad for me.

But we could start cooking rats in curry sauce, or sh*t in barbecue sauce, and say the same thing. The pig has been unclean and unhealthy since its appearance on the planet, and it will always be that way. It was never even meant to be used as food, after all.

Let's go over some basics:

☐ The pig has only one stomach and very limited excretory organs. Other animals, like cows, have much more in their bodies to help them digest their food. The pig doesn't. That means the pig is full of sh*t.

☐ The pig doesn't have any pores to sweat from. That's why it rolls in the mud or feces to keep cool. That's also why all of the filth in the pig stays inside of it.

☐ Every holy book and religion has put the pig down as filthy and unclean. From Ancient Egypt, to the Old Testament (Leviticus 11:7,8, Genesis 1:29, Isaiah 65:2-4, Isaiah 66:15-17) to the Qur'an (Surah 2:172-173, etc.), even down to the New Testament, where Jesus sends demons out of a man and into a herd of pigs.

☐ The Honorable Elijah Muhammad taught that the pig was used around 2000 B.C. to clean out the filthy caves where the Europeans lived then. In more recent times, pigs have been bred to clean the streets of early Spain, and the sewers of Chicago. This works, because pigs will eat anything nonstop, including feces, garbage, and poison, and not die.

☐ A diet heavy in red meat, especially pork, is one of the most significant factors behind the high rates of cancer, heart disease, high blood pressure, arthritis, and diabetes in the Black community. Want a cure for cancer? Stop eating bullsh*t (or more appropriately, porksh*t). That's a start.

☐ More Black men die from eating the wrong foods than they do from homicide. But when do these problems start showing up? When it's too late. At some point, you're just sick as hell, taking pills, until the doctor says, "stop eating red meat." Doctors tell woman the same when they're pregnant, which makes you wonder: if it's bad for you when you're pregnant, isn't it always bad for you?

Pig meat contains:

- ❑ Excessive quantities of histamine and imidazole compounds, which lead to itching and inflammation.
- ❑ High levels of dangerous cholesterol and saturated fat, which leads to gallstones, obesity, and heart disease
- ❑ Sulphur-containing mesenchymal mucus, which leads to swelling and deposits of mucus in tendons and cartilage, resulting in arthritis, rheumatism, etc. Sulphur also helps cause firm human tendons and ligaments to be replaced by soft mesenchymal tissues like the pig. The sulphur also causes the degeneration of human cartilage.

> **Did You Know?**
> Common parasites found in pork don't just stay in your digestive system. The worms and their eggs can migrate into your muscles (where they build homes), your lungs, your heart, your brain, and even into your eyes. If you Google *Scientific American's* article "Worms N Us" you'll find a slideshow that has pictures of some of this nastiness, including the "eggs in your eye" scenario. You can also look up a documentary called *Monsters Inside Me*, which is available via On Demand and on YouTube.

- ❑ The Taenia sodium worm, a tapeworm found in pig flesh. They also occur in human intestines and are not only capable of spreading to other organs, but are incurable after passing a certain stage.
- ❑ The Trichinae nematode worm – which causes trichinosis. Trichinosis is a disease one gets from eating pork that is undercooked. Then, there's the cramps, aches and stiffness – later followed by nausea and vomiting. And then, headaches and nervous disorders. The Trichinae worm is able to burrow through tissues and invade neighboring organs, or go straight into the bloodstream. After this point, they are often known to invade the brain or nervous system, as in the story above. Approximately one in six people in the U.S. and Canada have trichinosis, and may not know it.
- ❑ Plenty of other fun critters like the kidney worm, the lungworm, the thorn-headed worm, and the roundworm.

There are also diseases common to the pig, like:

- ❑ Genital papilloma (Note: This did not come from a man f*ckin' a pig...or did it?)
- ❑ Infectious porcine encephalomyelitis (or Teschen disease, porcine poliomyelitis, Talfan disease, or picornavirus)
- ❑ Swine erysipelas
- ❑ Hog cholera (or swine fever)
- ❑ Hemophilus influenza (or swine influenza, swine flu, hog flu)
- ❑ Swine plague, enzootic pneumonia, swineherd's disease, and swinepox

With some of these diseases, neither the animal, nor the humans consuming its meat, show any symptoms, at all.

This nasty, sick sh*t is a 10-billion-dollar-a-year industry. Why do you think that – even though there's thousands of Americans sick every day from eating it – we never hear how bad it is for us? It's simple: The FDA. (See "I'll Be Your Pusher: The FDA") FDA guidelines for packaged food allow:

- ❏ No more than 50 insect fragments or 2 rodent hairs per 100 grams of peanut butter.
- ❏ No more than 10 fruit fly eggs in 100 grams of tomato juice.
- ❏ No more than 150 insect fragments in an 8-ounce chocolate bar.

In fact, a December 2005, Ohio University research study found that Americans unintentionally eat 1 to 2 pounds of insect parts a year. Now, SOME of that is because, in the course of an average lifetime you will eat 70 assorted insects and 10 spiders while sleeping (and that's a fact). But even that disgusting number is NOTHING compared to what's in your food! And you can't do much about the crap that gets in your mouth while sleeping (except clean your nasty bedroom), but you can do a LOT about the crap you eat while wide awake (assuming you ARE awake by now).

Just ask yourself why, even though we know eating red meat, like beef and pork, leads to cancer and heart disease, pork is promoted as the "Other White Meat." Pork is NOT a damn white meat. These folks will sell you death on a platter and make you pay extra for the hickory smoked flavor!

"I ate, like, the tiniest piece of meat, and I woke up violently sick….It was vicious pain. I was throwing up. And I realized meat's become a poison for me now." – Mike Tyson, after becoming vegan

If you still don't believe that pork (and beef) is that toxic, try quitting them for a month and then have nice big serving after the month is up. If you can't even make it a month, then that should tell you how addictive those chemicals are. If you DO make it a month, you might not even want anymore, because you've kicked the addiction. But if you still do, try a nice juicy pork chop or bacon cheeseburger. And just watch how sick you become. If that doesn't tell you something, nothing will.

People can get sick by what they eat, think, or do, and do not know it!

WHAT IS LARD?

BY DR. J. H. KELLOGG [13]

It seems to be considered that pork is such a delicacy that not a particle should be wasted. In the case of no other animal is so much of the dead carcass utilized as food. The fat and lean portions are eaten fresh, or carefully preserved by salting or smoking, or both. The tail is roasted; the snout, ears, and feet are pickled and eaten as souse; the intestine and lungs are eaten as tripe or made into sausages; black pudding is made of the blood; the liver, spleen, and kidneys are also prized; the pancreas and other glands are considered great delicacies; while even the skin is made into jelly. In fact, nothing is left of the beast, not even the bristles, which the shoemaker claims. Surely it must be quite an important matter, and one well deserving attention, if it can be shown that an animal which is thus literally devoured, and that in such immense quantities, is not only unfit for food, but one of the prime causes of many loathsome and painful maladies. Let us examine the hog a little, and see what can be determined respecting his real nature, and his office in the economy of nature, if he has any.

If you can possibly sacrifice your taste in the cause of science, pork-loving friend, just climb over into the reeking sty, and take a closer view of the animal that delights the taste buds of some of your friends, perhaps your own. Make him straighten out his fore legs. Now observe closely. Do you see the open sore a few inches above his foot on the inner side? Do you think it is a mere accidental wound? Find the same on the other leg; it is rather a wise and wonderful provision of nature. Grasp the leg high up and press downward. Now you see its purpose, as a mass of corruption pours out. That opening is the outlet of a sewer. Yes, a sewer of disease; and hence the offensive, pungent matter which discharges from it. Should you fill a syringe with mercury or some colored injecting fluid, and drive the contents into this same opening, you would be able to trace all through the body of the animal little pipes communicating with it.

What must be the condition of the body of an animal so foul as to require a regular system of drainage for its teeming filth?

[13] Dr. John Harvey Kellogg was born in 1852 in Michigan and raised in a Seventh Day Adventist church, which instilled in him a lifelong interest in health and proper diet. He travelled the world and studied among the foremost medicine men and naturopaths of his day. He promoted vegetarianism, which led to his development of the "corn flake" and other breakfast cereals that still bear his name. Kellogg let his brother run the company that bore his name, but did not approve of the sugar content of their bestselling Corn Flake breakfast cereal. This article is based on excerpts from Kellogg's book, *Pork: The Dangers of Pork-Eating Exposed* published in 1897, and available free (in full) online at www.HoodHealthHandbook.com

Sometimes the outlet gets closed by the accumulation of external filth. Then the pungent stream ceases to flow, and the animal quickly sickens and dies unless the owner cleanses the parts, and so opens anew the feculent fountain, and allows the festering poison to escape.

What dainty morsels those same feet and legs make! What a delicate flavor they have, as every gourmet asserts! Do you suppose the corruption with which they are saturated has any influence upon their taste and healthfulness?

Perhaps you are thoroughly disgusted now, and would like to leave the scene. Pause a moment. Now let us look at the inside of this wonderfully delicious beast! Do you imagine that the repulsiveness of this loathsome creature is only on the outside? That within, everything is pure and wholesome? Vain delusion! Sickening and disgusting as is the exterior, it is, in comparison with what it covers, a fair cloak, hiding a mass of disease and rottenness which grows more and more filthy as we penetrate deeper and deeper beneath the skin.

What is Lard?

Just under the foul and putrid skin we find a mass of fat from two to six inches in thickness, covering a large portion of the body. Now what is this? "Lard," says one, "animal oil; an excellent thing for cooking; a very necessary kind of food in cold weather." But where did all that fat come from, or how did it become so heaped up around that poor hog? Surely it is not natural; for fat is only deposited in large quantities for the purpose of keeping the body warm in winter. This fat is much more than is necessary for such a purpose, and is much greater in amount than ever exists upon the animal in a state of nature. It is evidently the result of disease.

So gross have been the habits of the animal, so great has been the foulness of its body, that its excretory organs – its liver, lungs, kidneys, skin, and intestines – have been entirely unable to carry away the impurities which the animal has been accumulating all its life. And even the extensive system of sewerage with its constant stream, which we have already described, was insufficient for purging so vile a body of the debris which abounded in every organ and saturated every tissue. Consequently, this great flood of disease made its way through the veins and arteries into the tissues, and there accumulated as fat! Quite a delectable morsel, a slice of fat pork, isn't it? Concentrated, consolidated filth!

Lard, then, obtained from the flesh of the hog by heating, is nothing more than extract of a diseased carcass! Who that knows its character would dare to defile himself with this "broth of abominable things?"

What Shall We Do With the Hog?

Stop raising him. Turn him loose. He will soon find his place, like the five thousand which ran down into the sea in the days of Christ. If he must be raised, use him for illuminating our halls and houses. Lubricate our car and wagon with his abundant fat. Do anything with him but eat him. **It would be dangerous to adopt the principle that we must devour everything which is in the way, or which cannot be otherwise utilized.** Adam Clarke thought of one appropriate use to make of the hog. He said that if he was going to make an offering to the devil, he would employ a hog stuffed with tobacco.

The Mohammedans, as well as the Jews, abstain entirely from the use of pork. Such is also the case with some of the other tribes of Asia and Africa. Readers, what will you do? Can you continue to use as food such an abominable article as pork?[14]

No part of that pork belongs on your fork. Health wise, it's useless and can do you no good.

WHY SHOULD YOU CARE ABOUT PESTICIDES?
BY SUPREME UNDERSTANDING

One of the reasons why people buy organic food is to avoid pesticides and other chemicals. Even small doses of these can cause long-term damage to our health, especially in the womb and during early childhood. Think about it. A pesticide is literally a poison used to kill living things. And some fruits and vegetables get sprayed with dozens of 'em. For example, **studies have found that some apples have as many as 36 different pesticides on them!** These pesticides have been linked to a variety of health problems, including nervous system toxicity, cancer, hormone system effects, and skin, eye and lung

---

[14] Here's another old school commentary on pork (and meat-eating in general) from *The Ministry of Healing*, written in 1909 by Ellen G. White, a prolific Christian author who helped birth The Seventh Day Adventist Church and whose push for vegetarianism inspired Kellogg:

"Flesh was never the best food but its use is now doubly objectionable, since disease in animals is so rapidly increasing. Those who use flesh foods little know what they are eating. Often, if they could see the animals when living and know the quality of the meat they eat, they would turn from it with loathing. People are continually eating flesh that is filled with tuberculosis and cancerous germs. Tuberculosis, cancer, and other fatal diseases are thus communicated. The tissues of the swine swarm with parasites. Of the swine, God said, "It is unclean unto you; ye shall not eat of their flesh, nor touch their dead carcass." This command was given because swine's flesh is unfit for food. Swine are scavengers and this is the only use they were intended to serve. Never under any circumstances was their flesh to be eaten by human beings. It is impossible for the flesh of any living creature to be wholesome when filth is its natural element, and when it feeds upon every detestable thing."

irritation.

Still, nobody is trying to scare you off fruits and vegetables. At least WE're not. The health benefits of eating a plant-based diet are a LOT stronger than the risks from those chemicals. So it's very important that you eat at LEAST 5 fruits and vegetables a day, but if you only eat the ones on the "Dirty Dozen" list below, you should know that you're also eating an average of 10 pesticides a day. But you can easily cut that down to nearly nothing if you eat the "Clean 15" or simply buy organic. Of course, everyone can't afford to buy organic, so this list can help you decide which fruits and vegetables you can buy "regular" when money is tight.

> **Did You Know?**
> The Pesticide Action Network reported that Americans can experience up to 70 daily exposures to residues of a class of toxic chemicals known as persistent organic pollutants (POPs), including such chemicals as DDT and dioxin, through their diets. The report, "Nowhere to Hide: Persistent Toxic Chemicals in the U.S. Food Supply," analyzes chemical residue data collected by the FDA and finds persistent chemical contaminants in ALL food groups.

Will Washing and Peeling Help?

You should always wash your produce. However, washing reduces pesticides but doesn't get rid of em altogether. Especially if the produce has a thin skin (like hot peppers) or has been heavily sprayed (like apples). Peeling helps, but valuable nutrients often go down the drain with the skin.

The Dirty Dozen		The Clean 15	
The MOST Contaminated Foods – Buy Organic		The LEAST Contaminated Foods – No Need to Buy Organic	
1. Celery (Most)		15. Onions	7. Cabbage
2. Peaches	8. Spinach	14. Avocado	6. Eggplant
3. Strawberries	9. Kale	13. Sweet Corn	5. Cantaloupe
4. Apples	10. Cherries	12. Pineapple	4. Watermelon
5. Blueberries	11. Potatoes	11. Mango	3. Grapefruit
6. Nectarines	12. Grapes (Imported)	10. Sweet Peas	2. Sweet Potato
7. Bell Peppers		9. Asparagus	1. Honeydew Melon (Least)
		8. Kiwi	
Produce that isn't listed above is somewhere in between. The full list of 49 fruits and vegetables, ranked by pesticide contamination, is available at www.foodnews.org			

Tips for Buying Organically

Buying organic foods can be expensive, and some produce is less likely to be contaminated than others. In order to stay within budget, many of us may have to focus on buying organic only those foods on the Dirty Dozen. Below are some more useful tips:

- [ ] Purchase from your local farmer's markets, not your supermarket.
- [ ] Join a community-supported agriculture program if one is available near you (it allows you to buy produce, meats and other foods directly from the farm)
- [ ] Plant a garden; even a small space can produce a lot of fresh food
- [ ] If you must shop in a supermarket, look for locally grown items, which are likely to be fresher than other foods

Follow the steps above to get the most out of your produce, health wise and financially.

JUNK FOOD IS CRACK

BY SUPREME UNDERSTANDING

Junk food is almost as addictive as heroin. That's not my *opinion*. That's what science has found. In a series of studies conducted over the course of three years and published in the journal *Nature Neuroscience*, scientists Paul Johnson and Paul Kenny have shown that an unrestricted diet of junk foods like burgers, fries, and sweets will actually reprogram your brain into craving even more foods that are high in sugar, salt and fat, and these junk foods can eventually become a substitute for happiness, leading binge eaters to become addicted. This is one of the first studies to suggest brains react the same way to junk food as they do to drugs like crack and heroin.

In the study, one group of rats got normal amounts of healthy food to eat. Nothing bad happened. Another group was given limited amounts of junk food. Again, nothing major. The third group was allowed access to unlimited amounts of junk, including cheesecake, fatty meat products, and cheap sponge cakes and chocolate snacks. This group quickly became very fat and started binging. When the researchers electronically stimulated the part of the brain that feels pleasure, the mice on unlimited junk food needed more and more stimulation to register the same level of pleasure as the ones on healthier diets. Typical symptoms of drug addiction. **Other studies have shown that consuming excess sugar eventually lowers the body's ability to produce its own endorphins, which can result in depression.**

How Addictive?

Johnson and Kenny also discovered that a diet including unlimited amounts of junk food can cause rats to become so addicted to the unhealthy diet that they will starve themselves rather than go back to eating healthy food.

Having established that the junk food rats had become addicted, Johnson and Kenny wanted to know how far this addiction would push them. So they took both junk-food addicted rats and rats that had not previously been exposed to such food, and exposed them to electrical shocks whenever they ate junk. Rats that had just been introduced to junk food quickly stopped eating it, while the addicted rats ignored the discomfort and kept eating.

Perhaps, the most shocking finding came when the researchers took away the addicted rats' access to junk food and started feeding them only healthy rat chow again – the same diets the rats had eaten as pups. When junk food was no longer available, the rats simply refused to eat for two weeks.

"They actually voluntarily starved themselves," Kenny said. "It's almost as if you break these things, it's very, very hard to go back to the way things were before. Their dietary preferences are dramatically shifted." It's like what happened to the Indian children from *Slumdog Millionaire* who didn't want to live in India anymore after being exposed to McDonald's in America (during their trip to the Oscars). Research strongly suggests many modern humans also suffer from junk food addictions. **"Food can be highly addictive,"** said author and nutritional supplement producer Jordan Rubin. **"When people describe overeating and weight loss as a battle, this is why."**

Don't starve to eliminate all the bullsh*t. Add positive foods and lifestyle choices as you go along.

SLOW DOWN...FAST FOOD VS. SLOW FOOD
BY C'BS ALIFE ALLAH

"When you see the Golden Arches you are probably on the road to the Pearly Gates." – William Castelli, MD, Director of the Framingham Heart Study

Our mamas all told us to slow down and chew our food. But we grew up and started eating at places called "fast food" restaurants, where chewing is optional. America is on some "hurry up and do...get it done like yesterday" daily living. The only two things that people say that they don't have time for – eating and sleeping – are the only two things that people NEED to do. There is currently a movement called the Slow Food Movement. This movement is good in that it puts your diet in its proper perspective and will help build your food community. People, in the past, didn't used to get all of their food from thousands of miles away. **By concentrating on food that is closer to you, the quality of your food will immediately improve.**

Fast Food

"Fast food" is basically food that can be prepared and served quickly. It is mass-produced. Therefore, the quality of the ingredients is sub-par, plus the preservative levels are off the chart. It is meant to be eaten "on the run." If you observe nature, animals don't eat food "on the run." **They find a place to cop a squat and get into their meal. Fast food is sending people to a fast grave.** This is happening all over the world. In fact, you can tell if a country has been neo-colonized by how many fast food chains they have. If a country is "anti-West," you best believe that the West is trying to win them over with their food and entertainment. **Colonizers used to send the missionaries in first. Now, they send in McDonald's.** But, nowhere is fast food more prevalent than in the United States. 30% of American adults eat at least one meal outside the house daily, most of which are fast food. Between all the carbs, calories, cancer-causing chemicals, fat, and artificial ingredients, we've become a LOT sicker, now that "eating faster." **Not only are six out of ten Americans either overweight or obese** (including 15% of 6 to 9 year olds), **the rates of diabetes, cancer, and other diet-related diseases have gone through the roof ever since the fast food diet takeover.** Not only that, but fast food franchises are routinely involved in unethical practices in order to make their brands more prominent and profitable. **Even Anthony Bourdain, who travels the globe and eats all kinds of unimaginable foods for his job** as host of *No Reservations*, **does NOT eat fast food!** This man will eat roasted crickets, but not Chicken McNuggets. What does that tell you? In his words:

> They know exactly when and how to start building brand identification and loyalty with brightly colored clowns and smoothly tied-in toys. From funding impoverished school districts to the installment of playgrounds, McDonald's has not shrunk from f*cking with young minds in any way it can. But I want my little girl to see fast-food culture as I do. As the enemy.

But, beyond ALL of this, you know that fast food meal don't taste scrumptious like the meals your mama or grandmama used to make!

Slow Food

Did You Know?
Living within half a mile of large numbers of fast food restaurants can raise the chances of becoming obese by a third, a new study shows. The findings come on top of previous studies which showed that areas with a high number of fast food outlets also had a greater number of heart attacks. Large numbers of fast food restaurants in an area can also push up the stroke risk by up to 13%.

Slow food is basically a way to get more "bang for your buck" in terms of the overall nutritional value of the food you're eating. **Also, it's a** way to preserve the regional/traditional foods of your area, while assisting local farmers. In reality all indigenous cultures lived off of the slow food model. In this era of "frankenfoods," it's wise to know where your food comes from.

So, How Can I Be Down?

Here are some ways to help you get in-tune with the "slow food" in your area:

☐ Get in tune with the farmer's markets in your area. They bring food directly from the farms. That stuff is fresh and is the food that is in season. This site will hook you up: www.localharvest.org

☐ Support your regional or local seed bank, which preserves heirloom varieties of vegetables and fruits. Heirloom vegetables and fruits are varieties of food that were grown in the past, yet declined in production with the coming of large scale agriculture. For instance there are dozens of varieties of tomatoes yet when you go to the store, you generally only find a couple of types.

☐ Plant your own garden. Teach gardening among students and/or prisoners. Learn about the benefits of local farms, the dangers of fast foods, pesticides and genetically modified foods.

☐ Learn about the benefits of organic foods.

☐ Educate others.

☐ Organize a local food feast to highlight the local fare and make it an annual event.

Slow down and smell the local flowers. Your body will thank you.

WHAT'S IN A CHICKEN MCNUGGET?
BY SUPREME UNDERSTANDING

If you didn't already know, a McDonald's Chicken McNugget is less than 50% chicken. The majority of the ingredients are corn and corn by-products. Of course, there is *some* chicken broth added in there (or else there wouldn't be any chicken flavor after all the processing it goes through). But there's some more chemicals in there you probably should know about. As one author has written:

> These chemicals are what make modern processed food possible, by keeping the organic materials in them from going bad or looking strange after months in the freezer or on the road. Listed first are the "leavening agents": sodium aluminum phosphate, mono-calcium phosphate, sodium acid pyrophosphate, and calcium lactate. These are antioxidants added to keep the various animal and vegetable fats involved in a nugget from turning rancid. Then there are "anti-foaming agents" like dimethylpolysiloxene, added to the cooking oil to keep the starches from binding to air molecules, so as to produce foam during the fry. The problem is evidently grave enough to warrant adding a toxic chemical to the food: According to the *Handbook of Food Additives*,

dimethylpolysiloxene is a suspected carcinogen and an established mutagen, tumorigen, and reproductive effector; it's also flammable.

But perhaps the most alarming ingredient in a Chicken McNugget is tertiary butylhydroquinone, or TBHQ, an antioxidant derived from petroleum that is either sprayed directly on the nugget or the inside of the box it comes in to "help preserve freshness." According to *A Consumer's Dictionary of Food Additives*, TBHQ is a form of butane (i.e. lighter fluid) the FDA allows processors to use sparingly in our food: It can comprise no more than 0.02 percent of the oil in a nugget. Which is probably just as well, considering that ingesting a single gram of TBHQ can cause "nausea, vomiting, ringing in the ears, delirium, a sense of suffocation, and collapse." Ingesting five grams of TBHQ can kill."

So TBHQ comes from petroleum (oil) and is basically a cousin to lighter fluid. What about that dimethylpolysiloxane (the anti-foaming agent)? Guess where else you can find that one? Silly Putty. **So you're basically eating corn, lighter fluid, silly putty goo, chicken broth flavor, and some chicken scraps.**[15]

Oh, yeah! As far as the actual "chicken" in the McNugget? The 2004 documentary, *Super Size Me*, states that McDonald's Chicken McNuggets, originally made from old chickens no longer able to lay eggs, are now made from chickens with unusually large breasts. These chickens are stripped down to the bone, and then "ground up" into a "chicken mash," then combined with a variety of chemicals, pressed into familiar shapes, breaded and deep fried, freeze dried, and then shipped to a McDonald's near you. What's this "chicken mash" you ask? Just keep reading!

The Meat Mash

Guess what this is a picture of? Whatever you guessed, just keep it in mind as you read the following.

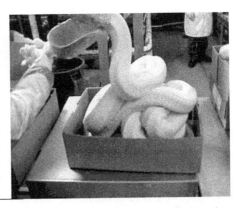

The kind of meat you find in hot dogs and chicken nuggets probably isn't what you think. These products are usually made from "meat slurry" and/or "mechanically

---

[15] As one blogger writes: "That begs the question: If those ingredients are so safe, then why are neither of them used in the Chicken McNuggets sold in Britain? McDonald's says the differences are based on "local tastes" (like I said, petroleum and Silly Putty, yum!). But it likely has more to do with Europe's stricter food regulations. For the record, British McNuggets are healthier all around with 170 calories, 9 grams of fat, and 1 gram of saturated fat for 4 pieces. (Stateside McNuggets have 190 calories, 12 grams of fat, and 2 grams of saturated fat for 4 pieces.)"

separated meat." Meat slurry (also known as reconstituted meat or emulsified meat) is a liquefied meat product made from the leftover pieces of the animal. (See "Nasty Fast Food Stories You'll Love To Tell") Why? It's cheaper, easier to distribute, and easier to shape into cute little products. Since it can't be sold alone, it is used in cat food, dog food, chicken nuggets and hot dogs. Yup. Just think about that. Mechanically separated meat is a little different, but not by much. It's a "paste" made from the stripped carcass of the animal. "Stripped" as in all meat has been removed and the only thing left is the tissue, some unwanted organs, and bone. They take the skeleton and push it through a high-pressure, high-temperature sieve. Then this paste (in the picture) is used for all the meaty food products that no longer look like meat, from Campbell's Cream of Chicken, to most frozen meatballs, some deli meats, just about all franks and sausages, and even turkey bacon. If you hadn't already guessed, it's also the main ingredient of Slim Jims, Spam, hot dogs, and chicken nuggets. This is common with pork, chicken, and turkey, but not beef. Why? Because after the Mad Cow disease outbreak, people found out that most cases of Mad Cow Disease were coming from ground up cow spines (yes spines), which is where the disease is most concentrated. So after that, mechanically separated beef was declared "inedible."

Some things are so processed they are unrecognizable and contain ingredients that belong nowhere near food.

THE "FOOD" THAT NEVER SPOILS
BY SUPREME UNDERSTANDING

The chemicals that were named in the article above are the same that make it possible for McDonald's food (and some others) to sit still for four or more years, without ever spoiling or getting rotten. You heard me right. Four years. You haven't seen the videos on Youtube? Just look them up (try searching "four year old McDonalds"), or better yet, do it at home for your child's next science fair project. I'll sum it up for you though. **Several individuals have been keeping a McDonald's cheeseburger** (just bread, patty, and cheese, no toppings) **and French fries, anywhere from 12 weeks to FOUR YEARS, and documenting what happens. Unlike burgers and fries from a real restaurant, they never went bad.** They never even changed color. And food is SUPPOSED to go bad pretty quickly. As Norma Joann writes in her Baby Bites blog, titled "Happy Birthday to My Happy Meal":

My Happy Meal is one year old today and it looks pretty good. It NEVER smelled bad. The food did NOT decompose. It did NOT get moldy, at all. This morning, I took it off my shelf to take a birthday photo. The first year is always a milestone...Because Colorado has an arid climate, over the year the moisture has been slowly pulled from the Happy Meal. The bread is crusty and if you look closely, you will see a crack across the top. The hamburger has shrunk a bit and still resembles a hockey puck. Yet, the French fries look yummy enough to eat. I never

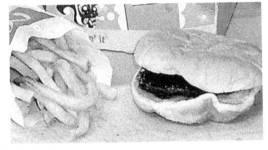

had an odor problem, after a couple of weeks, I couldn't even smell the fries...Food is SUPPOSED to decompose, go bad and smell foul...eventually. When I was a kid, I remember our garbage pail for the leftover food scraps was kept by our back door. After a couple of days, flies deposited their larvae (maggots) in the meat. When I would lift the lid, I would see the recently hatched maggots wiggling on the putrid mess. A fly never bothered to land on the tiny hamburger patty on my office shelf. Food is broken down into its essential nutrients in our bodies and turned into fuel. Our children grow strong bodies, when they eat real food. [If] flies ignore a Happy Meal and microbes don't decompose it, then your child's body can't properly metabolize it either. Now you know why it's called "junk food." I think ants, mice and flies are smarter than people, because they weren't fooled. They never touched the Happy Meal. Children shouldn't either.

Again, try it yourself. It would be a great science experiment for children to try at home, comparing the aging process of a homemade burger and fries to a McDonald's meal. It would be a great learning experience, pushing them to investigate the role of chemicals in the "food" we eat. In fact, some of us adults could use the same education!

One of our authors, SciHonor Devotion, did this project with her two children. They compared McDonald's to Burger King and a local diner. They expected the two fast food spots to do the same and for the local diner's food to mold as it naturally should. Her daughter, SciDey, and son, El Adon, reported:

The McDonald's cheese burger is completely intact with no mold whatsoever. Even the pickles, onion and cheese look like we just bought them. The Burger King French fries have white mold all over them...The Burger King Whopper Jr. however, has absolutely no mold on it, including the lettuce, tomato and onions. **The local diner's cheese burger and fries, to our surprise, look like they are brand**

new. There is no mold on either the cheese burger or the French fries. If this stuff is not breaking down due to all of the preservatives on it, can you imagine what it is doing inside of your stomach? Our mother wouldn't allow us to open the jar to take the pictures of our results, because of the smell, but the pictures we were able to take (and our full report) will be online at www.HoodHealthHandbook.com

Wow. So we're not demonizing McDonald's alone, because obviously other fast food spots share their practices (and problems). But as Morgan Spurlock (the star of *SuperSize Me*) explains in *Don't Eat this Book*, the reason people focus on McDonald's is because it represents the industry as a whole. No other franchise compares, not in terms of media influence, not in terms of destruction of the environment, and definitely not in terms of who is making the most people sick, throughout the world. This is why, even though I'll occasionally hit up a Taco Bell or a Subway when I'm on the road, I no longer go to McDonald's for anything. I won't even get a coffee there. Even *that's* probably got some chemicals in it to keep me coming back like a junkie. **Quitting McDonald's in large numbers sends a message to everybody, even the people who decide what kind of food is acceptable in this country.** Other nations have done it, or at least started the resistance. Join in.

> **Don't eat anything that won't spoil. Meat, vegetables, and fruits can barely last a week without spoiling. Never mind months or years!**

> **Did You Know?**
> Extra Virgin Olive Oil may be more than just a good substitute for margarine. It also appears to boost long-term memory. Olive oil is a top source of oleic acid, an omega-9 fatty acid that is converted during digestion to oleoylethanolamide (OEA), a hormone that helps keep brain cells healthy. In a new study from the University of California, Irvine, rodents fed OEA were better able to remember how to perform two tasks than those that didn't eat it. Researchers hypothesize that OEA signals the part of the brain responsible for turning short-term memories into long-term ones.

BUTTER VS. MARGARINE
BY SUPREME UNDERSTANDING

Speaking of ants, mice and flies not touching a Happy Meal, you know what else those critters won't touch? Margarine. Why? Because **Margarine is closer to plastic than it is to food.** Margarine is made by a process called hydrogenation, in which cheap, poor quality vegetable oil (some of which has already gone rancid) is converted into solids, or semi-solid grease, through the use of high heat, pressure and a toxic catalysts, such as nickel.

In the jargon of the chemicals industry, this process of turning liquid oils into solids, or semi-solids, is called plasticization. That's right, plastic.

At the end of the process, the resulting product is GREY and foul-smelling! You wouldn't spread some funky grey sh*t on your toast, so the margarine gets bleached, deodorized, dyed yellow, and artificially flavored. Then, they sell it to you as a "healthy alternative" to butter. But is it healthier? Butter is full of saturated fats. Margarine has less of these, though it's full of trans fats. Which kind of fat is worse for you? All the recent studies (except the ones funded by the margarine people) point to trans fats, which are now known to cause heart disease, obesity, diabetes, cancer, fertility problems, low birth weight, and other degenerative diseases. And when we talk about margarine, we're not talking about naturally occurring trans fats. We're talking about some grey plastic, so we're talking chemical byproduct sh*t. On the other hand, saturated fats may not be so bad for us. For more on that, check out **www.stop-trans-fat.com.** When it comes to butter vs. margarine, plain, unsalted butter is the healthier choice. And if you're stuck on margarine, Earth Balance (vegan) and Smart Balance (non-vegan) are the healthiest brands.

> Did You Know?
> 33% of kids eat fast food daily, much of it fried. The French fry is toddler's first finger food and 21% of toddlers eat French fries every day. A study published in the International Journal of Cancer discovered that early consumption of French fries by children was linked with adult breast cancer. Children in the study (ages 3 to 5) who regularly ate French fries were associated with a cancer increase of 27%. All it took to raise the risk was one serving a week!

If you can't make it yourself, you probably shouldn't eat it. Anything that takes industrial ingredients to make is not food.

WHAT ARE TRANS FATS?
AND HOW THEY'RE KILLING YOU NOT-SO-SOFTLY
BY MARCEL MALEKEBU

Tran-saturated fats, or "trans fats," are artificial fats. They're the more challenging members of the fat family. Found in virtually everything on the McDonald's menu, and in many fried foods (for example, French fries, doughnuts, pastries, etc.), **trans fats are the most difficult fats to rid your body of.** Sticking to your love handles and thighs, they are nearly impossible to burn off. The fat deposits in your hips are the most dear to your body. Meaning, only when the human body is starved of calories does it pull from these deposits for energy. This means that in order to eradicate these fats from your body, you must either starve yourself after each time that you eat them, or stop eating them entirely, and wait for them to leave your system.

Trans fats also lower your HDL cholesterol levels, and raise your LDL cholesterol levels. HDL (or High-Density Lipoprotein) cholesterol is commonly known as "good" cholesterol because it has been proven that high levels of this cholesterol seem to prevent cardiovascular diseases. LDL cholesterol (or Low-Density Lipoprotein), on the other hand, is known to increase the risk of cardiovascular disease. **To get technical, LDL particles are so lethal because they cannot only transport cholesterol into your artery walls, but can also become oxidized by free radicals** (e.g. cigarette smoke), **leading to heart disease.** Trans fats have not only been proven to promote cardiovascular disease and obesity, but have also been connected to Alzheimer's Disease, cancer, infertility, and even liver disease. As a result, trans fats have been banned in cities and countries all over the Earth.

So what do you do? Read the labels. No matter what sneaky name they're using in the ingredient label, the amount of trans fats is listed clearly on the "Nutrition Facts" label, on every food product you buy.

When you see anything besides 0g of trans fat, it's best you think twice about buying. This includes the fast food menu.

NASTY FAST FOOD STORIES YOU'LL LOVE TO TELL
BY SUPREME UNDERSTANDING

I'm sure you remember that disturbing video of the forty or fifty rats running wild in that West Village KFC/Taco Bell in New York. If not, you've got to see it to believe it. But what's more disturbing is this: **The day before news cameras caught 30-50 rats scampering playfully through a combo KFC/Taco Bell in the West Village,** the restaurant passed a NYC Health inspection. The so-called inspection was performed in response to complaints about rats in the restaurant, and yet the inspector couldn't find any. If you've ever worked in fast food or had a friend 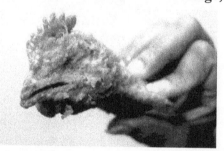 who did, you've heard exactly how filthy those places can get...while still maintaining a great score on their health inspection reports.

You've probably also heard those crazy stories about what can end up in your food: roaches, fried mice, severed fingers, cleaning agents, used condoms, etc. Some of those are myths, but many of them are 100%

true! The following is a selection of stories that made the news…and, in some cases the victims won the lawsuits they filed. **Next time you get a craving for some fast food, just remember this article!** It may help persuade you to stick to eating food that you've prepared yourself.

1994: A firefighter in Virginia Beach found two used bandages in his quarter pounder from McDonalds.

1995: A man in Alabama was dining at McDonalds when he found a condom in his burger.

2000: A woman purchased a box of chicken wings at a local McDonald's, only to find that one of the chicken pieces was actually a chicken's head! FYI: Deep fried chicken head is not on the McDonald's menu.

2002: A woman eating a bowl of clam chowder at a McCormick and Smicks's seafood restaurant in Southern California found a condom in her chowder, which she originally mistook for calamari. She sued the restaurant and won an undisclosed settlement amount.

2003: Pastor Tony Hill was enjoying a three-piece combo at a Popeye's Chicken in Baltimore, and as he took a bite out of his chicken, he noticed that a mouse had apparently lodged itself between the skin and the meat of the chicken. Various news media outlets have reported Popeye's refused comment, but the city health commissioner has stated that particular outlet has had rodent infestation problems before, and has been closed two other times for infestation or unsanitary conditions.

2004: A study conducted in Durban, South Africa (where Ludacris filmed the video for "Pimpin' All Over the World") concluded that 20,000 food outlets, including popular fast food joints, inspected by the City Health Department, failed to meet minimum health requirements. Health officials found hair, insects, cigarettes, weevils and fingernails in the food at these places.

2004: An Ohio man found skin, apparently from part of a thumb, in his sandwich at Arby's.

2005: A man found the whole finger – a different one – in some Kohl's frozen custard.

2006: Employees at an Oregon Jack in the Box decided to "amuse themselves" one day by adding a variety of disgusting things to customers' burgers, including acid, soap, phlegm, hair, and staples.

2007: 50-year-old Renaldo Ramirez contracted a disease called *cysticercosis* (either caused by employees not washing their hands after going to the bathroom, or from pig feces mixed in with the pork) after eating regularly at mobile diners (food trucks) in Houston. His food was contaminated with tapeworm eggs which nearly killed him. The larvae spread to his brain causing him to have persistent headaches that wouldn't go away with Tylenol. Doctors at a clinic gave him medicine for high blood pressure. A few days later he passed out and didn't wake up for eight days. Ramirez was the fourth patient treated for the disease in that area within a few months. During his recovery, Ramirez learned to cook and now prepares his own food.

2008: A Nebraska policeman was awarded $40,000 after he sued a Taco Bell/KFC that served his family food containing an employee's spit and urine. His son was hospitalized with gastroenteritis and dehydration.[16] The employee who did it was fined $100 but kept his job.

2008: A Youtube video shows a Burger King in South Beach, Miami where the bread is kept outside, for pigeons to eat.

2009: A Youtube video shows employees at a Domino's Pizza in North Carolina making "booger bread," farting on salami, and washing dishes with a sponge used to scrub genitals. In the video, a Health Department score on the window gives that Domino's Pizza a 96.5, an "A" rating.

2010: A Toronto man found a batch of dead ants in one of his two McDonald's breakfast burritos, after he'd already eaten the first one. According to the man and his girlfriend, there was no apology when he returned to the store with the contaminated food. Instead the store manager offered to replace the couple's burritos.

I hope you're sufficiently grossed out. Remember the point of this book is not to scare you into eating NOTHING. The point of this book is to inspire you to question EVERYTHING. So think twice about where you eat, and what you might be (unknowingly) eating there. **In fact, some of the WORST ingredients you'll encounter are the ones that you can find right on their ingredient lists!** Stuff like chemical fertilizer in Subway sandwich rolls (listed as ammonium sulfate), human hair and/or duck feathers in Noah's Bagels (listed as L-cysteine or cystine[17]), and straight up SAND in Wendy's Chili (listed as silicone dioxide). If THIS is the stuff they'll actually list on their

---

[16] However, the illness was more likely caused by the spit (containing bacteria or viruses) than the urine (which is actually sterile and relatively non-toxic when it leaves the body). Go figure!

[17] Artificial cysteine is available, but more expensive to use, so it's mostly used to create kosher and halal products

nutritional info, just imagine what you DON'T know.

Is KFC Chicken or What?

More like what. Factory farming is what most large-scale producers of meat (like Tyson or Perdue) and big franchise restaurants (like KFC and just about any other fast food chain) use to pump out meat fast and cheap. **Factory farming means that most of the "chickens" you'll eat actually don't look much like chickens at all.** Don't believe me? **Watch a documentary called *Meet Your Meat* (it's free online) or visit www.kentuckyfriedcruelty.com.** Here are a few things you may observe about those so-called "chickens": They don't have beaks or claws (so they don't poke each other while confined 30 deep to a tiny cage). They may not have eyes, or are blind, because they have lived their entire lives in dark boxes and cages. The chickens are huge. In fact, the latest methods have these birds at twice the size in less than half the time, reaching adulthood in about 39 days! Most importantly, it doesn't matter if they are clearly sick or diseased. They still go straight to processing. Enjoy.

Chances are this has happened to you already! You've had the beakless chicken, liquefied meat, and contaminated soda!

STUFFING YOUR FACE AIN'T ATTRACTIVE
THE CULTURE OF GLUTTONY IN AMERICA
BY C'BS ALIFE ALLAH

In that cartoon movie *Wall-E*, it shows a future where humans are in space, fat and overweight slumming around in hover-scooters. But think about it for a second, and then think about how the number of obese people has "skyrocketed" during the past few years…and think about how many of those people you see riding in those little scooters nowadays. Sounds like the movie should've been called *Wal-Mart* instead.

America, to many, is the land of opportunity, yet it's also viewed as the land of excess and gluttony. If you check the political cartoons of many countries when they choose to personify America it is usually as an overweight, fat man depicting 'Western' consumption.

Man vs. Food (one of my favorite television shows) follows a man that travels all around the United States entering the eating challenges/contests of various restaurants. The monstrosities that they come up with are unending. Literally sometimes there are pounds of different types of meat smothered in a variety of different sauces and deep fried three different ways. There are desserts with mountains of cream, hills of sugar, glaze from Monday to Friday. **But what most people don't know is that the host, who travels all around the U.S. to do these challenges, is under constant medical observation. When he is not doing these contests, he is an extremely healthy eater.** He says that he has to be, because what he does (as his job) puts extreme stress on his body.

I remember when I was young there was the famine in Ethiopia. There were a million and one "Ethiopian jokes" going around in my school. The jokes were cruel yet the other level of the cruelty is that we take more than our share and flaunt it to the whole world.

Colleges and fast food places throw out tons of food garbage on the daily. A few donate some portion of their products to homeless shelters yet most dispose of the food. I know of many fast food places that pour bleach in their food that they place in the garbage so that the homeless cannot get to it. There is more than enough food on the planet to feed all its people.

Indigenous cultures never wasted food. The food that was left over was preserved in some manner. It was canned, pickled, dehydrated, etc. Look into preparing meals that are in proportion and ways that you can preserve the food that you buy, such as freezing and storing it.

See if your local bakery or small food business would be into donating food to a homeless shelter. Don't be a glutton.

BEETLE JUICE
BY SUPREME UNDERSTANDING

We couldn't wrap up a chapter about "The Wrong Foods" without talking about candy. Now, I'm sure you're wondering why this article is titled "Beetle Juice" if it's about candy. Don't worry. We'll get to that in a minute. Let's start with the basics though. You're a grown-ass man or woman. Why are you still eating candy? Okay, maybe I shouldn't ask that, considering that many of us never grew up, and the rest of us are chemically-addicted to sugar. So I guess it's not a fair question. After all, I was still eating candy until I began work on this book, and I'm still having a hard time letting go of my chocolate snacks. But it's a reasonable question, and it should at least get you thinking about the nature of what you put in your system. **Indigenous people have sweets and snacks, but nothing of the "pure sugar + color" variety, like we have in the West. Instead of eating a fake, gummy version of a strawberry, we'd just eat the strawberries! Or we'd have dried fruits if we were goin for the gummy taste.** But now, you're only getting that "gummy" taste thanks to an ingredient called gelatin, which is a perfect reference point to illustrate what's wrong with most of the crap we eat.

As Marni, author of the "La Vegan Loca" blog writes:

> I am often surprised when I'm having a conversation with someone about being vegan and despite starting with lots of questions for me, we quickly get to a point where they ask me to stop telling them the truth about what they eat. When I realized what was really happening in the meat and animal byproduct industry, I was horrified. I was disgusted. I was flaming pissed. I was eating that stuff! Why didn't I know sooner? Why doesn't everyone know?

> Gelatin is a great example. Mmmm...who doesn't love jello? Harmless, wiggledy jiggledy jello. It's fun. It's colorful. Adored by kids everywhere. They even give it to you in the hospital when you are at your most vulnerable. What could be wrong with it?

> How 'bout the fact that gelatin is manufactured from the boiled hooves, bones, and skins of animals, for starters. That's just wrong. Do you think kids (or anyone for that matter) would be so excited about eating jello if they knew it was really manufactured from some demented witch's brew of slaughter house dregs? Yum! Appetizing, right? Who comes up with this stuff, anyway?

And it doesn't stop at gelatin. **Food and candy manufacturers use crushed bugs as red food coloring** (listed in the ingredients as carmine or carminic acid, but sometimes listed only as "natural color"). **They use beetle secretions in sprinkles and candies** (listed as shellac, which is also used in wood varnish). That's some real "Beetle Juice" for ya! **There's sheep secretions in bubble gum** (lanolin), **beef fat in ALL Hostess snacks, and even COAL TAR in many red-colored candies. Just so you understand, coal tar is listed as #199 on the United Nations list of "dangerous goods,"** but that doesn't stop people from using it as "Allura Red AC" in red-colored candies, sodas and other sweets. **Even pig intestines are used to make malt liquor and pig blood is used in cigarette filters, but don't think your snooty red wine is safe.** "Fining" is a process used by wineries to remove particles and impurities from wine. Fining agents include isinglass (from sturgeon bladders), gelatin (from pig bones), and ox blood. **And when grapes are gathered for wine, they're often crushed along with everything else on them, often**

including **sticks, insects, rodents, and even larger mammals.**
Wine-makers label this "ingredient" MOG, or "Material Other than
Grapes." Mmm…good old rat wine. Perhaps **the worst ingredient,
castoreum, an extract from beaver anal glands, is extensively
used in perfumes and…brace yourself…sometimes food!** And as
usual it's labeled under "natural flavors." (See the "Animal Derived
Ingredient List" for more examples and healthy alternatives.)

**The reality is not as sweet when you know the truth. Don't be
fooled by what pleases your sweet tooth.**

MADE IN CHINA

BY SUPREME UNDERSTANDING

Is there any difference between stuff made here and abroad? Possibly.
Because of lighter regulations, the difference can be quite significant
and dangerous to your health. Nowhere is this a bigger concern than
with China. **The super-cheap stuff from China, the kind you find
in every aisle of the dollar store can be downright toxic.** From
toxin-tainted candy canes to lead-painted children's toys…down to
safety recalls on infant car seats…you might be putting your family in
danger when you shop TOO cheap.

Cheap, imported food products can be just as risky. **In 2010, a
Chinese regulatory agency said 152,000 food plants and retailers
were shut down last year due to unsanitary and substandard food
being sold.** We're not talking about roaches and rats, folks. We're
talking ingredients like formaldehyde, anti-freeze, paraffin wax, and
industrial oil. We're also talking about 'recycled, expired, or already
used' food…whatever that means! US inspection records show that,
for years now, products like these were being sent back to China and
then shipped right back to the US (sometimes more than three more
times). By that time, these products are so old they can only be sold –
where else – in the hood. And guess what? **99% of imported food
doesn't even get inspected by the FDA or USDA!**

While conservatives believe this is all part of some subtle "attack on
Americans" plot from Communist China, I think it's just plain
capitalism at work. After all, **China sends us bullsh*t because some
large American company is paying…and then put it where they
put all the other crap nobody wants** – including American-made
crap – **the hoods, the barrios, and the trailer park communities.**
(See "11 Things Not To Get From The Dollar Store")

EATING RIGHT

THE IMPORTANCE OF NUTRITION
BY QUEEN GENIALLY GREEN EARTH

Nutrition is the process of nourishing or of being nourished. Nourish means to sustain with food or nutrient, to supply with what is necessary for life, health, and growth. Proper nutrition is absolutely necessary for balanced brain function; this we know by our day-to-day living, with no detailed scientific proof necessary. **We must seek to be our own chefs and our own doctors, in order to experience the highest level of physical body functionality.** There is no chef that should be able to set the standard of what is quality food for you. There is no doctor that should know your physical body better than you do.

"Let our food be our medicine and our medicine our food."

The way we live our lives shows through the way we choose, what we eat and so forth. We must choose a way of life that promotes sustaining life as well as foods that are in tune with that life sustaining culture.

If born healthy, we are templates of the UNIVERSE. We are in perfect harmony with the universe, our body itself from head to toe, inside and out, replicates the perfection of the universe over and over. **Through our cellular structure, molecular structure, and genetic DNA, we reflect the template of the universe.** As such, we are connected to the universe as a whole and receive our most vital nutrition from the universal body itself.

"By eating we become sick, by digesting we become healthy." – Old Arab Saying

Each time we consume food we are absorbing instructions. Each bite is exact instructions to the body of how it is to be used. This is our main interaction with the Earth. We must strive to consume instructions that are life promoting and life sustaining.

Ingestion/consumption, digestion, and proper elimination is the process of creating and maintaining optimal physical wealth.

Enzymes break down complex carbohydrates into simple sugars, they break down heavy fats and oils into simple fatty acids, and they break down large protein molecules apart into their constituent amino acids.

Our body contains enzymes that break down food and foods provided by nature also have enzymes that assist in the digestion process when consumed. The natural enzymes in the body interact perfectly with the natural enzymes in food provided by the Earth. **When we consume food that is not in its natural form, the vital instructions are altered and/or destroyed.** If most of our diet consists of food that is not in its natural state, we are extremely taxing our body through eating. Eating this way causes:

- mal-nutrition
- deficiencies
- toxemia
- smaller brain size
- glandular damage

- weakened immune system
- enlargement of pancreas, kidneys, liver, and heart
- disease

- poor elimination
- mental illness
- untimely death
- eventual deterioration of the entire body and mind

Like the roots of a tree drawing liquid and nutrients from the Earth our intestinal organ draws nutrients from the food we consume. All that we eat must be broken down and liquefied in order for nutrients to pass through the intestinal organ into the bloodstream.

The body contains eliminative channels that remove and relieve the body of toxic waste after digestion. Proper elimination is absolutely necessary for optimal physical health. As our body replenishes, rebuilds, and renews dead old cells and toxic waste must be released from the body. **The eliminative channels in the body are...**

Liver: Major detoxifier in the body, all waste from digestive tract goes directly to the liver. It filters blood, Regulates water levels, pH levels, mineral levels, blood pressure.

Lungs: Site of oxygen intake and carbon dioxide discharge. The lungs can be used to eliminate excessive toxins through: bad breath, sneezing, coughing, and mucous discharge.

Skin: Regulates body temperature and water levels by giving off up to one quart of fluid per day. Used to excrete excess toxins in the body that create body odors, salts, oils, blemishes, boils, sores, etc.

Lymphatic System: Involved in both the immune and elimination system and carries waste products away from cells.

Mind: Mental and emotional stress suppresses the process of the immune system, interferes with digestion, and utilizes oxygen or adversely assists in proper elimination.

Colon: Major eliminative organ, receives waste product from the digestion process, the liver, the sinuses, the throat, the lungs, and the blood and lymph systems. Has a role in water regulation in the body and some nutrient absorption, maintains friendly bacteria that provide lubrication for waste removal, produces vitamin B-12 and vitamin K, produces enzymes, and displaces harmful bacteria.

Food should be thoroughly digested before reaching the colon. Food that is not thoroughly digested in the colon can be toxic. Leading to physical blockage, unhealthy harboring of bacteria, and toxemia.

The best way to maintain optimal health is to be conscious of all the processes in the body. In being conscious of our bodily functions we learn to listen and respond. **All eliminative channels must be properly maintained to prevent toxemia and in order to maintain direct connection with the universal body/ALLAH (the most high).**

"God created the law of free will and God created the law of cause and effect. And he himself will not violate the law. We need to be thinking less in terms of what God did and more in terms of whether or not we are following those laws." – Marianne Williamson

We must choose a culture that best fits our nutritional and mental needs. Whether it centers on meat and animal by-products, Pescetarian (centering on fish, fruits, vegetables, no meat and little dairy products), vegetarian/vegan (See "What Is A Vegan?"), or a Raw Foodist/Living Foods Lifestyle, where you avoid all cooked foods, meats and animal by-products, and mainly eat raw fruits and vegetables, sprouted or soaked grains, beans, nuts, and seeds.

It's important our diet matches our standard of living and consciousness. In my own experience no one could tell me what was best for me, I had to walk myself and do the knowledge to myself along the way. The transformation is not easy, but that is why our own personal goals must be a part of the process, in order to motivate us and assist us as we travel the path to complete purification.

Develop your own culture of healthy living. Consisting of healthy eating, thinking, and actions.

THE MEAT VS. VEGETABLES TRUE-FALSE QUIZ

AN EXCERPT FROM HOW TO HUSTLE AND WIN, PT. 2

Take this quiz and see how much you know. Answers below. Don't cheat!

1	T	Millions of people get sick each year from eating
	F	contaminated meat and fish, and thousands die. For

		example, 98% of all broiler chicken carcasses have levels of E. coli bacteria that indicate fecal contamination (meaning there's sh*t in your chicken).
2	T F	Meat-eaters are more likely to have parasites, worms, and bacterial infections, some of which can survive in even well-cooked meat.
3	T F	Every product that is put into the animal's system becomes a part of the meat-eater's system, which leads to diseases, chemical imbalances, and hormonal problems, such as how girls are beginning puberty younger and younger each year.
4	T F	Well-planned vegetarian diets provide us with all the nutrients that we need, minus all the saturated fat, cholesterol, pesticides, dioxins, hormones, antibiotics, bacteria, and other contaminants found in animal flesh and by-products.
5	T F	Meat-eaters are 9 times more likely to be obese than vegans.
6	T F	Vegetarians are 50% less likely to develop heart disease than meat-eaters.
7	T F	Vegetarians have a cancer rate 60% lower than meat-eaters, even if they're smokers.
8	T F	Scientists haven't yet proven that animal fat and cholesterol cause heart disease, or that animal protein causes cancer.
9	T F	Consumption of meat, eggs, and dairy products has not been strongly linked to osteoporosis, Alzheimer's, asthma, and male impotence.
10	T F	Vegetarians have stronger immune systems than meat-eaters, which further reduces their risk of disease.
11	T F	Vegetarian children grow taller and have higher IQs than their meat-eating classmates.
12	T F	Older people who switch to a vegetarian or vegan diet cannot prevent and even reverse many chronic ailments.
13	T F	Experts agree that healthy vegetarian diets support a lifetime of good health and provide protection against numerous diseases, including our country's three biggest killers: heart disease, cancer, and strokes.
14	T F	Meat-eaters are typically stronger than vegetarians, and better fighters and athletes.
15	T F	Vegetarians and vegans live, on average, 6 to 10 years longer than meat-eaters.[18]

---

[18] All the statements are true, except numbers 8, 9, and 12.

WHAT IS A VEGAN?

BY AFYA IBOMU

AUTHOR OF THE VEGAN SOULFOOD GUIDE TO THE GALAXY

Vegetarianism has been around for thousands of years and is documented as being practiced by the ancient Egyptians and Ethiopians in Africa, Hindus in India, Buddhists in China and is even talked about in the Bible. (See "We Started This Captain Planet Thing")

> **Did You Know?**
> When someone is dealing with a serious disease, one therapy is to fast, cleanse and detoxify because your diet plays a key role in whether or not you contract diseases such as cancer, diabetes, heart disease, high blood pressure, obesity and more.

There hasn't been a 100 percent vegan society in recordable history so this concept is fairly new to human beings. **Even ancient cultures that were primarily vegan would consume in very small amounts** (less than 3 percent of their total diet) **either some fish, insects or fermented dairy products.**

Why Vegan?

Now that we have discussed what a vegan is, let's discuss why someone may want or choose to become vegan.

The leading causes of death in the U.S. are cancer, heart disease, diabetes, and obesity. Traditional soul food, poor diet, malnutrition, smoking and drinking cause the majority of these diseases. Luckily, all of these health problems can be prevented and probably cured on a healthy vegan diet. **You don't have to be a vegan to be healthy but eating a 98% balanced vegan and organic diet is optimal for good health and longevity.**

What are the Health Advantages of a Vegan Diet?

Introducing whole grains, fresh fruits and vegetable, nuts and beans will regulate and increase your energy and put less of a stress on your immune system, keeping you supplied with ample energy every day. Eliminating meat, dairy, soda, candy, sweets, poor quality oils, processed white sugar, white flour, and white rice, then incorporating whole grains, fresh fruits and vegetables, nuts, seeds and water helps your body begin its healing process. **Improvement or Total Elimination of Chronic Illnesses.** I suffered from asthma, allergies, irritable bowel syndrome and frequent colds my entire life until I became a vegan. my mom had Asthma and MS (Multiple sclerosis).

After eliminating toxins from her body through abstaining from cooked foods, consuming medicinal herbs and then adopting a healthy vegan diet, her asthma has disappeared and her MS has improved so much so that she no longer has to take MS medication

Weight Loss/Weight Maintenance. Having a healthy balanced vegan diet enables you to maintain a comfortable weight. Initially you may lose weight once you change your eating habits, primarily due to detoxification, try different foods to see what works for you and your ideal size.

Regulated and Eased Menstrual Cycle. As a woman and health counselor I can bear witness that many of my female clients' menstrual cycles have eased up. They experience milder cramps (or none at all), reduced blood flow and a reduction in PMS symptoms. **Growth hormones from dairy products attack and settle in a women's reproductive organs and may show up as fibroids, cysts and endometriosis.** Processed foods, meat and dairy can also congest your intestines causing constipation, which can worsen cramps.

Longevity and Vitality. Studies have shown that vegetarians have a lower incidence of cancer, heart disease, high blood pressure, obesity, and diabetes. This is primarily due to their food choices. The longest living people in the world have a whole food, organic, and 97 percent vegan diet (3 percent comes from seafood, insects or fermented goat or dairy products).

The Environment. By becoming a vegan or significantly reducing your meat intake, you are helping to protect the environment. The waste of land, water and energy it takes to raise, feed and produce livestock is contributing to global warming, soil destruction and water depletion (less available drinking water). At the same time, the antibiotics and growth hormone laced manure from farm animals is seeping into the earth's soils and water. This spreads toxins to us through the water we drink and seafood we eat, which destroys animals and throws off the balance of nature.

For more on how to make the switch, as well as incredible recipes to make the transition ten times easier, check out *Vegan Soulfood Guide to the Galaxy.*

If you experience any of the above symptoms, it'd be wise to consider a vegan lifestyle.

HOW TO BECOME VEGETARIAN

BY MENTAL SUN AND AIYA ABRIHET

Do Your Research

Learn as much as you can about the vegetarian/vegan diet. Study the human body and the immune system. Learn about everything you are now putting into your mouth, as well as all the foods that you're leaving behind. By taking in as much as you can on the topic, the change will become an informed and genuine one and you won't have to rely solely on willpower. **Don't simply stop eating something because someone told you not to.** Get hands-on, do the research and learn the information for yourself. Fortunately, this book should help you with most of that process, but don't stop here.

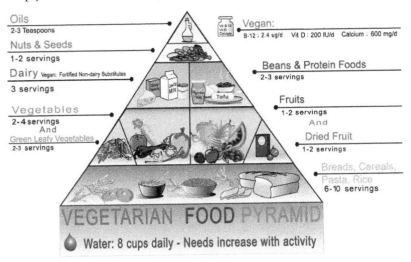

Oils
2-3 Teaspoons

Nuts & Seeds
1-2 servings

Dairy Vegan: Fortified Non-dairy Substitutes
3 servings

Vegetables
2-4 servings
And
Green Leafy Vegetables
2-3 servings

Vegan:
B-12 : 2.4 ug/d   Vit D : 200 IU/d   Calcium : 600 mg/d

Beans & Protein Foods
2-3 servings

Fruits
1-2 servings
And
Dried Fruit
1-2 servings

Breads, Cereals,
Pasta, Rice
6-10 servings

VEGETARIAN FOOD PYRAMID

Water: 8 cups daily - Needs increase with activity

Swap Out Old Choices for New Ones

Transitioning is all about getting healthier, not simply eliminating things. Many people find it easy to transition by eating vegetarian meat alternatives like vegan burgers, hot dogs, and even "chunks" for stir-fry dishes, and those may help you kick the "meat" addiction. However, don't get stuck there, and think eliminating meat is all it takes to be healthy. Remember to switch white rice, for brown rice, quinoa or black rice. Switch white bread to whole grain bread or spelt bread. And instead of white sugar, try agave nectar or maple syrup. For those transitioning away from dairy, look for a vegan product called Daiya cheese. Replace cow's milk with almond, hemp, coconut or rice milk. You can even make your own in a blender with almonds and water.

It's also important to constantly add new foods to your diet. Meat-eaters typically have very limited food choices (which makes it especially ironic when they ask vegetarians, "So what DO you eat?"). As a vegetarian, you'll need to expand your tastes. Not only should you try the cuisines of other cultures (Indian, Thai, and Ethiopian are good places to start), but you should start trying new fruits and vegetables. Add a new fruit, vegetable, or grain to your diet every week. Learn how to prepare it and work it into the new recipes you're learning. To really eat healthy, color-coding can help. Set a goal of eating 4 or 5 different colors (natural colors, not food coloring colors!) at every meal, and you'll be getting the full range of nutrition you need.

Don't Be a Starchetarian

People transitioning often make the mistake of becoming starchetarians. Make sure that you don't attempt to make up for the meat you're not eating with more bread, pasta and potatoes (or "veggie meat" made from wheat or soy). **A diet overemphasizing starch is almost as dangerous as a meat-based diet.** Replace meat with more fruits and vegetables, preferably leafy greens. Remember to be strong like the cow (or bull), don't eat the cow, eat what the cow eats (in its natural environment of course).

Make Smoothies

Get in the habit of starting your day off with a smoothie. Use lots of frozen fruits, bananas, nuts and one of the milk alternatives mentioned above. Smoothies are a great way to increase your fruit intake and because everything is blended up and easy to digest, you can get a lot of ingredients down that you probably wouldn't be able to eat whole in one sitting. Also, look into the benefits of juice fasting. (See "Living The Fast Life")

Don't Bring Junk into Your Home

If you control what comes into your kitchen and refrigerator, don't allow unhealthy food to enter your home. What often happens is people end up eating whatever they're surrounded by

Try Not to Go Hungry

It's usually when we're hungry that we'll cheat on our diet. By eating before you go out you'll avoid any temptation to stop for fast food. This is especially important before grocery shopping. (See "Spending Less to Feed More")

Eat Out

Try out local veggie spots in your neighborhood.[19] It's a great way to keep you motivated and help you get creative when it comes to preparing your own food. Research what restaurants offer vegetarian/vegan options. Call a restaurant ahead of time if necessary. Learn to analyze menus, there are always options, even if you have to get something customized for you.

Stay Strong

No matter how good you feel or how good you think you're doing, be prepared because there will always be someone there to scrutinize your actions. Usually these people mean well, but for the most part they are usually mis-informed when it comes to proper nutrition. Don't let someone who doesn't share your discipline, talk you out of doing the right thing.

Find and surround yourself with as many healthy people as you can. Join online vegetarian/vegan social networks, a great place to meet people with common interests, ask questions and look for new recipes. The greater the support system around you, the greater your chances for success.

For more ideas on how to become vegetarian, and over 1,000 of the world's best vegetarian meal and drink recipes, check out *A Taste of Life: 1,000 Vegetarian Recipes from Around the World*, available from Supreme Design Publishing.

Set yourself up for success, and you will be successful. Know what you are doing.

SUPER FOODS AVAILABLE AT THE CORNER STORE
BY SINCERE JUSTICE ALLAH

Super foods. What do you think of when you hear the word, "Super foods"? What are the kind of mental pictures that first come to mind? Are they expensive and exotic foods that only rich white folks can afford? Are they foods that you know you'll never get because you live in the hood...or because they're simply too "weird" for your tastes?

Actually, real Super foods are common and you probably have had at least a few of them in recent meals. **Super foods are simply powerful foods that are packed with nutrients that build up your resistance to disease.** They are a good investment because they literally add value to your life, rather than take away from your life.

---

[19] Check out www.happycow.net for a world-wide listing of vegetarian/vegan restaurants, health food stores and more.

Super foods include fruits, vegetables, legumes, whole grains, and seeds (which include nuts). Here are some reasons you gotta make some power moves with these power foods:

- ☐ They can strengthen your immune system
- ☐ They can keep your heart healthy
- ☐ They can build resistance against disease
- ☐ They can improve digestion
- ☐ They can provide you cancer-preventing antioxidants
- ☐ They can encourage weight loss
- ☐ They can help improve your vision, skin, muscle tone, etc.
- ☐ They can boost your energy

Let's start locally

And you don't need to buy exotic stuff that's delivered from 9,000 miles away to get these benefits. While those "trendy" super foods are cool too, some of them are being promoted because people are just trying to make money off the "next big thing." Real super foods include apples, oranges, bananas, carrots, spinach, garlic, oats, legumes tomatoes, seeds and nuts. (See "The Healing Power Of Fruits/Vegetables," "Herbs-Medicine," "A Simple Guide To Legumes," and "An Essential Guide To Grains" for detailed information.

Also, another thing to do is to always check the ingredients of the foods you eat at the corner store cause you might find some Super in 'em. For instance, I found a jar of mole sauce that contained pumpkin seeds. Pumpkin seeds are good for your prostate, lowers cholesterol, keeps your blood pressure on point and has magnesium for muscle and nerve function in your body.

Some of you may say, "I can get these same nutrients from a pill." You can do that, however, where do you think the pill manufacturers extracted the nutrients from? And which form do you think is gonna work better with your body's chemistry? Food...or a pill?

There are way too many Super foods for me to mention here, however here are some others that I recommend you to check out for yourself: Blueberries, Strawberries, Pomegranate, Avocado, Beets, Broccoli, Kale, Green Tea, Olive Oil, Sea Vegetables, Chia Seeds, Goji Berries, and the list goes on. Super foods are just one way to superb health because living without health insurance ain't a joke. It's a matter of everyday survival.

Nature has and will continue to produce the best food supply. Don't stray away from what is natural to us. Accept no substitute.

A Simple Meal Plan

BY JUSTICE RAJEE

One of the easiest ways to take control of your diet and get more bang for your buck is make a meal plan. The hard part is developing a habit of sticking to the plan. I am going to break down a simple method that you can use to get started. You will need a notepad or a couple of pieces of paper and something to write with.

☐ On your paper, create a column splitting the page in half down the middle.

☐ Draw lines across the page to create seven rows, one row for every day of the week.

☐ At the top of the page on the left, write "Meals." On the right, write "Groceries."

☐ Under each day of the week, write down three categories: Breakfast, lunch and dinner. And what you are going to eat for each meal..

☐ In the grocery list, write down what you will need to create the meals you have listed.

☐ If this sounds confusing, you can download or print a free meal plan chart at www.HoodHealthHandbook.com

☐ Place the completed chart on your fridge or a kitchen cabinet so you can see it clearly.

The first step in changing behavior is creating a means to hold yourself accountable to the new standard. Writing This down allows you to remember what you promised yourself you would do. **By changing what you eat into something you plan instead of something that's an impulse, you'll become motivated by your choices.**

When you go shopping with a list and menu, you are less likely to come back with items you did not plan to purchase. Stores are designed to get you buy things you never wanted. The layout, coupons, signs, and even the lighting are all focused on getting you to think with your stomach. When you have a counter to the emotional cues found in the store, you have a better chance of limiting your spending to just what you need. This is also why you include days you intend to eat out. Eating out in our world of fast food dollar menus and cheap processed snacks can quietly lead to far more spending than you may notice. Creating a plan and sticking to it will give you a leg up in changing your eating culture.

When you have a plan and you condition yourself to follow your plan, you get a better hold of what you're eating, how much you are spending, and how fast you go through those items. (See "Spending Less To Feed More").With a greater understanding of your eating habits you will be able to make comfortable and sustainable adjustments to meet your ultimate diet goals.

There are far more complex meal planning methods you can use, from Excel spreadsheets to detailed food logs – you name it (you can find many examples online).

Whatever you do, start out simple and work your plan.

WHEN ALL ELSE FAILS: HEALTHY FAST FOOD?
BY SUPREME UNDERSTANDING

We understand that it's unlikely you'll cook EVERY meal at home, and will eventually have to eat out at some point. This can be a daunting task for vegetarians. In many cities, vegetarians have the option of dining at a number of exclusively vegetarian restaurants or establishments that are especially vegetarian-friendly. **To find out what's in your city, we suggest the online guide to vegan, vegetarian, and veg-friendly establishments at www.happycow.com.** You may even find a few that only serve raw and living foods. **But what about when your budget or time constraints make those options unlikely? Or what about when you're brought along on a lunch or dinner date to a place you'd never expect to find healthy food?** We understand those concerns, so we've created the following guide to vegetarian dining at non-vegetarian food franchises.

Before we begin, there are a few things you should be mindful of at ANY place where you eat:

☐ Is this place clean? Does it have a good rating from the Health department? (See "Food Poisoning")

☐ Do they cook meatless items separately? Or is everything cooked on the same grill (or in the same wok) and cut with the same knives? Do they clean the grill or wok for meatless dishes? Is this enough for me?

☐ Does the server appear knowledgeable about which items contain animal products? Do I need to consult a manager? Does the manager need to call their manager?

☐ Finally, can I replace the meat in an entrée with extra vegetables? And are meals discounted when meat is eliminated? For example, Burger King charges less for a Veggie Whopper (a Whopper without the beef patty), but McDonald's charges the same price for a burger with or without the meat! T.G.I.Fridays normally takes $2-3 off entrees without meat, but Johnny Carino's charges full price.

With that said, the following information should help you make an informed choice when eating out.

Burger Joints

There are several popular establishments where you can now order veggie burgers. These include: Backyard Burgers, Bennigan's, Burger King, Cheeburger Cheeburger, Cheers, Claim Jumper, Coco's, Denny's, 5 and Diner, Flamer's Grill, Hard Rock Café, Hard Times Café, Harvey's, Houston's, John Harvard's, Johnny Rockets, Kelsey's, Mimi's Café, Pyramid Brewery, Rainforest Café, Ruby Tuesdays, Shari's, and Village Inn franchises. Many of these restaurants also offer side items such as cooked vegetables, in additional to the traditional carb-heavy French fries.

Bagel/Bread/Breakfast Shops

Most restaurants catering to breakfast food, whether it's bagels or pancakes, have a decent selection of items fit for vegetarians. Again, be aware of how and where these items are prepared. At places like Einstein Bros. and Manhattan Bagels, nearly all the bagels are vegan, except for the cheese and egg varieties. At some shops, like Einstein Bros., hummus is offered as a healthy (and tasty) alternative to cream cheese. At Manhattan Bagels, the Manhattan Grille and Vegetable Garden sandwiches can be made on a bagel, a roll, or a tortilla, and are vegan if you omit the spreads and cheese. Panera Bread has a wide selection of soups and sandwiches, but many of their soups are made with a chicken stock, and our readers have reported difficulty with getting straight answers from the people who work there. Be careful about uninformed workers! Just because the big girl with the gold tooth told you its "vegetarian" doesn't mean there's not chunks of chicken waiting for you to discover (many people don't think chicken or fish, or animal byproducts, are the same as "meat")

IHOP and Waffle House are gradually becoming more mindful of the needs of vegetarians, but you should still ask if your eggs and hash browns will be cooked on the same grill as items prepared with meat. Denny's vegan foods include oatmeal, English muffins, bagels, grits, applesauce, fresh fruit, vegetable plates, seasoned French fries, baked potatoes with several vegetable toppings, garden salads with light Italian or oil-and-vinegar dressing, and sandwiches that can be made with several vegetable options.

East Asian Restaurants

Asian restaurants, like the continent of Asia itself, are not homogenous in any way. In spite of the great diversity between, for example, Thai eateries and Japanese Steak and Sushi joints, there are some things to look for wherever you go. For beginners, many East Asian cultures are familiar with sects of Buddhism that avoid eating meat entirely, or at least for particular periods of time. Thus, most servers will understand your request for vegetarian food. However, with Japanese food, you should also be clear that you are not interested in katso bushi, or the fish stock/powder that makes it into a great deal of their otherwise "vegetarian" dishes. Out of the East Asian countries, Vietnamese and Mongolian cuisine rely heaviest on meat dishes, and are thus least likely to have cookware set aside for vegetarian fare. Chinese restaurants may offer more tofu (sometimes called bean curd) and vegetable dishes, but depending on the size and quality of the restaurant, your food may be cooked in the same wok as the meat dishes. If you're at a place called "Mr. China King, home of the $2 Lunch Special," I would think twice before ordering. Finally, Thai food is often one of your best bets for good vegetarian food, as Thailand has a long-standing vegetarian (Buddhist) tradition that is recognized everywhere in the country. This is reflected in Thai restaurants, nearly all of which offer some sort of "tofu curry" dish.

Ethiopian Restaurants

Most Ethiopian restaurants offer vegetarian entrees like Allicha Kik and Meser Wot, wonderfully seasoned lentil or vegetable dishes that are sopped up in the traditional Injera flatbread.

Greek/Middle Eastern Food

There's much more at these places than lamb gyros. Most of the side items, like the tabbouleh, baba ghanoush, hummus, cous cous, and stuffed grape leaves, are vegetarian (and in most cases vegan). You can assemble a full meal from these items or order a falafel wrap (or veggie wrap) as your entrée.

Indian Restaurants

With a population of nearly 1 billion, and recognized by many as its own "subcontinent," India is also home to great diversity in both culture and cuisine. For beginners, North Indian cuisine is much more reliant on meat than South Indian cuisine, and Hindu-owned eateries are more mindful of vegetarians than their Muslim-owned counterparts. With this in mind, it's still good to know that most servers will understand your request for a meatless dish, and nearly all Indian restaurants will have something to satisfy you.

Jamaican/Caribbean Restaurants

Because of Rastafarian influence on the cuisine and culture of many Caribbean islands, one can usually find some vegetarian items at any Caribbean restaurant. While some only offer baked patties filled with spinach, callaloo (a plant similar to collard greens), broccoli, or mixed vegetables, others offer entrees based around curry tofu and the like.

With vegetable sides however, it is best to ask what kind of stock they've been cooked in. In fact, if you're not at the type of place that serves tofu, it's best to ask about the status of any item, especially if you're vegan. One of the few Caribbean food franchises, Pollo Tropical, offers several vegan options such as the Vegetarian TropiChop entrée, the Balsamic Tomatoes and Bananas Tropical. The chain's black beans, French fries, white rice, yellow rice, boiled yucca, and corn are vegan too.

Mexican Restaurants

Many Mexican restaurants can substitute beans for meat on their items, but it is important to know what the beans and tortillas were cooked with, because in more traditional restaurants, it may have been lard. This is less common in franchises, particularly those restaurants that serve somewhat Americanized versions of Mexican fare. Many such franchises, Chili's for example, offer vegetable quesadillas, burritos, and fajitas on their menu. Others, like Moe's or Willie's Mexicana Grill, offer tofu as a meat substitute. Chipotle offers a vegetarian fajita burrito, but be sure to order it with black beans—the pinto beans are cooked with bacon. Finally, Taco Bell may not seem like a healthy choice for a vegetarian, but they now offer the opportunity to make any item "vegetarian" simply be requesting it as such. They will then replace any meat in the item with refried beans, which – like everything else at Taco Bell – is now cooked without lard.

Pizza Places/Italian Restaurants

Though it isn't the healthiest option, cheese pizza is a common resort for new vegetarians. Enjoying pizza can be a little more complicated if you are vegan. However, both the pizza sauce and dough at Chuck E. Cheese, Little Caesars, and Papa John's are vegan. Pizza Hut uses vegan sauce, and only its Thin 'n Crispy and dessert crusts are vegan. Thus, by omitting the cheese and choosing your favorite vegetable toppings, you can easily make a delicious vegan pizza. With Cici's you should ask about the vegan status of each item on your pizza, but they also offer a pasta-and-salad buffet with many vegan options. Regarding Italian restaurants in general, it's usually pretty easy to order a vegetarian meal featuring pasta, vegetables, and sauce (just make sure the sauce is meatless). Ordering vegan requires that the noodles aren't made with egg and the sauce isn't made with dairy, but a knowledgeable server should be able to assist you. A number of popular Italian-based franchises are vegetarian-friendly. Macaroni Grill has several vegetarian options, including all the pastas with garlic and oil (vegan), the Capellini Pomodoro (vegan), and many options including dairy, such as the Tomato Bruschetta and Penne Arrabbiata.

Vegans can ask for these dishes without cheese.

As a side note, pizza (and most pastas) are actually not traditional Italian innovations, but are actually "borrowed" from China.

Sub/Sandwich Shops

Vegetarian subs, sandwiches, and wraps are available nearly everywhere nowadays, including: Blimpie, Cousin's Subs, Firehouse Subs, Jason's Deli, Jersey Mike's Subs, Quizno's Subs, Roly Poly, Subway, and World Wraps. You can also make a vegetarian subway sandwich "meatier" by purchasing vegetarian "lunchmeat" and putting a few slices into your sandwich. In fact, most supermarkets with a deli counter can prepare a vegetarian sandwich, and a trip to the nearby health food aisle should provide you with the "meat" to put inside. For people trying to avoid "fake meat," extra mushrooms can also provide the substance and texture of a traditional sandwich or sub. Keep in mind that it's typically the sauce that gives the sandwich its flavor. With this in mind, however, also remember that "vegetarian" doesn't always mean "vegan" and many sauces contain dairy products.

Miscellaneous Fast Food

At Arby's, vegans can have the hash browns, baked potato, garden salad or side salad with Italian dressing, and an apple or cherry turnover. Burger King has the BK Veggie (which you can have "your way" – that is, with mushrooms, Buffalo sauce, etc.). Just ask how it is prepared. Some places run it through an oven, others microwave it, and a few others fry it with the meat! You can also order a Veggie Whopper, which is a Whopper minus the meat, for about $1.49 at most places. At Carl's Jr., the french fries, hash-brown nuggets, breadsticks, English muffins, and CrissCuts are all vegan. In the restaurant, there is an all-you-can-eat salad bar that offers a variety of fresh vegetables and a three-bean salad. They also offer baked potatoes, which can be ordered with all-vegetable margarine.

McDonald's, as you know, secretly used beef powder and beef fat on their French fries for years, until vegetarians complained. So they stopped, but the fries weren't as "flavorful" (meaning addictive), so they secretly snuck beef powder back in until a vegetarian association launched a huge lawsuit against them. Now they've stopped, but considering their corporate practices throughout the world, as well as the chemicals in their food, they're hard to recommend for anybody trying to eat healthy or vegetarian. **In fact, McDonald's website now says that NONE of their items can be guaranteed 100% free of animal ingredients.** You can learn a lot more about McDonald's elsewhere in this book.

Years back, Taco Bell also sold a Vegetarian Fajita that was made with clam and oyster sauce. However, since then, Taco Bell has made a significant transition in meeting the needs of vegetarians. **You can now order any item at Taco Bell "vegetarian," which, as said earlier, simply involves them replacing the meat on an item with vegan refried beans.** At Wendy's, vegans can have the plain baked potato, the Deluxe Garden Salad with red Italian dressing and no cheese, or French fries. You can also ask for a veggie sandwich, which is pretty much the same as Burger King's Veggie Whopper.

To reiterate my first point however, being healthy is not JUST about "avoiding meat." You can avoid meat and still eat at Mickey D's every day and damn near die like dude on *SuperSize Me*, except you'll be experiencing the vegan version of fast food death. So think of fast food as a last resort. This guide is here to help you make the best of that last resort.

There IS another alternative, however. According to Dr. Joe Esposito:

> Yes, healthy fast food does exist...and not only fast food, but "traveling fare" is also at your fingertips...There is the obvious, (or maybe not so obvious), healthy choices such as fruit bars and trial mix. These are usually my first choices, they are inexpensive, don't need to be refrigerated and will help keep you healthy while under the stress of traveling...Sesame sticks made with wheat or spelt are always a hit. Dried pineapple or dried papaya are high in digestive enzymes and will satisfy your sweet tooth. Dried ginger has been shown to help with motion sickness, is great for circulation, and has been claimed to be an aphrodisiac (so be careful with this one!) What if you want something a bit more exotic and more like a meal? Dried, packaged hummus is a great choice. Just add water and you have hummus! How about dried, packaged tabouli? Again, just add water and eat them as they are or put them on a baked chip or baked cracker. If you don't mind your "traditionally hot foods" a little on the cool side, how about dried refried beans... just add water. A can of room temperature baked beans, no meat chili, soups, rice and beans or even a can of organic veggies are good choices. If you are going camping or on an overnight trip and you want a "traditional" breakfast, bring along powdered soy milk and dry, healthy, organic cereal or granola, add water to the powdered soy milk and enjoy your All American breakfast of cereal and milk. These ideas are quick, light weight, healthy and will save you a bundle on restaurant bills. Not to mention the convenience of having your choice of quality food where you want it and when you want it.

Carefully observe WHERE you're eating and you'll make a better choice about WHAT you're eating.

WHERE TO COP THAT GOOD HERB

INNER CITY RESOURCES FOR HERBS, ROOTS, AND
NATURAL SUPPLEMENTS

BY C'BS ALIFE ALLAH

After you had some bad side effects from some over the counter medicines you pledged to get back to nature. You're ready yet, live in the hood. There is no forest of herbs in your hood. There are no hippie-ran holistic food stores on your block. So where in the hell do you get these herbs if you've made a personal commitment to take it back to a more natural way of dealing with your health? You might not have a Whole Foods Store or Trader Joe's around you yet I bet you that you have one of these spaces right near you.

Botanica: I know, at first you have images of Santeria, Voodoo, and other things spring up in your mind. The first thing that you need to do is get those white Hollywood images out of your mental. **These are just African religions that have been transplanted to the New World and given a bad rep by your former slave master.** Most people identify botanicas only with the religions. The reality is that they are also an herb shop. You can find a whole bunch of dried and fresh herbs at any botanica. Don't think that they only sale things that are about the religions or magic.

Rasta Spot: You know the spot. The spot where you go to buy black soap, incense and reggae music. **The Rastafarian I-tal lifestyle promotes a back to nature approach.** Nine times out of ten this spot will carry a host of herbs that will benefit you. It's an extra bonus because a lot of them are herbs that aren't found stateside.

Chinese Emporium: If you're on the west coast you're familiar with the Chinese Emporium. If you have huge Chinese communities near you there's one. Most big cities have some type of Chinese or Asian Emporium near them. Ethnic groups within the United States ALWAYS have a place where they can buy their own foods. These places have a huge selection of herbs and natural items. **You may need to ask a lot of questions regarding translations because everything will NOT be in English.**

Latin Market: Trust me. You have a Latin/Spanish market somewhere near you. That's because you know of a barrio near you. Whether you are on the East coast with the high Puerto Rican/Dominican/Cuban population or on the West coast with the high Mexican population. These spots have what you're looking for. Get up in there.

Desi-Mart: If you have a whole bunch of Indian restaurants near you then you have one of these spots. If you live near an Indian/Pakistani population you definitely have one. I live in New Haven, CT and there are like seven of them. A few of them are in the cut so you might not notice at first.

Grow yourself: If you have any plot of land around your dwelling you can just grow your own herbs. It's not hard. **Even if you don't have any land you can grow many herbs inside your house.** Some of the easiest to grow in small pots inside are mint, rosemary, bay leaf, savory, oregano, chervil, and thyme. Experiment and try for yourself. Don't just take my word on it.

Not only can you pick up a new language, but visiting these spots will make you well cultured, and with the right herbs, healthy.

FOOD COMBINING
IT AIN'T JUST WHAT YOU EAT, BUT HOW YOU EAT IT!
BY JAMIL SULEMAN

Studies have shown that the more you chew, the easier it is for your body to absorb nutrients and actually use it for energy (remember, that was the point of eating in the first place).

So let's take a staple American dish... meat and potatoes. **Turns out that carbohydrates in complex carbs or starches** (like wheat, bread, rice and potatoes) **take different enzymes to digest than meat, and the interaction of both can cause some serious mal-absorption problems.** Usually, this means a backup in the system, resulting in an overpopulation of inflammatory bacteria that stick around and tear up your gut. **You may not feel it completely, but your body does, and over time it will show with various dis-eases and cancers.**

It's best to eat your meat with vegetables, and a lot of them at that. This will provide the necessary fiber to help the meat pass through the digestive track and allow for nutrients to actually be absorbed for energy. **That means you can't just jump to dessert right after dinner. Give it a minute, preferably an hour or so.** Here are some simple guidelines to think about next time you sit down to enjoy dinner with your friends and family:

Remember to always chew your food (turns out Mom was right about that one). Chew your food at least seven times and take in the flavor before you swallow. This helps digestion and keeps you from overeating.

Sit down and relax with a few deep breaths before you eat. This will relax your digestive track, making it easier to handle the food.

Avoid drinking while you are eating. If you have to drink something, take half a glass of water, but try and drink less during the meal. This allows the enzymes to thoroughly assimilate the food before being washed out.

Don't eat your proteins with carbohydrates. That means chicken and rice is gone, burgers, sandwiches… pretty much a lot of food you eat at the same time. Hey, I never said it was easy did I? Don't worry, the more you eat consciously, the less you'll crave those foods over time.

Eat fruits by themselves. Fruits contain a lot of sugar, and are quickly digested. When you mix that with heavy cream or sugary carbs (cake, I'm looking at you right now), the result is hard times for the gut. Feel free to mix different fruits, but try and keep them separate. And try eating fruits before the big meal instead of after (otherwise they'll sit on top of the longer-to-digest food and ferment and bubble up)

Avoid dairy products. Drinking milk from any other source, especially as an adult, is unnatural. Cheeses and yogurt tend to be less harmful, but try and cut down on the dairy. (See "Get Off The Cow Titty")

Give yourself a couple hours between meals and snacks, and try to limit the variety of foods you eat to 2-3 in one sitting. **Tibetan monks usually eat one type of food per meal, and needless to say, they tend to be pretty healthy.** At the very least, don't just mash down on everything at the buffet. **And give yourself time to digest, particularly when it comes to your last meal for the day, which shouldn't be at 11 pm.** Night-time is when your body should get a break to slow down its metabolism.

Listen to your body. This is sound advice, whether it's about eating food or self-healing a dis-ease state. Your body has intuitive wisdom that your conditioned mind may ignore. Try to tap into the feeling of your body while you eat or even when you are deciding what to eat at the grocery store. You might be surprised by what you hear.

Enjoy your food! Research has shown that people who enjoy what they eat, savor the taste, and appreciate their meals live longer and end up choosing healthier foods naturally. Take a moment to be thankful for your meal, and spread the wealth when you got the chance.

Follow these guidelines for improving digestion.

Juice Ain't Supposed to be Blue

by C'BS Alife Allah

When we were young we use to switch the bottles of spray-on insect repellent with sugar water so our friends would be attacked by a swarm of mosquitoes during the hot summer months. Not too long ago, children at a pre-school were fed car coolant as a fruit drink. (Fortunately they just got sick and recovered) The reason? Because most adults nowadays grew up on 'fruit drink' that is just colored, sugary, syrupy, water. The current generation wouldn't know what real fruit juice looks like... sad to say.

Fruit Punch ain't Juice

One of the main problems with sodas is that they are saturated in sugar and sugar substitutes. Unfortunately bottled water and fruit punch nowadays ain't that much better. Read the ingredients on your bottled beverages. **Many bottled waters (like Vitamin Water and Snapple Agave Melon Antioxidant Water) have up to 8 teaspoons of sugar in each bottle!** If you are drinking water, common sense tells us that the only ingredient should be water. And if it is supposed to have other 'herbs' in it, then alongside those herbs there shouldn't be a bunch of sugar. **A lot of the bottled teas and juices have levels of sugar that surpass any soda out there.** A great book that outlines how drinks line up against each other is *Drink This Not That! The No-Diet Weight Loss Solution* by David Zinczenco.

Juice Ain't Supposed to be Blue

Look at the 'flavors' listed for your "fruit punch." First off, the fruit punch is always red. So much that children (and adults) just refer to it as "RED flavored." **But check the 'fruit flavors' listed, (usually it's apples, pineapples, oranges, etc) It's a whole bunch of fruit that won't turn any juice red!** Make your own fruit punch and you tell me what color it ends up being. Try not to drink those punches, period. If the color is so thick you can't see through them, it ain't good for you. Try the straight 100% juices or the 100% mixes that are clear, like apple juices or apple/cranberry, apple/raspberry, etc. They are closer to the root. And what's up with blue juice? The only juice made from nature that would be close to a 'blue' would be pure blueberry juice, and that would be closer to purple than blue.

Recommendations

☐ When you're ready to upgrade from a blender, purchase a juicer. There are plenty of models available, and many are very affordable now. The Champion brand juicer is more expensive but does a better job, and is very easy to use and easy to clean.

- ❑ Try to avoid mixing vegetables and fruits in the same juice on a regular basis. (See "Food Combining")
- ❑ Try to do more vegetable juice mixtures than fruit juices.
- ❑ Develop a habit from the beginning of diluting all juices with 50% juice and 50% spring water. It will be difficult to get used to at first, but after a while undiluted juice will seem much too strong.
- ❑ If you buy juice from a grocery store, look for juice that is: (A) juice and nothing but juice (look for 100% on the front, but still check the ingredients in the back); (B) unfiltered; (C) organic; (D) uses filtered water.
- ❑ Apple cider is also good. Look for it without any sweeteners or preservatives.

Make sure you get the pure thing or as close as possible to it.

MADE FROM THE BEST STUFF ON EARTH?
BY SUPREME UNDERSTANDING

Snapple might have a clever marketing campaign, but it's definitely not REALLY "made from the best stuff on Earth." In fact, that's why they were hit with a lawsuit that argued Snapple shouldn't label itself "natural" since it is sweetened with High Fructose Corn Syrup, which is not found anywhere in nature. Not to mention that their juices aren't necessarily "juices," but just "flavors." For example, their acai blackberry juice drink, which contains neither acai nor blackberry juice.

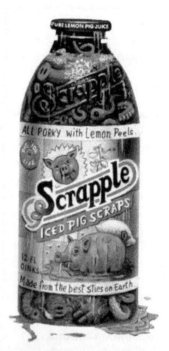

What Are the Healthiest Drinks?

You mean, besides water? After all, water is really the only "drink" the human body actually needs. Everything else is extras. Fortunately, some of it is good for you. Contrary to popular belief, Snapple is NOT made from the best stuff on Earth, so it's not on the list. This list is mostly fruit juices, but vegetable juices can be incredibly healthy as well. Only thing is, you'd be hard pressed to find any juice made JUST from vegetables (except maybe carrot juice) in your supermarket. You CAN, however, find healthy juices and smoothies made by brands like Odwalla,

Arden's Garden, and Naked. These are usually made from a mix of fruits and vegetables, with no "added ingredients" (like sugar). Even better (and often cheaper), you can buy the fruits and vegetables yourself and make your own drinks with a juicer or blender. It's actually very easy. The hardest part is actually cleaning that damn blender. Anyway, here's the top 9 healthiest drinks, according to our research:

9. Apple Juice: Apples contain a variety of essential nutrients and vitamins that may help protect the body from certain illnesses, including the common cold. Some scientific research shows that apple juice may help improve brain function, protect the heart, and inhibit various types of cancer.

8. Tea: Whether black, green, white, or South African Rooibos, as long as it comes from tea leaves, it's probably good for you. Green tea may reduce the risks of heart attack, atherosclerosis and memory loss. White tea may offer some protection against colon cancer. Both green and black teas may help prevent diabetes and its ensuing complications, including cataracts.

7. Orange Juice: As you know, it's all about Vitamin C here. OJ neutralizes harmful elements within the body, reduces iron deficiency, and strengthens your immune system. Not to be confused with OJ Simpson or OJ da Juice Man, who don't really do much of anything useful.

6. Cranberry Juice: Cranberries or Cranberry Juice are high in antioxidants and vitamin C. Cranberry tannins have anti-clotting properties. Cranberries, or cranberry juice, are recommended by medical professionals to help reduce urinary tract infections as well as potentially being effective against dental plaque-causing oral bacteria. Cranberries also have many of the health benefits identified below with blueberries.

5. Açaí Juice: Açaí is naturally rich in Omega fats, amino acids, electrolytes, antioxidants, protein; as well as vitamins A, B1 and E. Açaí berries/ juice are used in holistic treatment regiments for various health concerns, including digestive problems, skin irritation and insomnia.

4. Black Cherry Juice: Not only is this juice high in antioxidants, but there is evidence that black cherry juice can help with exercise-induced muscle injuries, gout and and other forms of arthritis. Cherries or cherry juice may also significantly reduce your risk for colon cancer.

3. Blueberry Juice: Blueberries have notably high levels of the essential dietary mineral manganese, vitamin B6, vitamin C, vitamin K and dietary fiber. Blueberries also have the potential to limit the development and severity of certain cancers and vascular diseases, such as atherosclerosis, ischemic stroke and neurodegenerative diseases of aging. This stuff is pretty expensive to buy, but you can always get some blueberries, cherries and a blender and make a hell of a smoothie.

2. Concord Grape Juice: Concord grape juice is a valuable source of potent antioxidants that are heart-protective and may help reduce blood pressure.

1. Pomegranate Juice: This is number one for a reason. At least 47 scientific studies have addressed the benefits of 100% Pomegranate juice on human health, including everything from prostate and cardiovascular health to erectile dysfunction. Pomegranate juice is available in most supermarkets near the produce section.

What about Red Wine?

Sure, studies have found that moderate alcohol consumption can reduce coronary heart disease risk, but malt liquor and Jack Daniels will do you more harm than good. It's red wine that can help your heart the most, as well as inhibit tumor development in some cancers. Red wine is high in antioxidants and anthocyanins, which are powerful pigments that help prevent cancer, heart disease, aging, diabetes, inflammation, and other degenerative diseases. **Researchers found that the best wines – those with the highest amount of flavonoids – were Cabernet Sauvignon, followed by Petit Syrah and Pinot Noir, followed by Merlots and Red Zinfandels, followed by white wines.** The general rule is that the sweeter the wine, the lower the levels of flavonoids and the less healthy it is for you. However, not everyone agrees that wine is good for you. As Dr. Fuhrman has written:

> Alcohol is not actually heart-healthy; it simply has anti-clotting effects, much like aspirin. Researchers have found that even moderate consumption of alcohol, including wine, interferes with blood clotting and thereby reduces heart attacks in high-risk populations, such as people who eat the typical, disease-promoting American diet. Thinning the blood with alcohol or aspirin is not life-span enhancing unless you are eating the typical heart-attack inducing diet. Once you are protected from heart attacks and strokes with nutritional excellence, the blood thinning only adds to more risk your life, in the form of gastrointestinal bleeding or a hemorrhagic stroke. Moderate drinking is defined as a maximum of one drink per day for women and two drinks for men. Consuming more than this is associated with increased fat around the waist and other significant health problems.

Even a moderate amount of alcohol may also increase the risk of breast cancer in susceptible women.

So, if you're not interested in drinking, you should know that 100% purple grape juice and non-alcoholic red wines (as well as grapes, raisins, and just about any fruits with dark red or purple skins) provide the same benefits.

Reach for one of these options instead of a soda or "fruit" punch. Better yet, try the fresh fruit.

DRINK TO YOUR HEALTH
BY WALASIA SHABAZZ

Whether starting/ending a fast, or supplementing your meals, there are plenty of simple & healthy beverages to be made at home with everyday ingredients.

Water
Try adding fresh mint to your pitcher of water, or slices of citrus – lemon, lime, orange or a combination of all three, or cucumber slices & fresh basil. These "tonics" have little or no calories, no added sugars, and will boost the taste for those who find water boring to drink. (See "The Fuel Of Life")

Juicing
Most juicers come with some recipes, but here are a few combinations to set your juices off right. Fresh is best, but in winter months or cities where fresh fruit is not abundant, break out your blender & use some of the fruits from your frozen fruit aisle (make sure no sugar has been added to the package!) Tasty combinations include:

- ❑ Orange-Carrot
- ❑ Watermelon-Lime
- ❑ Pineapple-Ginger
- ❑ Orange-Mango-Peach
- ❑ Strawberry-Banana-Apple
- ❑ Blackberry-Blueberry-Cherry

4 Roads Trini Peanut Punch
28 oz of chilled soy or almond milk

¾ cup of smooth peanut butter
Turbinado (raw) sugar to taste

Blend until peanut butter is evenly distributed. For a spicy punch add a dash of ground nutmeg, cinnamon, allspice and/or ground ginger.

Rich Vegan Horchata
1/3 cups long grain Brown rice such as Basmati

½ cup plus 2 tablespoons blanched almonds

A 3-inch piece of cinnamon stick

1 ¼ cups hot water

½ cup turbinado sugar, plus more to taste
1 cup cold vanilla or plain almond milk
Dash of Mexican or Tahitian Vanilla extract

In a large bowl, combine the rice, almonds, cinnamon stick and water. Cool, cover and refrigerate overnight. Pour into a blender, add sugar and blend on high for several minutes, until the mixture is as smooth as possible. Strain through a sieve or colander lined with cheesecloth, pressing on the mixture until only a dry pulp remains. Pour into a pitcher then add the almond milk. You may add more sweetener or vanilla to taste, if needed. Serve "on the rocks" or chilled.

Irish Moss

This is a specialty of the Caribbean (especially Jamaica), so if you want to make it yourself, you may have to visit a Caribbean grocery or order the Moss online from an importer. Irish Moss is said to increase the virility and stamina of men.

½ lb Irish Moss	2 tbsp. Vanilla Extract
½ cup Hemp Oil	½ teaspoon Nutmeg
1 can. Coconut Milk	4 quarts Water
2/3 lb Turbinado Sugar	

Wash the moss in the sink to remove sand or foreign matter. Bring water to a boil and then add moss and hemp oil. Let the ingredients simmer at a low temp for about an hour. Strain the liquid into another container and separate the boiled Irish moss from the drink, discard. Add the rest of the ingredients to the mix then allow it to chill in the fridge for at least four hours.

Note: Because the thickness of the drink may vary, you may have to dilute this mixture with more water to suit your liking. Some flavor the drink with peanut butter, strawberry nectar or ground nuts such as cashews. Don't be afraid to experiment!

Sorrel (Jamaica)

Brewed from the dried blossoms of red Hibiscus, Jamaica (pronounced Haa-My-Kuh) is a deliciously tart beverage enjoyed in many countries. Mexicans and other Spanish speakers call it Jamaica, while in Jamaica and other Caribbean cultures, it's called Sorrel. The drink was popular in ancient Egypt, even among the Pharaohs. Today in Egypt and Sudan, the drink is called Karkade and is used to toast at weddings. In Senegal it's called Bissap and is the national beverage. Sorrel or Jamaica is sold in "Hispanic" markets either in bulk or with the packaged spices, or in bulk at Caribbean shops.

1 pound sorrel	2 quarts water
2-4 oz. fresh ginger, peeled and grated	Turbinado sugar to taste
	8 allspice grains

Wash sorrel thoroughly, using the fingers to lift it from the water so any sediment falls to the bottom. Put into stainless steel container. Scrape the ginger then grate it and add to the sorrel along with the allspice grains. Boil water and pour over sorrel mixture. Allow to sit 4-6 hours. Strain it & discard the sorrel, then sweeten to taste and serve over ice.

Ginger "Beer"

Made popular in the states by the brand "Reeds" ginger beer which is a sparkling Ginger soda sweetened with Pineapple, the original Ginger Beer or Ginger Brew of the islands is a 'flat' beverage but can be mixed with sparkling water to recreate the soda-style if you like.

| 8 tablespoons of Turbinado sugar | 2 ½ quarts water |
| 1 pound fresh ginger | |

Puree ginger and water in blender. Let it sit for a day. Add sugar to your taste, mix thoroughly then serve over ice.

Coconut Water

If you've ever seen the green coconut (still covered with its husk) or "young coconut" in the store & wondered what it was & how to use it, the water inside is fragrant & healthful. Using a large, sharp knife, cleaver or machete, the top of the coconut is hacked off, water poured into the blender, shell cracked in half, inside "jelly" scraped out with a spoon then blended with the water for a unique and delicious treat. The coconut water is cooling, easily digestible, cleanses the urinary tract & bladder, rehydrating, rich in mineral salts and is said to improve mental concentration. Coconut water can be blended with almond or rice milk and honey to relieve fatigue, nervousness, constipation, male sterility, or to protect against osteoporosis. When the water is mixed with lemon juice only, it can prevent nausea or vomiting, loss of appetite, and even eradicate gastrointestinal worms.

Herbs/Teas

There are a few herbal remedies every household should have on hand for everyday health troubles. Avoiding aspirin, acetaminophen, products such as Pepto-Bismol etc. will increase your overall health – and there are natural ways to prevent or alleviate the symptoms you'd normally take an over the counter substance to treat. Most of these ingredients can be found at your health-food grocery store or you can certainly order the dry herbs online.

Ginger Root (fresh). Prepare with hot water (peel it first) and take as a tea for stomach trouble, nausea, sore throats, flu symptoms & colds. Can be taken with garlic for really tough colds/flu symptoms.

Parsley (fresh). Can be brewed like a tea for muscle relaxation.

Raspberry Leaf (dry). Great for pain relief.

Plantain Leaf (dry). Cleanses the urinary tract & bladder for men and women who experience bladder infections or painful urination. (If symptoms persist for this, see a doctor right away!)

Passion Flower (dry). Relaxes the body & helps alleviate insomnia.

Valerian Root (dry). Another sleep aid of the natural kind.

Chamomile (dry). Helps ease stomach ailments, in large quantities it is a sleep aid.

For more ideas, and over 1,000 of the world's best vegetarian meal and drink recipes, check out *A Taste of Life: 1,000 Vegetarian Recipes from Around the World,* **available from Supreme Design Publishing.**

Know that you have choices. It's bigger than just water, fruit and vegetable juices.

RED BALLS...ANY BETTER THAN BLUE BALLS?
GOING FROM ENERGY DRINKS TO HEALTHY DRINKS
BY C'BS ALIFE ALLAH

Did you know that so-called energy drinks like Red Bull can cause sexual dysfunction in men? Right. Red Bull can cause Blue Balls! The high caffeine content works against the muscle relaxation needed for a healthy erection. Viagra does the opposite, causing the smooth muscle cells in a man's reproductive tract to relax to allow the needed blood flow.

Energy drinks are a billion dollar business, making 6.9 billion dollars in 2009 alone. Of course, the biggest winners were popular brands like Red Bull and Monster, but nowadays there are more new energy drink companies than there are stores to put them in. You even have Black-owned energy drinks like Lil Jon's Krunk Juice, Nelly's Pimpjuice, and Pitbull Energy Drink. **But are they safe? Not if you ask Cheryl James, a Florida mom whose teenage son, Drew, died after drinking an energy drink with a ridiculously high amount of caffeine.** They don't say which drink it was, but it could've been one of the new brands, like Cocaine, which has three and a half times more caffeine than Red Bull. **In her county, poison center reports of adverse reactions to energy drinks have gone up more than 400%**

in one year. The medical examiner determined that Drew died of a cardiac arrhythmia due to ischemic cardiomyopathy, which is rare for 19-year-olds. She later told Cheryl, "taking into consideration the amount of caffeine he consumed, I would say caffeine played a large part in your son's death."

More recently, ALCOHOLIC energy drinks, like Four Loko (otherwise known as "liquid cocaine" and "blackout in a can"), hit the market. These drinks were being marketed directly to young Black and brown people, promoted as a way to get drunk while remaining alert. Of course, that's not what happened. The horror stories led to a ban against drinks that mixed the two. Yet you can still order a Red Bull and Vodka at any bar.

While all the vitamins and herbs on the labels may suggest that energy drinks are HEALTHY, we probably should be asking if energy drinks are SAFE? And if not, what's a better alternative?

The Original Energy Drinks

The first "sodas" started out as health tonics created by – who else? Long ago, Original people discovered natural 'soda' in mineral water. **During the Middle Ages, Arab chemists were experimenting and mixed up drinks made of mineral water, herbs, fruits and flowers.** These drinks traveled throughout the Islamic world and into Europe via the Moors who instituted the Renaissance in Europe. These drinks became famous later in Paris and England and eventually traveled to the Americas.

In North America the connection between health was made more apparent as the mixing of mineral water and herbs into a tonic was seen as a health drink. **In fact, pharmacists were the first ones to have soda fountains where people would come drink these tonics daily.** They started adding and experimenting with herbs and barks that are still used today in flavoring such as birch and sarsaparilla. **Soda was said to cure headaches, help with digestion, and provide energy.**

The Modern Soda

As mentioned earlier, sodas were first presented as healthy, the same way that cigarettes were presented as healthy herbs to help with meditation and relaxation (ads in the 50's for cigarettes used to be done by doctors). Many of the items in sodas were very natural such as the kola nut in Coca "Cola" (pure kola nut drinks are a staple in many parts of Africa. It works as a stimulant like coffee, tea, yerba mate. It ups physical energy, mood, and one's alertness. It also suppresses appetite.). As many of us know, cocaine provided the "Coca" part of the original Coca Cola formula. Yet overall, sodas WERE a healthy drink. The problem came in the beginning of the 20th century where they started to be mass produced and started to have many unhealthy artificial ingredients added to them along with an unhealthy amount of sugar in the form of corn syrup and other sweeteners.

The second thing is that soda corporations started to be formed. **The two major corporations are Coca-Cola and PepsiCo. These corporations, as they grew, became full manifestations of white supremacy in the form of unbridled white capitalism.** Especially in third world countries both companies have a record of using intimidation and even murder against the indigenous populations in their quest for profits. In addition they have been major violators of the environment in said regions where they set up shop, especially in reference to their effect on a region's drinking water supply. For more, visit www.KillerCoke.org.

The Modern Energy Drink

Being a country fueled on soda and coffee it was only a matter of time before America wanted to up the ante. The fast life of business and play is something that is worshiped in America. The first attempt at this that people recognize was probably Jolt Cola that came out in the mid 80's. It's tag line was "all the sugar and twice the caffeine"! It was the first soda in the modern era that was advertised as a stimulant. This fascination with stimulants (legal and illegal) characterized the 80's from cocaine to nodoze to crack. This connection between energy drinks and crack was made by the comedian Dave Chappelle in a skit comparing Red Bull to liquid crack (a charge brought in the past against the alcoholic beverage Cisco, by the way) as a parody drink, Red Balls.

Energy drinks unnaturally speed up your heart and blood circulation then they drop your metabolism significantly below its normal level. This unnatural stimulation is related to the same spike and drop in illegal drugs such as cocaine, crack and meth...even in medicines like Viagra! This is why the issues that people have with these items are insomnia, nervousness, headaches, dehydration and, in some extreme cases, heart attacks. **Ingestion of one Red Bull has been shown to temporarily raise the cardiovascular risk comparable to a person with coronary artery disease.** Other energy drinks such as Monster and Rockstar have had similar results. **After traces of cocaine were detected in some samples, Red Bull was banned in France, Denmark and Norway.** It has now since been made legal in Denmark and Norway yet it is still illegal in France. For more on the health risks related to caffeine and energy drinks.

Currently there are also "anti-energy drinks" hitting the market that aren't any better. If energy drinks are "crack and cocaine" than these "anti-energy drinks" are "heroin and opium." They have herbs that in the right doses and properly prepared are good for calming, like chamomile, melatonin, and valerian root. The problem is that these drinks are also saturated in sugar and sugar substitutes. So what do you do when you need an energy boost, and you're not trying to kill yourself with caffeine?

If you need to increase your energy rest and eat well. If you need the caffeine get you some tea. Energy drinks ain't worth a heart attack.

OILS ARE NOT HEALTH FOODS

BY SUPREME UNDERSTANDING AND DIVINEGOD B ALLAH

Just because you ain't cookin with lard don't mean you cookin healthy. **First, if you RECYCLE your oil by putting it back in a jar after you fry something, you're creating carcinogens in that oil that will give you CANCER. Most oils can't even be heated past a certain point without going bad, so imagine what we're doing when we keep reheating the same oil!** Beyond that, most of us use too much oil in our food to begin with. So the least we can do is use the good stuff.

What's the best? Well, since we're talking about the hood, where we choose "cheap" over "good" we should first answer, "What's the worst?" And that depends on who you ask. Some say the unhealthiest oil you can use (also the most common) is "vegetable oil," which is really just heavily refined soybean oil (or a mix) processed under high heat, pressure, and industrial solvents. Canola oil is a little better. But just like so-called "vegetable oil" is really made from any combination of other oils, there's no such thing as "Canola oil." What's called "Canola oil" is really "Rapeseed oil" (guess you can see why people wouldn't buy that). But it ain't just the name. **You see, rapeseed oil naturally contains a high percentage (30-60%) of erucic acid, a substance that was not considered safe for human consumption until 1974. Up until that time, Americans only used it as a lubricant for Navy ships during WWII.** Since then, they've made it a lot safer, but Canola oil, vegetable oil, corn oil, and soy oil (along with all oil-based spreads and partially hydrogenated vegetable shortenings) are still highly over-processed.

According to Dr. Andrew Weil:

Canola oil is monounsaturated and thus healthier than saturated or polyunsaturated oils, but I still consider it a distant runner-up to olive oil. Unlike olive oil, canola oil doesn't contain oleic acid, the fatty acid our bodies process best. I've always cautioned against buying canola oil found in supermarkets. These products have been extracted with chemical solvents or high-speed presses that generate heat. Both methods alter the oil's fatty acid chemistry in undesirable ways. Furthermore, canola oil producers use a lot of pesticides on their crops, and I suspect that residues find their way into the finished product.

> **Did You Know?**
> According to Dr. Douglas Graham, the author of the book *The 80/10/10 Diet* (who recommends we get only 10% of our calories from fat), "Higher than healthy levels of fat in the bloodstream forces fat to precipitate out and stick to arterial walls, a condition known as "atherosclerosis" (hardening of the arteries). This leads to HBP, heart attacks and strokes. Of course, this happens over time when breakfast, lunch, and dinner consistently contains fat.

Canola oil is a step above vegetable oil, which itself is a big step above cooking with lard...but if you can afford to step up higher, do so.

What's the best? Depend on what you're doing. **Non-processed and organic saturated fats** (the kind that are solid or semi-solid at room temperature) **are typically the best for cooking at high temperatures, as they will not go rancid nor oxidize** (which contributes to cancer). **That category includes coconut oil, sesame oil, or straight-up butter.** When using a low flame, or baking – monounsaturated cold-pressed, organic, extra virgin olive oil is the best choice. Yeah, look for all those words.

When buying oil, it's important that you look for these three terms on the label: cold-pressed, organic and extra virgin. This ensures that the process in which the oil was made did not use harsh chemicals (like hexane) nor high heat (which robs the oils of their naturally occurring nutrients). **Ideally, though it's best to limit your oil consumption altogether. After all, oils are dense forms of fat.** And eating a diet that is 100+ grams of fat each day is not a healthy diet, even if you're eating healthy food, cooked in tons of oil. Fat is fat! If you are taking in more than 20% of your calories from fat each day, then you are creating poor health and opening the door to unwanted health problems long term.

Fat is needed in our diet, but the best sources are from whole food sources like avocados and raw, unsalted nuts and seeds. Consuming 2,000 calories a day, you would eat a maximum of 120 calories per day of fat, which equates to one of the following: (a) 1 cup of nuts or seeds, (b) 4 avocados, or (c) ONE tablespoon of oil. Just ONE?! I doubt there's many of us with an oil intake that low. But you can at LEAST step your game up in terms of WHAT you're using.

SOMETHING'S FISHY

BY C'BS ALIFE ALLAH

But this time it's a good thing. If you aren't fully sold on a vegetarian diet, yet still want to make a step in the right direction, get rid of the pork and red meat. With that done, one of the things that can give you a good balanced diet is fish. **Having a steady diet of fish will allow you to really streamline your overall weight and health.** As a rule of thumb though, it's best to cut back on deep frying. Try different ways to prepare fish, such as baking or sautéing.

The key element that makes fish good for ya is what is called Omega-3 fatty acids. Those acids are good for your heart and circulation. It is found especially in those oily fish like mackerel, herring, and sardines. It has been shown to prevent certain types of heart disease also. Omega 3s also help in the development of the brain, so they are good for the youth.

One of the reasons that pork and beef can be bad for you is because of the tremendous amount of fat in the meat which isn't good. Fish is lean and has low fat, plus the fat it does have is good for you – the type that assists in the development and upkeep of muscles and body tissue.

Seafood, in general, is rich in the minerals of iodine, zinc, iron, and selenium, which are all good minerals to have coursing through your body. All the vitamins that assist in the upkeep of a healthy nervous system are found in fish. Also those that help with maintaining strong bones, teeth and good complexion.

Wait...there's still a problem?

Did You Know?

In 1997, EWG concluded that fish from more than 1,660 U.S. waterways were so contaminated with mercury that they should be eaten sparingly or not at all. Soon after, the EPA confirmed that more than 1.6 million women and children could face serious health risks from mercury-contaminated food. In fact, a Bush administration study found that one in six women has mercury levels so high that she cannot hope to have a child without significant risk of neurological damage. But it took two more years for the EPA and the U.S. FDA to issue warnings to women to limit fish consumption during pregnancy to 12 ounces a week, while still failing to warn about the dangers of tuna. EWG unearthed internal FDA transcripts in which agency officials noted that canned tuna contained enough mercury to harm the developing brain of a baby in the womb. In January 2004, EWG released an interactive Tuna Calculator to help people figure their own safe doses of tuna, based on weight. It advised women of child-bearing age and children under 5 not eat albacore tuna at all.

Fish live in the water. As a result, they absorb all the pollution that ends up in our water, and some fish absorb more than others. What's number one on the list of toxins found in fish?

Mercury. Yes, that silver liquid that you see in old school thermometers. It's toxic. There's so much mercury run off in our waters (coming from big factories) that all fish contain trace amounts. But this amount isn't enough to usually harm anyone. **Other fish though contain huge amounts that can harm young children and fetuses. So, to be on the safe side, children and pregnant mothers shouldn't be eating fish more than twice a week and they should only be eating fish that has that low mercury level, which we'll detail below.** And mercury doesn't pass through your body on its own, so it can build up in adults to the point that it causes damage to the brain and kidneys. Studies show that avoiding fish eliminates half of all mercury exposure.

So wait...you said to eat fish and now you're saying don't eat fish?

No, what we're saying is that you need to be selective as to which type of fish you're eating. In our article about scavengers, we mentioned that some sea food you don't need to eat under any circumstances. The main reason why is because the types of sea food listed concentrate the most toxins. And though we are focusing on mercury the same fish and seafood that carry a lot of mercury in their bodies also hold a lot of other toxins. So as a base rule, cut out shellfish (clams, lobster, crab, oysters, crawfish, etc), catfish), and the larger fish. Why? Bigger fish tend to eat anything, and live longer, so they build up more toxins in their bodies. Below are some lists of general mercury ratings for commonly eaten fish.

Low Mercury (2-3 times a week)		Moderate Mercury (6 or less/month)	High Mercury (3 or less/month)	
Anchovies	Sole	Bass	Bluefish	
Flounder	Tilapia	Carp	Sea Bass	
Haddock	Trout	Cod	Tuna (Canned Albacore, Yellow fin)	
Herring	Whitefish	Halibut		
Mackerel		Perch	Highest Mercury (just don't eat it)	
Pollock		Snapper		
Salmon		Tuna (canned chunky light)	Marlin	Tuna
Sardine			Shark	(Ahi)

Though we put listings all the way up to the highest level of mercury and still suggest amounts that you should eat, you really should consider not eating the ones rated "above moderate" at all. You can go to www.epa.gov/waterscience/fish/states.htm and check the mercury content of fish caught in your area.

Too much of anything is bad for you. Fish can help you balance your diet but eat the ones low in mercury!

FISH...WITH EXTRA OIL

BY SUPREME UNDERSTANDING

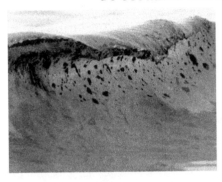

If you're like Common, who went vegan but later added fish to his diet (because he felt he needed something extra)...Or if you want to cut back on meat, but still eat fish...go for it. It's definitely healthier than eating pork fried rice and Big Macs. But don't forget that you're not just eating a fish. You're eating everything that fish has in its system. **And while an Environmental Working Group (EWG) study found that 72 out of 73 people have mercury in their system, mostly from eating fish, that's not ALL we're consuming.** Just think about how polluted our water is. As Dr. Joe Fuhrman has noted: "People who would be disgusted at the thought of drinking polluted water don't think twice about eating polluted fish with 1000 times more pollution in it." And this has been known for quite some time now. In 1909, Ellen G. White (whose work led to the development of the Seventh Day Adventist Church) wrote in *The Ministry of Healing*:

> In many places fish become so contaminated by the filth on which they feed as to be a cause of disease This is especially the case where the fish come in contact with the sewage of large cities The fish that are fed on the contents of the drains may pass into distant waters and may be caught where the water is pure and fresh. Thus when used as food they bring disease and death on those who do not suspect the danger.

That was over 100 years ago. Imagine how much more polluted our waters are today! For example, **there are now industrial pollutants known as PCBs, which accumulate in fish and in the body tissues of people who eat fish regularly.** As you've read elsewhere, PCBs cause cancer. Fuhrman continues:

In some cases, such as with the PCBs in Great Lakes trout and salmon, it can be shown that a person would have to drink the lake water for 100 years to accumulate the same quantity of PCB present in a single half-pound portion of these fish.

Yes, you read that right: trout and salmon, the "good fish." **Highly toxic PCBs were found in 43% of salmon, 50% of whitefish, and 25% of swordfish.** The National Research Council reports that PCBs are found in virtually every site where fish or shellfish are tested, even in spots as remote as rural Alaska, the Virgin Islands, and Hawaii.

Extra Oil

There's more. For example, a 1992 *Consumer Reports* survey found that half of the flounder sampled in New York contained pesticides. What else is in our fish? I've got two letters to help you figure it out: BP. **Did you forget about the BP oil spill? All that oil in the water is affecting every living creature in that ecosystem, even those hundreds of miles away.** Why do you think restaurants as far as Maine stopped serving shrimp? Look it up, because it's deeper than what you may have heard. In fact, it goes quite a bit deeper than we can explore in this book. You'll have to read *Chemical Genocide* for more, but let's just say this much: **This wasn't the first time BP was involved in something like this. In July of 2007, BP was issued a government permit to dump mercury into Lake Michigan.** Yes, a government permit. The permit exempted a BP plant 3 miles southeast of Chicago from a federal regulation limiting mercury discharges into the Great Lakes. "The permitted levels will not affect drinking water, recreation or aquatic life," Environmental Commissioner Thomas Easterly told the *Chicago Tribune*. If you believe THAT, you've probably got that brain damage we're talking about here.[20]

In fact, those aren't the only cases you need to know about. In the Summer of 2010, hundreds of thousands of

---

[20] Another fact to consider: The Company responsible for cementing the oil rig so it wouldn't blow? Halliburton. If you know your politics, you know who these folks are. Halliburton workers had just finished cementing the well when the rig blew, leading experts to wonder what happened, and leading me to wonder why nobody can figure it out. Halliburton was also responsible for cementing a well off the coast of Australia that blew in August of 2009, leaking oil for ten weeks before it was plugged.

gallons of oil were also spilled into the waters of Kalamazoo, Michigan; Salt Lake City, Utah; and who knows where else?[21] That same summer, federal agencies and the Illinois Department of Natural Resources spread Rotenone, a chemical toxic to fish, along the Little Calumet River on Chicago's South Side on Thursday. Over 100,000 pounds of dead fish soon washed up soon after. Months later, over ten thousand dead fish washed up on the shores of Massachusetts, followed by over ten thousand more on the shores of New Jersey. The most telling fact? Even the seagulls wouldn't eat them. **A month later, in September of 2010, *hundreds* of thousands of dead fish, crabs, stingray, and eel hit the surface of a Louisiana waterway. It looked like a gravel road.** You couldn't even see water, only dead sh*t. They even found a dead *whale* in there. Yet nobody's investigating why!

Radioactive Fish

Remember the little three-eyed fish that kept popping up near the nuclear plant on The Simpsons? That's real. In fact, there are plenty of reports of fish being caught with radioactive chemicals in their system. For example, in February of 2010, a fish caught in the Connecticut river, four miles upstream from a Vermont nuclear reactor, tested positive for radioactive strontium-90, which has been linked to bone cancer and leukemia. Makes sense, since the water (and soil) is full of it. Radioactive tritium also turned up in the water at levels 100 times higher than the EPA's safety limit for drinking water. Other radioactive isotopes were found as well, including cesium-137, zinc-65 and cobalt-60. So we're not saying fish is completely healthy, but we're also not saying you can't eat any fish at all. What we ARE saying is that every decision you make should be an informed decision. For example, would you eat fish that came from the Gulf Coast? The Connecticut River? The Great Lakes? What about the kind of fish that – no matter where it comes from – is gonna be full of mercury? Exactly. So if you're going to eat fish, follow these recommendations, in order of difficulty:

☐ Stick to the ones in the "low mercury" category. (See "Something's Fishy")

---

[21] In case you didn't know, 706 MILLION GALLONS of oil end up in the earth's water every year. 52 million gallons of that come from oil spills and offshore drilling leaks, which are both more common than you think. In the the Niger Delta (the US's 5th-biggest source of oil) alone, there have been 7,000 oil spills between 1970-2000. That's roughly 300 spills per year and over 13 million barrels of oil…yet the people who live in the region (and who are becoming sick) suffer from fuel shortages! Talk about dirty. The rest of the 706 million gallons comes mostly from industrial giants regularly pouring oil "down the drain" (yes, on purpose).

- Buy fresh instead of frozen.
- Instead of frying, try raw (sashimi/sushi), marinated (ceviche), steamed, grilled, baked, broiled, or smoked (as in salmon and trout).
- Eat sparingly. Two to three servings a week is enough.
- If possible, find out where the fish came from. Cheaper doesn't mean better. A good example is those inexpensive fish sticks people buy for their children. What are they made of? Tilapia? Salmon? Nope. Albacore Tuna, one of the cheapest (and most toxic) fish you can eat. Well, that plus a mix of other fish parts and other special ingredients... but that's another story.
- Try to get fish that were actually caught by fishing (like wild Alaskan salmon) instead of "farmed" fish (like "Atlantic salmon"). Farmed fish contain pesticides, antibiotics and other drugs used to control diseases that occur when fish are crowded together in the pens of fish farms (for more details, visit www.avianweb.com/fish.html).

As for me personally, I don't eat fish because I just gave up on the idea of eating anything with a face. Just seems nasty. But I also respect that many of us aren't ready to give up eating meat, so I normally support "pescetarianism." (See "The Importance Of Nutrition")

So I'll leave it up to you to take your own steps at your own pace. But I'll leave you with the words of Neal Barnard, M.D., of the Physicians Committee for Responsible Medicine:

> Fish diets are certainly nothing like diets based on vegetables, fruits, grains, and legumes. Vegetarian diets, along with an otherwise healthy lifestyle, can actually reverse existing heart disease, with none of the stroke risk that fish oils can bring. And while you can buy organic, pesticide-free produce, there is no such thing as "organic fish" – fish are loaded with chemical contaminants.

The toxins within fish reflect the contamination of our oceans, as our bodies reflect the toxicity of our lifestyles. Let's stop polluting both.

IS SALT BAD FOR YOU?
BY TESNIM HASSAN

Salt was a major stepping stone in the building of civilization. Because salt is an excellent food preservative, (especially when used to preserve meat), people gained the ability to travel farther distances. The use of salt as a food preservative also decreased people's dependence on food that, before, was only seasonally available.

Salt was highly valued by many cultures and became a very important product. Many salt roads were established because of its' frequent trade. **Some of these roads were established as early as the**

Bronze Age (6050 BCE). **From salt mines in prehistoric China** (c. 6000 BCE) **to the ancient West African salt trade** (which is why some African tribes traveled so much), **salt was of serious importance to Original people.** The ancient Egyptians made funeral offerings of salt, salted fish and salted birds. **The ancient Egyptians also exported salted fish to the Phoenicians, who then traded Egyptian salt fish with their neighbors. This is probably how Europeans picked up on the value of salt.** Before long, there were salt roads all up and down Europe. The word, "salary"

actually derives from the Roman word, "salarium," which loosely translated means, "money given to soldiers so that they can buy salt." As things normally go, the Romans soon controlled the availability and price of salt. They would raise the price to fund wars, or lower it so that the poor could afford it, since it was an important part of the diet. In fact, the word "salad" comes from the ancient Roman practice of eating lettuce leaves with salt. (Not a recommended recipe for you to try now, however.)

Why We Need Salt

Salt is made mostly of sodium chloride. In small amounts this mineral is necessary for animal and plant life. **The body needs it to regulate blood pressure, blood volume, water balance and cell function.** However, in large amounts, sodium chloride is harmful to animal and plant life.

Four main electrolytes are found in the human body; sodium, potassium, calcium and magnesium. **All of these are found in unrefined (or raw) salt.** The proper balance of these electrolytes is necessary for the survival of all higher forms of life. Why? Because Sodium, potassium, calcium and magnesium are found inside of your cells (intracellular), as well as outside of your cells (extracellular). They move back and forth across your cell walls as they attempt to stay balanced on both sides.

Think of this process as being similar to a scale, or a see saw. For example, if there is more sodium inside of your cells than outside of your cells, the sodium will move out of your cells. If there is more sodium outside of your cells than inside of your cells, then the sodium will move into your cells.

These electrolytes are necessary for nerve and muscle function. **Too little, or too much, sodium chloride in the diet can cause muscle cramps, dizziness, problems with brain function and renal failure. A sodium chloride imbalance can even be fatal.** Both nerves and muscles are considered "electrical" tissues. This means that a slight electrical charge is needed for these organ systems to work properly. This is why electrolytes are needed; to carry this charge. The heart, being one of the most important muscles, is immediately affected when your electrolytes are out of balance.

Electrolytes can become imbalanced when the body is dehydrated or overhydrated. **Sports drinks, such as Gatorade and Powerade contain essential electrolytes. Pedialyte works to correct the electrolyte imbalance in a child that is vomiting or has diarrhea.** Children quickly become dehydrated and it's important to keep them hydrated when they're sick. If dehydration is severe enough, and you find yourself in the Emergency Room, you will quickly be given electrolytes and fluids through an IV. **Dehydration can occur due to vomiting and diarrhea, exercise which leads to sweating, and liquor intoxication or starvation.**[22]

Sodium Deficiency

For the reasons given above, avoiding salt may lead to more bad than good. **Studies show that only 9% of the population suffers from sodium sensitivity, meaning that blood pressure increases in response to increased sodium consumption.** The remaining 91% of the population appears to be sodium resistant, meaning their blood pressure does not rise consuming excess sodium, though this may change over time. **What appears to be more important than how much salt you eat is how your diet is balanced between sodium and potassium. New research suggests that the real cause of high blood pressure is a diet low in calcium, potassium and magnesium.** This means the lack of other electrolytes, instead of an overabundance of sodium, may lead to high blood pressure.

---

[22] By the way, it's possible to make your own electrolyte drink by using the right amounts of water, sugar, salt, potassium substitute and baking soda. Another organic recipe for a home-made electrolyte drink is: pure organic fruit juice, water or green tea, and organic sea salt.

Sea Salt

Sea salt is obtained by evaporating sea water in shallow beds that are warmed by sunlight and blown by the wind. It can have a bitter taste because it contains minerals other than sodium chloride. Some of the most common sources for sea salt include the Mediterranean Sea, the North Sea, and the Atlantic Ocean. Sea salt is much healthier than traditional table salt because of the trace elements that it contains, other than sodium.

Coincidentally, many of the minerals that are found in the blood are found in sea salt. This is the reason that sea salt is a better dietary alternative than refined or table salt. **As many as eighty minerals that are necessary for human life may be found in raw sea salt.** Some of these minerals are iron, manganese, zinc and iodine. Sea salt has many necessary nutrients, without the unnecessary chemical additives found in refined salt.

Rock Salt

Rock salt forms when bodies of water, (such as enclosed lakes and seas), dry up, leaving evaporate minerals. These underground salt beds are found throughout the United States, Canada, in the United Kingdom, Austria, China and Northern Africa. Salt is extracted from these underground rock beds by mining.

Refined Salt

Refined salt is the most common type of salt found in the average person's kitchen and in restaurant salt shakers. Refined salt usually comes from the rock salt mines that were mentioned above. **The refining process rids the salt of the essential trace elements, leaving mostly sodium chloride.** Later in the refining process, other chemicals are added. During the 1940s, the British began to add various chemicals to salt brine to prevent the salt from caking. Some of these chemicals are sodium ferrocyanide, tricalcium phosphate, calcium and magnesium carbonates, fatty acids, magnesium oxide, silicon dioxide, calcium silicate, sodium aluminosilicate and calcium aluminosilicate. Once the refining process is complete, the finished product contains about 3% of ingredients that are NOT sodium chloride.

"Standing at my podium, I'm tryin to watch my sodium/ Die of high blood pressure, or either let the Feds get 'cha" – Young Jeezy, Kanye West's "Amazing"

High intake of refined salt (table salt) **has been shown to lead to many health complications,** including strokes and cardiovascular (heart and blood vessel) problems such as hypertension (high blood pressure), cardiac enlargement, heart attack and heart failure. Other health problems that are associated with the intake of refined salt are edema, ulcers, stomach cancers and kidney failure. **Unfortunately, studies have found that 1 in 10 people have a moderate consumption of sodium, with the rest of us getting way too much.** It's not just salt from the salt shaker, either. **With 70% of our salt coming from processed foods, most of which contain generous amounts of refined salt.** Check the food labels to see for yourself.

Why Iodize?

Currently salt is cheap, readily available and often iodized. American salt manufacturers began to iodize salt in the 1920s

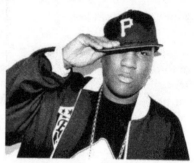

in cooperation with government requests. **Still, iodine deficiency affects many millions of people worldwide and is a major, yet preventable, cause of mental retardation among both children** (Cretinism) **and adults** (myxedema). Cretinism causes physical and mental growth to be stunted in children. Along with mental retardation, symptoms associated with myxedema may include depression, fatigue, a slow heart rate, low body temperature and hair loss. **Iodine deficiency may also cause thyroid problems, including the formation of non-toxic goiters.** A goiter is a swelling of the thyroid gland, and sometimes, also the neck and voice box.

Iodine is added to salt in the form of potassium iodide, sodium iodide or sodium iodate. The United States adds up to four times more iodine to the salt than other countries, like the United Kingdom. To maintain good health, less than 225 micrograms of iodine need to be consumed on a daily basis. Sea food and some forms of sea salt contain iodine naturally, and so it is unnecessary to eat an iodine supplement if you already eat sea food and/or the correct form of sea salt.

What's Best?

The best alternative to your ordinary "refined" table salt with its aluminum additives, **is to use roasted sea-salt** (you can buy it this way or roast the cheaper kind yourself for 30 min. at 375 deg. F and leave the kitchen to avoid chlorine vapors). **You can also use Miso with active Aspergillus culture** (miso promotes beneficial bowel flora, and was used effectively by the Japanese after atomic bombing for minimizing radiation damage to digestive tract).

SWEETENERS

BY TESNIM HASSAN

Living in the United States, it's easy to develop an addiction to sweets. For this reason, there are a number of different ways to sweeten up your diet and some definitely aren't as healthy as others. Below, we'll discuss a few natural and unnatural sweeteners, starting with the most "unhealthy" alternatives, and ending with the most "healthy."

Aspartame

NutraSweet, Equal, AminoSweet and Canderel are all aspartame. Aspartame is 2,000 times sweeter than sugar, without the nutritional value. The makers of aspartame say that aspartame can be found in 6,000 products, throughout the world. Aspartame was developed by the pharmaceutical company, G.D. Searle in 1975. When aspartame was tested on rats and mice, they developed brain lesions, tumors and seizures, with some even dying from consumption of the substance. For 16 years, the FDA refused Searle's applications for approval, with the FDA eventually asking the Department of Justice to prosecute Searle for submitting falsified evidence, in an attempt to get aspartame approved. Even the National Soft Drink Association had objected to the use of aspartame because it is very unstable in its' liquid form, and breaks down into various substances, including FORMALDEHYDE. When Donald Rumsfeld, (yes, HIM), CEO of G.D. Searle at the time, was made part of Ronald Reagan's presidential transition team, a new FDA commissioner was appointed, who quickly approved the use of aspartame. Since the FDA's approval of aspartame, the FDA has compiled a list of 92 symptoms that are linked to eating aspartame.

Aspartame is a chemical that is known to be carcinogenic (cancer causing), and which contains excitotoxins. Excitotoxins cause the neurons in your brain to fire in spasms. Because of this, the neurons are damaged and may eventually burn out and die. This leads to painful, crippling headaches. With up to 90% of migraine headaches being caused by food allergies, it's no surprise that aspartame tops the list of allergens. In fact, aspartame may trigger migraines in 50% of people that suffer from migraine headaches. In some cases migraine headaches may lead to convulsions and grand mal seizures. It has also been found that aspartame may also be responsible for causing nausea, dizziness, shakiness and diminished vision, deafness, weight gain and

DEATH.

When looking for aspartame on a product's ingredient list, bear in mind that the ingredient, "phenylaline" is a component of aspartame. If the product contains phenylalanine, it contains aspartame.

Saccharin

Sweet 'N Low is saccharin. Saccharin is an artificial sweetener that is much sweeter than sugar, but has an unpleasant aftertaste that may be described as bitter or metallic. It does not contribute to food energy, at all. In fact, saccharin goes through the human body's digestive system WITHOUT BEING DIGESTED. Saccharin is used to flavor numerous products including drinks, candies, toothpastes and medicines. Saccharin is often used along with aspartame in diet sodas so that each chemical can hide the other's off-taste. Also, aspartame has a pretty low shelf-life in comparison to saccharin, so even when the aspartame breaks down into formaldehyde and other chemicals, the saccharin remains.

Saccharin was first produced in 1878 by a chemist who was isolating coal derivatives. Saccharin is a coal tar product that is made using anthranilic acid, nitrous acid, sulfur dioxide, chlorine and ammonia. Sugar shortages during World War I caused for saccharin's use to become widespread. It became more popular during the 1960s and 1970s when dieters began to use it.

In October of 1989, the Office of Environmental Health Hazard Assessment (OEHHA) added saccharin to a list of known carcinogens, or cancer-causing agents although it was taken off of this list in April of 2001. The United States' position on saccharin has repeatedly changed ever since 1908. Saccharin has been banned in Canada since 1978. Although there has been shown a causal relationship between laboratory rats who are fed saccharin and bladder cancer, it has been argued that the rats' consumption of saccharin far exceeds human consumption. Because no definitive studies show a carcinogenic effect resulting from saccharin consumption, in 2000, the US government repealed a law stating that saccharin packages had to be labeled with a warning. It still sounds suspect to me.

Sucralose

Splenda, SucraPlus, Candys, Cukren and Nevella are all sucralose. Sucralose is a non-sugar, non-nutritive sweetener that is 600 times sweeter than sugar. Sucralose is found in 4,500 products. Because it is more stable than aspartame when heated, it is used for baking. Sucralose is often used in combination with other sweeteners like aspartame and high fructose corn syrup. Sucralose was developed by a multi-national agri-processor in 1976. It was approved for use in the United States in 1998.

It is manufactured by chlorinating sucrose using any of a number of chlorinating substances, including phosphorous oxychloride. It belongs to a class of chemicals called organochlorides or chlorocarbons. Some chlorinated substances are known to be toxic to plants and animals. It has been stated, however, that sucrose is not toxic in small amounts.

However, eating just seven Splenda packets affects the amount of good bacteria in the intestines, with regular consumption killing up to 50% of the good bacteria that we carry. This may have to do with the fact that it increases the pH level in the intestines, which causes an alkaline environment. It also causes for an increase in body weight. Sucralose limits the use of medications in cancer patients, AIDs patients and heart patients by sending the medications back to the intestines, instead of allowing the body to absorb them. James Turner, chairman of Citizens for Health, has been quoted as saying that using sucralose "is like putting a pesticide in your body."

Acesulfame-K

Sweet One or Sunnet is Acesulfame-K or Acesulfame potassium. It is 200 times sweeter than sugar, and has a somewhat bitter aftertaste that is similar to saccharin. It is more stable than aspartame when heated, and is found in baked goods and products with long shelf lives. This product was first developed in 1967 by Hoechst AG, a German pharmaceutical company. Its' use was approved by the FDA in 1988. Acesulfame-K is often mixed with other sweeteners like aspartame and high fructose corn syrup. The safety concerns about acesulfame-K are related to the results of animal studies. At high levels, rats were found to develop cancer. It has also been shown to affect the thyroid in rats, rabbits and dogs. There have not been enough studies of this product although it is found in a number of products.

High Fructose Corn Syrup

Fructose is usually processed from corn or fruit. High fructose corn syrup, or HFCS, is made from cornstarch. The glucose in cornstarch is converted to sucrose, and then fructose. This is done through a series of steps which involves the use of three different enzymes, bacteria and fungus. By the end of the processing, HFCS has a fructose content of 55%. The body does not process HFCS in the same way that it processes sugars from cane or beets. HFCS contains empty calories and has no nutritional value.

HFCS has been linked to obesity, diabetes and metabolic dysfunction for two main reasons. First, although it can be said that anything is harmless "in moderation," this rule does not apply to the use of HFCS. When shopping at the grocery store, 75% of processed foods contain HFCS including yogurt, bread and cough syrup. In 1966, Americans consumed absolutely NO HFCS. In 2001, the average American consumed 62.6 pounds of HFCS per person. Second, HFCS affects the body's natural ability to control hunger. Leptin and ghrelin are the two main hormones that regulate your appetite. Leptin tells your brain when your stomach is full. Ghrelin tells your brain when your stomach is empty. HFCS limits your body's ability to produce leptin. This means that your brain does not receive the message that your stomach is full. Additionally, HFCS never limits ghrelin production, and so your brain constantly receives the message that your stomach is empty. The end result is that the body never gets the message that the stomach is full, and this causes you to eat more.

There are strong links between HFCS and heart disease because it raises triglyceride levels. When triglycerides are present in the blood in high amounts, they cause the walls of the arteries, (blood vessels that carry blood from the heart), to become thick. Thickened arterial result in a condition called atherosclerosis. Atherosclerosis causes for the heart to have to beat harder as it tries to push blood through narrow arteries. For this reason, eating too many triglycerides is linked to heart disease and stroke.

White Sugar

When people say, "sugar" what they're talking about is a sweet, edible substance that may be sucrose, fructose, glucose, etc. The sugar that's found in food is usually sucrose. Sucrose is usually called saccarose or "table sugar." Refined white sugar is 99% sucrose. In industrial foods they may use a combination of sucrose, gluctose and high fructose corn syrup.

Sucrose comes from either sugar cane or sugar beets. Sugar cane is a tall, perennial grass that is native to Southern India and can be only be grown in tropical and temperate climates. Brazil currently produces most of the world's sugar cane, followed by India. Sugar cane has six times more output than sugar beets. Sugar cane is used to produce molasses, rum and ethanol, among other products and by-products. Sugar beets are grown in nations with colder climates and more advanced farming techniques, for example the United States and the European Union.

White sugar is made by bubbling sulfur dioxide through raw sugar. To further refine sugar, the raw sugar is first combined with heavy syrup and then centrifuged (this is called affination). Phosphoric acid and calcium hydroxide are then added in order to remove "impurities" which are skimmed off the top. Another similar process uses carbon dioxide and calcium hydroxide. The remaining product is then filtered through activated carbon. The sugar is then crystallized and re-crystallized in vacuum, finally producing white sugar. In order to produce brown sugar, the above process is followed by blending the white sugar with the washings from the affination process, and then crystallizing the sugar, again. Meaning that brown sugar is even more processed than white sugar.

We all know that too much sugar causes tooth cavities, but maybe more importantly, sugar's been linked with obesity and Type 2 diabetes. According to the FDA, women should eat no more than 25 grams of sugar a day, and men should eat no more than 37 grams of sugar a day. But one can of soda has 39 grams of sugar, so it isn't hard to believe that most Americans eat three to five pounds of sugar A WEEK!

Turbinado
Sugar in the Raw is one example of Turbinado sugar. Turbinado, or turbinated, sugar is made from sugar cane extract. Freshly cut sugar cane is crushed and then heat is used to evaporate the juice, which is later crystallized. The crystals are then spun in a turbine to remove extra moisture and molasses. This leaves behind large, brown crystals. Turbinado sugar is similar to brown sugar, but has larger, dryer crystals. Most of the Turbinado sugar that is sold in the United States is produced in Hawaii and is often sold as an organic product.

Stevia
Stevia is an herb that is in the sunflower family and grows in North, Central and South America. Stevia is also known as sweet leaf or sugar leaf. The leaves can be eaten fresh off of the plant, or can be added to teas or food. It is 300 times sweeter than sugar, but some of its extracts have an aftertaste that is similar to licorice.

Since sugar has proven to be such an unhealthy part of diet, many people have turned to stevia as a low-carbohydrate alternative. It has a very small effect on blood sugar, and for this reason is an excellent alternative for diabetics. Medical research has shown that stevia may even have some benefit in the treatment of obesity and high blood pressure. Most studies have found stevia to be absent of harmful effects, with no link to either cancer or birth defects.

The Japanese have used stevia as a sweetener since the 1970s. They use stevia more than any other country, with stevia making up 40% of their sweetener market. Although some countries have restricted or banned stevia use, it used widely throughout Asia, South America and in Israel. The United States banned stevia until the early 1990s, unless it was labeled as a dietary supplement. It is suspected by some that the FDA's stevia ban was an effort to protect the interests of the artificial sweetener industry. In 2008, the United States allowed for the stevia-derived Rebaudioside A to be used as a food additive or a sweetener. However stevia must undergo a rigorous extraction and refining process which includes ethanol, methanol, crystallization and separation, in order to produce Rebaudioside A. Rebaudioside A is currently sold under the trade names Only Sweet, PureVia, Reb-A, Rebiana, Sweet Leaf, or Truvia. In recent years, stevia has grown in availability, worldwide.

Agave Nectar

Agave nectar is a natural sweetener that is produced in Mexico from a number of agave plants, including Blue Agave, Salmiana Agave, Green Agave, Grey Agave, Thorny Agave and Rainbow Agave. They are large, spiky plants that look like cactus. It is made of mostly sucrose and glucose. Some say that agave is sweeter than honey, but it is not as sticky. There are different methods for extracting sugars from agave based on the species. One type of agave nectar is produced when the sap is squeezed from the core, and then heated at low temperatures until it forms simple sugars. Another type of nectar is produced when the agave stalk is cut from a newly growing plant, leaving a hole where sap accumulates. This sap is then processed using enzymes. Agave nectar does not cause the same "sugar-rush" or spike in blood sugar that is caused by many other sweeteners. There are light, amber, dark and raw varieties of agave. This nectar is frequently used by vegans. Agave can also be used as a healing balm and to dress wounds.

Honey

Honey is made by bees from flower nectar because bees use honey as a food source. The nectar is regurgitated by the bees and stored in honeycombs in the bees' hive. Beekeepers encourage overproduction of honey and collect it, making it available for sale. Its' sweetness is similar to sugar because of its' carbohydrates. These carbohydrates are mostly fructose and glucose. Aside from simple sugars, honey also contains vitamins, minerals and antioxidants. International food regulations say that honey must be a pure product, which does not allow for the addition of any other substances.

Because of its' low water content, honey is an antimicrobial, meaning that most microorganisms do not grow in honey. Honey can be used to treat skin infections associated with MRSA and diabetic ulcers. Honey is also used to reduce wound odor, swelling and scarring. It reduces the amount of time that it takes for a burn to heal. It is also an effective treatment for sore throats and coughs.

Clostridium botulinim (which causes botulism) is, however, sometimes found in raw honey, and for this reason, it should not be fed to infants younger than a year old, because their intestines are not fully developed.

If you must sweeten your food or drink, use the sweeteners least likely to give you diabetes or cancer!

SPENDING LESS TO FEED MORE
BY SCIHONOR DEVOTION

In this day and time, food is expensive. For those of us who have children, grocery bills could really add up. Some of us have larger households than others, so here are some ideas to help shop for healthy foods on a budget.

Determine a Budget. Make sure it is compatible with all your other household needs. **Consider your light bills, travel expenses, phone bill, etc.** It may be a good idea to look back at old receipts and do some calculating to see how much you spend on these bills, determine what is unnecessary (and can be cut) and how much you can spend on food. **Remember that food is a necessity, while cable TV is not.** Don't forget to include all of your non-food items like toothpaste, soap, shampoo, feminine hygiene products, paper towel, toilet tissue, cleaning supplies, etc.

Plan Ahead. Make a meal plan for the next 2 weeks. This will help you to find out what ingredients you need to shop for. Scan your cabinets, refrigerator and freezer to see if you already have the things you need, so that you don't spend money unnecessarily. (See "A Simple Meal Plan")

Look for Savings. Cut coupons. I know you don't feel like sitting there cutting coupons like an old woman, but hey, you gotta do what you gotta do. Get to clipping. Keep the coupons organized (perhaps clip them to your list), and don't cut coupons for products that you don't use. You'll end up spending money on something you don't need, just because it's on sale. But returning to the last tip, plan your meals around what's on sale. **If what you buy usually doesn't have a coupon in the Sunday paper, check the store circulars.** Some stores offer discounts on cases of items, such as rice milk or water. **Some have a scanner guarantee program where if an item comes**

up at the wrong price at the register, you could get it for free. Ask around. Read the signs. Their policies may even be listed. Also, many health food stores now accept EBT/food stamp cards.

Shop at Wholesale Clubs. The cost of membership is well worth it when you calculate all of your savings. You can buy things in bulk there and the prices are usually really good. **If your family is not big enough to take advantage of the bulk quantities they offer, you can find a partnering family and split the cost of membership** (and even the products). I do this with a good friend of mine.

Travel. Another way to look for savings is to travel to different stores. I know this may seem time-consuming, but it could be well worth it if the stores are not really far away from each other. On the street where I do a lot of my shopping, there is a Whole Foods, a Trader Joes, and a Stop and Shop. I've been to them all so many times that I know which ones offer the best deals on which products. So, **when I go shopping, I organize my list by store and section.**

Stick to Your Script. When you go to shopping, stick with the items on your list. **Many stores place more expensive items on the shelves that are at eye level.** Don't get got. **Look high and low for savings, literally.** Be sure to not only check the nutritional value of the items but also the unit pricing. It's usually listed on the shelves below the item. This will tell you how much you are paying for each ounce or pound of that particular item. You can compare costs easily this way.

Farmer's Markets. Check out local farmers' markets when they are in town. Also, check out CSA's (Community Supported Agriculture). CSA's provide delivery of produce sometimes weekly to its members. For example, you may pay a certain amount for membership for a certain amount of produce in pounds. Whatever is harvested for that season is what you get. You may pay, let's say, $40 each month and twice a month, you may receive, 3 pounds of plums, 5 pounds of nectarines, 2 pounds of grapes, 3 pounds of tomatoes, and 2 pounds of broccoli and 1 pound of cauliflower. Now, this is just an example since you may not know exactly what you will get since you will get whatever is harvested and in season.

Food Co-ops. Food co-ops are like grocery stores except that they are basically owned and operated by their members. So, **if you join a food co-op, you will be able to get some good deals on food, but, you will be required to work in the store in some capacity.** Don't worry. **It's not like a full time job. You may have to do something like 6 hours a week.** Oh and the good thing is that anyone in your household can do the shift for you. So, if you have a large family, send one of the children who are old enough to do the shift. It'll be good for them. No, seriously.

Don't Eat Out. It costs way too much, whether you have a large or small family. Just add up what you spend every week and you'll see.

I suggest you wake up earlier than you usually do, cook at home for breakfast, and bring your own lunch from home as well. **Leftovers that wouldn't make a full meal may be good to bring for lunch.**

Or you can cook all day Sunday and freeze your meals so that you'll just have to worry about salad of some vegetables when you get home from work. And when I say cook, I mean from scratch. You will need to get used to taking more time to prepare meals, but as always, involve the children in the preparation. This will be good for them too.

Now, one box of instant potatoes is about $3. A 5 pound bag of potatoes is about $3 too. Which one do you think will feed most of you for the longest period of time? Of course the bag of potatoes. You can make mashed potatoes, baked potatoes, home fries for breakfast, potato pancakes, homemade French fries, Sheperd's pie, or even your own hash browns. You can make a ton of meals with that bag and only a side of a meal with that box. See the cost savings?

Other Things to Try. There are many things that you can try in order to cut back on spending and to make sure that your family is getting the nutritious meals that you all need. Here are some...

☐ Get a water filter – This way, you don't have to worry about always buying bottled water. (See "The Importance Of Water")

☐ Learn to eat new healthy things like cauliflower, cabbage, squash, zucchini, eggplant, and other things besides the popular veggies like broccoli, peas, string beans, and carrots.

☐ Avoid soda – it is not only unhealthy, but it is expensive and if you have children can be contributing to headaches, behavioral problems, and other issues.

☐ Use smaller plates, cups and bowls. We tend to overeat in this country. Don't worry. You will not cheat your family of their needed nutrition.

☐ If you can't afford fresh vegetables, buy frozen. You must have some sort of vegetables in your diet each day

☐ Keep Food Fresh – Be sure that when you close packages or containers, you get rid of the air in it first. Air is a breeding ground for bacteria to grow. Use the green bags made to keep produce fresher longer. They may sell them in your produce section. Keep onions away from other produce. The natural sulphur in them will ripen your stuff too soon.

- If you buy spoiled food, don't hesitate to return it. I've held on to stuff for 2 weeks just so I could get a replacement or get a credit or my money back when I returned it. Food is too expensive to literally just throw away.

- Avoid canned foods. But if you do get them, wash the cans with warm, soapy water, then rinse the food after you've opened the can. Rinsing will get all the added salt and sugar from syrup off of the food before you eat it.

- If you make burgers or some sort of patties, you can add things to it to bulk it up like oatmeal, beans, rice, cornmeal, cream of wheat, chopped vegetables, and other things laying around that will give it some weight.

- Don't eat out of the box or bag. You will probably eat more than if you just pour some out in your hand.

Finally, at www.EatDrinkBetter.com, Rachel Fox provides the following advice on saving money by storing and reheating food:

> The summer season provides us with bountiful farmer's markets and overflowing gardens. An easy way to save food dollars is to cook in batches. You can pre-portion meal servings and refrigerate/freeze them for later. Leftovers make for easy lunch planning and are a life saver when you have no time to make dinner. Remember these eight tips when enjoying your leftovers.

- Keep stored food cold. The bacterial danger zone is between 41-140 degrees Fahrenheit. Purchase a refrigerator thermometer to double check your temperature.

- Travel safely. If you need to bring your lunch to work, keep it in a cooler while in transit to your workplace. Maintaining the cold temperature is important in preventing bacterial growth.

- Don't save food forever. Leftover food should be kept in the refrigerator for 7 days or less. If you need to, put date labels on storage containers.

- When in doubt, throw it out! If your food looks funny, smells funny or feels funny...it's probably time to pitch it. (See "Food Poisoning")

- Reheat thoroughly. Your reheated food should be too hot to eat for 2 minutes after cooking. If you can eat your leftovers right out of the oven (toaster oven/microwave) you have not heated it hot enough to kill harmful bacteria.

- Don't reheat in plastic! Ever wonder why reusable containers turn red after heating tomato sauce? The sauce is melted into the container and yes the container melts into the sauce. Don't eat your plastic containers anymore; reheat in glass/ceramic.

Follow the above advice to get the most food for your money. Remember what is most important when creating a budget.

READING (AND UNDERSTANDING) FOOD LABELS

BY SATORI ANANDA

Knowledge of self is more than just the history of yourself; it also includes the *current* understanding of who you are as well. The old saying you are what you eat has proven to be true. Nutrition Labels can help us to determine what we are putting into our bodies when we choose to consume packaged food. **Taking nothing on face value is an excellent principle especially when dealing with food labels.** For example, **in 2003 the FDA permitted the manufacturers of food products sold in the United States to make health claims on food labels which are supported by less than conclusive evidence.** In other words a health claim can be made on very limited scientific facts. Keep in mind the best and healthiest choice of consuming fruits and vegetables requires no understanding and deciphering of complicated and misleading labels. (See "I'll Be Your Pusher: The FDA")

Popular trends of drinking "specialized" water or antioxidant drinks especially highlight the misleading labels. Knowing what is actually in drinks like Vitamin Water would have most of us putting that very "anti-healthy" drink right back on the shelf and saving money by drinking plain old H20. An actual ingredient list off one of those fancy waters reads: *Reverse Osmosis Water, Cane Sugar, Crystalline Fructose, Citric Acid, Vegetable Juice (Color), Ascorbic Acid (Vitamin C), Natural Flavor, Berry and Fruit Extracts (Acai, Blueberry, Pomegranate and Apple), Magnesium Mate (Electrolyte), Calcium Lactate (Electrolyte), Monopotassium Phosphate (Electrolyte), Niacin (B3), Pantothenic Acid (B5), Pyridoxine Hydrochloride (B6), Cyanocobalamin (B12)*

> **Did You Know?**
> Coca Cola's defense lawyers – when hit with a lawsuit about the (fraudulent) health claims of Vitamin Water – felt comfortable responding, "No consumer could reasonably be misled into thinking Vitamin Water was a healthy beverage." They really said that. Apparently, 50 Cent wasn't joking when he rapped, "I took quarter water, sold it in bottles for 2 bucks/Coca-Cola came and bought it for billions, what the f*ck?"

What it should say is simply: *water, sugar, colors, needless vitamins and minerals.* Oh and that Crystalline Fructose sounds so pretty! But it's just another form of sugar, derived from corn. Similar to high fructose corn syrup (HFCS) on steroids, as it is 98% fructose. One bottle contains 8 teaspoons of needless, useless sugar, at 125 calories.

So we have two methods of labeling that occurs. One method will not list all of the ingredients so as to mislead us and the other method will list all of the ingredients to well… mislead us. Frustrating I know. But **here are some tips to keep in mind to help understanding** language used in labels.

The Daily Values are based on a 2,000-calorie a day diet. Based on the calorie count of the meals you eat, it's important to know whether something is providing only 5% of something you need (like Iron), which means you'll need 20 servings to get your daily needs…or 30% of something you don't want (like sugar, cholesterol, fat, or sodium), which means if you eat 4 servings, you're ODing on something unhealthy.

Labeling deceptions include using words like "light" to mean light in color; flavor or texture, misleading us into thinking the product is low in calories or fat. **"Natural" means absolutely nothing, because there's no FDA standard for it, unlike "Organic" which has very specific standards.**[23] "Made with real fruit" often means fruit flavor is used. Not actual fruit. "Free" doesn't mean much either. **Words like "fat free" are allowed to be used if the product has less than 0.5 grams per serving**

Serving Size – All the information (from calories to vitamins) is based on a predetermined serving size. So the nutrition facts found on the label are based on one serving of the product, not the whole thing! For example, a 20 ounce bottle of Coke has 2.5 servings, so drinking the whole bottle means you are getting more than double the calories and sugar listed on the label.

Ingredients – The label lists ingredients from greatest amount to least. If you are trying to watch a certain ingredient such as sugar or salt make sure that it is not listed as one of the first three ingredients.

100% of anything can't have any other ingredient!! So if it says 100% wheat check the ingredients and make sure.

Fresh is used on poultry to indicate that the meat was not cooled below 26 degrees Fahrenheit.(6 degrees below freezing). Not very fresh if it was frozen.

Free Range is a label regulated by USDA and can be used if the animal had some access to the outdoors each day for some unspecified period of time, even a few minutes.

---

[23] The National Organic Program, enacted in 2002, restricts the use of the term "Organic" to certified organic producers. The term "natural" can, and is, used freely but isn't regulated like "Organic." If you don't see the word Organic – it's not.

The **Nutrition Facts** lists nutrients such as fiber and sugars. When you are eating carbohydrates (from the grain group), look for foods with high fiber. When you look at the fat content, all fat is not the same. Choose healthy UNsaturated fats. (See "Butter Vs. Margarine" and "What Are Trans Fats?") Choose foods and drinks low in sugar. Every 4 grams of sugar listed on the label is equal to 1 teaspoon of sugar. Picture how many teaspoons of sugar are in a bottle of Mountain Dew with 77 grams of sugar per serving! (You can check out www.sugarstacks.com to get a visual image using sugar cubes)

You should look for vitamin and mineral content as well, but don't weigh them heavier than the stuff above, because you can get fooled that way. **Chemically added vitamins and minerals doesn't mean you're eating healthier if you're eating something loaded with sugar and fat.** Now let's test what you've learned! Check out the Nutrition Facts labels here. Which label is a better choice? Why? (Think of 3 reasons.)

Nutrition Facts

Serving Size ¾ cup
Servings per Container 11

Amount per serving

Calories 100   Calories from Fat 10

	% Daily value*
Total Fat 1g	
Saturated Fat 0g	
Trans Fat 0g	
Polyunsaturated Fat 0g	
Monounsaturated Fat 0g	
Cholesterol 0mg	
Sodium 150mg	
Total Carbohydrate 26g	
Dietary Fiber 6g	
Sugars 6g	
Protein 2g	

Vitamin A 0%	Vitamin C 15%
Calcium 0%	Iron 1%

*Percent Daily Values are based on a 2,000 calorie diet. Your daily values may be higher or lower depending on your caloric needs:

Calories	2,000	2,500
Total Fat	Less than	65g	80g
Sat. Fat	Less than	20g	25g
Cholesterol	Less than	300mg	300mg
Sodium	Less than	2,400mg	2,400mg
Total Carbohydrates		300g	375g
Dietary Fiber		25g	30g

Calories per gram:
Fat 9 • Carbohydrate 4 • Protein 4

Nutrition Facts

Serving Size ¾ cup
Servings per Container 13

Amount per serving

Calories 170   Calories from Fat 30

	% Daily value*
Total Fat 3g	
Saturated Fat 0.5g	
Trans Fat 0g	
Polyunsaturated Fat 0g	
Monounsaturated Fat 0g	
Cholesterol 5mg	
Sodium 240mg	
Total Carbohydrate 29g	
Dietary Fiber 0g	
Sugars 18g	
Protein 6g	

Vitamin A 30%	Vitamin C 25%
Calcium 15%	Iron 25%

*Percent Daily Values are based on a 2,000 calorie diet. Your daily values may be higher or lower depending on your caloric needs:

Calories	2,000	2,500
Total Fat	Less than	65g	80g
Sat. Fat	Less than	20g	25g
Cholesterol	Less than	300mg	300mg
Sodium	Less than	2,400mg	2,400mg
Total Carbohydrates		300g	375g
Dietary Fiber		25g	30g

Calories per gram:
Fat 9 • Carbohydrate 4 • Protein 4

If you chose the first one, give yourself a pat on the back. You've learned a lot. The label on the left is higher in fiber, lower in sugar, and has no saturated fat.

Know what to look for when reading food labels. If you don't know what you're looking at, you don't know what you're buying.

TIPS AND TOOLS FOR HEALTHY EATING
BY BRYANT TERRY
AUTHOR OF VEGAN SOUL KITCHEN

Look, I won't pretend that I make every meal from scratch. I enjoy eating out and being served as much as the next man. But I do realize the costs (and I'm not just talking about money). Food eaten outside the home has more salt, more sugar, more fat, and almost twice the calories of meals prepared at home. Why, you might ask? 'Cause salt, sugar, and fat taste good and don't cost much to produce. So think about it, if you are selling food for mass consumption, overloading your products with inexpensive salt, sugar, and fat makes good business sense. Processed, packaged, and fast food is cheap to make; this type of food can last a long time without rotting once you add preservatives to it; and you can turn major profits by selling a lot of it. (See "The Food That Never Spoils")

Some Equipment to Help You Become a Better Cook
Baking Sheets: Whether you are heating frozen fries, roasting carrots from scratch, or baking canned biscuits, you should keep a baking sheet handy. And a good oven glove will keep you from burning your hands.

Blender: You can find a good blender for less than 20 bucks. Use it for making smoothies before and after workouts and blending soups made from scratch. Remember not to fill it more than halfway if you are blending hot liquids or you will get burned.

Colander: Keep a large colander (12-inch) handy for draining (and washing) vegetables, beans, grains, and pastas after cooking.

Cutting Board: I won't pretend I've never cut straight onto a counter before. But after getting cursed out by moms for scratching up her surfaces, I made sure I used a cutting board after that. In order to avoid getting food poisoning you should keep at least two: one for preparing fish and meat and another for vegetables. Use woodcutting boards since bacteria can't thrive on them and they won't make your knife as dull as other types of cutting boards.

Grater: Perfect for shredding cheese for tacos and vegetables for salads.

Knives: If you are serious about throwin' down in the kitchen you should invest in a good chef's knife. If you take good care of it, your knife should last for a couple of generations.

Measuring Cups and Spoons: Unless you already feel comfortable enough to freestyle when you are cooking, owning some plastic or metal measuring cups and spoons (for dry goods) and glass cups (for liquids) will help you follow recipes with ease.

Peeler: A solid Y-shaped swivel peeler is great for peeling the skin off potatoes and other vegetables and fruits.

Pots and Pans: Unless you choose to invest in a set of pots and pans, you should decide what a priority is and slowly build your arsenal. Here are a few options to consider:

❏ 10-inch fry pan	❏ 3-qt. sauté pan with lid
❏ 4-qt. saucepan with lid	❏ 7-qt. stockpot with lid

Salad Spinner: Assuming that you will be eating more salads after reading this book…invest in a salad spinner to wash your greens before dressing.

Spoons: Next to the stone axe, a wooden spoon is probably the oldest tool known to man. Get you one or two.

Tongs: Think of these as your metal fingers when cooking. Whether on the stove or the grill, a pair of tongs is great for frying, roasting and barbecuing.

There are tools for every job. If you are working towards better health, these are your tools.

BASIC COOKING TECHNIQUES
BY EBONI JOY ASIATIC

I understand that if we're going to recommend that you eat less fast and processed food, and microwaved meals…many of you will have a hard time because you think you don't know how to cook. Once you know a little about these techniques you'll be much less intimidated to try new things in the kitchen.

Boiling
To boil food is to cook it in liquid, usually water, that is boiling – rapid or "rolling" bubbling, breaking bubbles into steam – at a temperature of 212° F. With a lid on the pot the liquid will come to a boil faster, and prevent evaporation. If left uncovered, liquid will evaporate quicker increasing the risk of burning one's food. **If the pot is too full the liquid will boil over onto the stove top.**

The advantages of boiling one's food is that it is relatively safe (no chance of a grease fire) **and simple, and the best means to producing a flavored stock.** Tough leafy greens (like collards) become edible and still retain their nutritive value when not boiled for too long. The disadvantages, however, is that generally soluble vitamins are extracted out of the food and into the water it has been boiled in, also boiled foods can become limp and withered looking. When I do boil foods I strive to retain the water turned juice as a broth.

Steaming

Steaming works by allowing water to be heated to its boiling point, maintaining a rolling boil as the water vaporizes into steam. The steam then carries heat to the food that's typically placed in a circular metal or bamboo steamer basket and a lid placed on top during cooking. **By keeping the food separate from the boiling water, it's cooked by the steam, maintaining many of its nutrients, enzymes and moist, yet crunchy, texture.** The only food that cannot be cooked by steaming are mushrooms – they will get water-logged. Steaming veggies shouldn't take longer than 5 minutes, including time to sprinkle on a little sea salt and ground black pepper.

Frying

A technique of cooking food at high temperatures in oil or fat – difference being their melting point and fats are solid at room temperature. The crispy surface that develops in fried foods allows for moisture to be retained under the surface so that fried foods are both crispy and juicy. Shallow, deep, and stir frying, sautéing, and pan searing are all common frying techniques requiring more or less oil, and categorized based on what kind of pan or fryer the food is cooked in – a frying pan, deep fryer, griddle, or wok.

Shallow frying is placing food only halfway covered in pre-heated oil inside a shallow frying pan or skillet. In deep frying, the food is submerged in oil that has been pre-heated in a deep fryer. Some fried foods are battered or breaded before frying, allowing the outside to become golden and crispy, yet maintaining tender juiciness underneath.

Both frying techniques cook food relatively fast. Proper frying temperature depends on the thickness and toughness of the food being prepared (think sweet potato vs. eggplant), but most food is typically fried at 350–375° F.

Stir Frying

This involves frying quickly at very high temperatures, requiring the food be stirred continuously to prevent it from sticking to the wok and burning. This technique originated in China, and by cooking bite-sized chopped tofu and vegetables (or whatever you choose) in a wok very quickly and at high heat, followed by a quick steam-in sauce you can cook a complete one-pot wonder meal. When stir frying, your oil must be heated in the wok first, the foods that take longest to cook should be placed in the wok next – for instance, you would first fry your meat or meat substitute, then add onions and carrots after about 4 to 5 minutes, and then broccoli and squash for the last couple minutes of cooking. And when the food is about two-thirds done, add your sauce, cover the wok, and your food should steam for a minute or two.

All ingredients must be prepped before you start cooking to prevent burning and sticking. And because you're cooking at high heat, you'll need to use an oil with a high smoke point like peanut, safflower, corn or canola.

Sauté

Sautéing and pan frying (or searing) vary only slightly in that in searing you use less heat and cook larger portions of solid food like half an eggplant, a chicken breast, or a fish steak. In searing, you do not have to stir, toss or flip your ingredients as frequently as when sautéing. Because the heat is lower when sautéing, you can even prepare foods in butter – or a vegan butter – without fear of burning, but foods that require less cooking time must only be prepared with butter because it burns much more easily than oil. Non-stick pans are good for sautéing in light oil or butter, however, if you are creating a sauce a metal pan helps to create browning. Make sure your pan is hot enough before adding the fat/oil and cold ingredients or the juices in the food can be released as the pan heats up, and your food becomes dry.

Baking

In general, the term baking is used in reference to cakes, pies, pastries and breads; and means "immersing the object to be cooked in an environment of still, hot air." This is why we pre-heat our ovens before placing our food in it to bake, so that all of the air in the oven reaches the same temperature and the food being prepared cooks evenly. Baking in convection ovens require less baking time and less heat (25 to 50 degrees lower). Baking in high altitudes requires more time and higher baking temperatures.

Roasting

Roasting is the baking of food – not bread and desserts – in an open pan, uncovered. When roasting meat, the meat is usually placed on a rack that fits inside a fairly shallow pan, so that the meat does not sit in its "juices." The difference between roasting and baking is that you typically roast food that has structure already, like meats and vegetables. And baked foods are those that require rising, or whose structure changes during the baking process, like cakes, pies, breads, and casseroles.

Roasting is often considered a healthier method of cooking foods because of the need for less oil and fat in the preparation process – however, basting is often required to keep foods from drying out. Poultry should be cooked breast down to start and finished on the flip side so that the fat ("juice") drips into the breast meat. This can also be used to create gravies and sauces.

You must always pre-heat your oven before roasting, and in roasting your thermostat is usually set at a high temperature (375-450° F), this seals the outer layer of your food and prevents the loss of juices while also caramelizing the surface. After about 20 minutes, the temperature can be lowered to about 350° F for the remaining cooking time.

Choosing a roasting pan is of vital importance – if it is too big your food will burn, too small and your food will stick to the pan, too deep and your food will steam (not roast), and too shallow and the juices will splatter all over the oven causing a horrible mess and difficult clean-up job.

Braise

Braising is a cooking technique in which the main ingredient is seared, or browned in fat, then simmered in liquid on low heat in a covered pot for a relatively long range of time – from 1 to 6 hours – depending on what you're cooking. The best equipment for this process is a crock pot, pressure cooker or Dutch oven, and can be done on the stove top or in the oven. Braising is typically used as a means to cook less expensive, tough cuts of meat. The end result is said to be tender and flavorful. However, since we are building on "hood health" we recommend that you refrain from eating cheap, tough cuts of meat – as inexpensive cuts are almost always higher in fat which causes heart health problems, and tougher meats are harder to digest and begin to decompose in your intestines and colon before they can be digested – leading to colon cancer. Vegetables that are ideal for braising include squash, sweet potatoes, leeks, parsnips, carrots, beets, cabbage and onions.

Stew

People tend to think of stew as a dish rather than a cooking method, but it's actually both, and the dish itself is defined as "meat or fish and vegetables cooked by stewing." This cooking method, is "a moist heat cooking process by which meat and vegetables are slowly simmered in a flavorful liquid."

There is really very little difference between braising and stewing. In a braise the meat and/or vegetables are typically left whole, in a stew they are cut in chunks. In a stew the meat and/or vegetables are completely submerged in their cooking liquid, when braised, the liquid doesn't come further than halfway up the food being prepared.

Did you know that chili is a stew? And French Ratatouille is simply stewed vegetables. Vegetables ideal for stewing include eggplant, tomatoes, celery, celery root, leeks, cabbage, fennel, carrots, potatoes, onions, garlic and almost any tough greens, such as collard greens, chard, kale or mustard greens.

Grilling

All too often the terms grilling and barbecuing are used interchangeably, when they are quite different, and true barbecuing is rare. Traditional barbecue is done slowly, with low cooking temperatures, with lots of smoke accumulating over an open (preferably wood fire rather than charcoal) pit. A gas grill cannot accomplish this goal.

Grilling, however, requires a higher temperature to sear what's being cooked in order to preserve the food's juices. In fact, if you are comparing grilling to any other cooking method, the most similar would be broiling – as they both use a high heat source, however the grill's heat comes from below, whereas the broiler's heat comes from above. They are both ideal means of cooking tender cuts of red meat, poultry, fish and vegetables – and let's not forget our meat alternatives like seitan, tempeh and tofu. Whatever you're grilling, you want to ensure that it isn't too thick to cook properly on the interior otherwise be stricken with a food borne illness.

Although grilling is considered by many to be a healthier way to cook because the fat drips off of the food and into the fire, inhaling smoke is never good for the lungs, and the charring process isn't particularly good for our intestinal tract or digestive system. When grilling, you must also be careful to avoid flare-ups – don't want to burn your food or yourself!

Vital notes on grilling: **Bring your food to room temperature before placing it on the grill.**

Start with a clean grill. The best time to clean (remove residue from) a grill is immediately after you finish cooking and the grate is still hot.

Brush or spray the grill with oil to prevent food from sticking.

The grill must be pre-heated 15 to 30 minutes before food is placed on it.

Put all of your cooking utensils, seasonings and sauces near the grill before you put the food on it, and have a spray bottle filled with water on hand in case of flare-ups.

Every grill is different and will have different hot and cool spots. It's important for you to learn where they are and use them to your advantage. Marinating your food to be grilled for as long as possible is the best way to ensure a flavorful meal – but your food must be patted dry before being placed on the grill in order to reduce dripping which prevents flare-ups. Our favorite "hood" marinade – barbecue sauce – which is nothing more than the perfect combination of pureed tomatoes, vinegar, onion, mustard and brown sugar – it is so easy to create your own by also adding your preferred spices (mine are spike, with salt, and powdered jerk seasoning).

The time frame for which it takes your ingredients to grill differs – refer to your favorite cookbook for timing guidelines.

Broiling

Broiling is cooking your food in the bottom compartment of your oven, and allowing it to be cooked via infrared radiation from the oven's top burner, so your food is being cooked from above rather than below, as in baking and grilling. The downside to broiling is that lots of splattering occurs causing a clean-up mess and smoke can repeatedly set off the fire alarm. This is why most people prefer to grill, and why, when broiling, it's imperative to make sure the broiler pan, which catches excess liquid and grease, is always in place before you start to broil any food.

The upside to broiling if you are a meat eater is that the broiler does not have to pre-heat, and is a fast method for cooking meats, poultry and fish, and gives it a nice dark char. The broiler is actually located in a compartment beneath the oven, pull the drawer all the way out and it usually folds down for easy removal of the broiler pan or the flipping of food. Every oven's thermostat knob has a "broil" position.

Blanching

Blanching is a cooking term that "describes a process of food preparation wherein the food substance, usually a vegetable or fruit, is plunged into boiling water, removed after a brief, timed interval, and finally plunged into iced water or placed under cold running water (shocked) to halt the cooking process." Many fruits and vegetables can be frozen and preserved once blanched (I have done this with leeks, onions and celery). Blanching literally means "to whiten" but often, its purpose is to so soften a food, remove an overwhelming taste, or even preserve the original vibrant color of a food before cooking it in another manner. Upon blanching nuts, the skin of the nut becomes softened by blanching and can be removed once cooled.

Live/Raw

Yes, you're right, preparing live/raw food is not "cooking." So why mention it? Because it's an important aspect of food preparation, and eating fresh, uncooked vegetables, fruits, grains, nuts, seeds, and sprouts is necessary in acquiring health for ourselves, our families and our community. Incorporating raw foods into your diet doesn't require special tools or special knowledge (but a few recipes that go beyond salads can help!). You will find some raw foodists create amazing meals with a dehydrator that can heat food without cooking it. A seasoned raw foodist will also have a frequently used juicer and food processor in their kitchen as well.

Be Prepared

Finally, the last bit of best advice I can give as a professional cook is about *mise en place* (pronounced MEEZ ahn plahs), which translates from French as "to put in place" – which means before you start cooking have all of your ingredients prepared. Have them on hand for one (to avoid running to the grocery store at the last minute), and have them washed, peeled, deseeded, chopped, diced, andjulienned.), etc.

The times have been too frequent when I've delved into a recipe and halfway through the cooking process I realize I'm missing an ingredient and I have to substitute with another or run to the grocery store in mid process. I have also found my food burning uncontrollably as I cut vegetables while another ingredient is cooking and the entire dish is ruined. Trust me when I say you will save yourself a world of hurt by making a comprehensive list of ingredients before you start cooking, double check to make sure you have them on hand, and prep them as need be before turning on a single burner on your stove.

And keep in mind one of the greatest sayings in the culinary world – cooking is an art, so experiment with flavors and textures and turn your favorite recipe into your own unique creation; baking is a science, stick to the blueprint and you can't go wrong!

These techniques will have you preparing healthy meals in no time. You can start slow, by trying out one technique a week.

QUICK VEGETARIAN COOKING TIPS
BY SUPREME UNDERSTANDING

Smaller = quicker. Instead of trying to cook one large solid item, cut it or break it into very small pieces. (Instead of a baked potato, try potato cubes!) Likewise, thin spaghetti will cook faster than thick.

Frozen, not fresh. Sure, fresh is better, but often, you may not have made the time to prepare fresh vegetables. Frozen veggies can be stored for long periods and microwaved quickly in small portions on an "as needed" basis. They may not be as crunchy or as nutritious, but it's better than NO veggies!

Work vegetables into everything. Even an "ordinary" sandwich or burger could be improved by throwing in some spinach leaves or mushrooms. And adding green and yellow/orange veggies (most of which are easy to freeze and store) to a meal is always good nutritionally.

Sauté Substitute. You can heat chopped onions, green peppers, etc. for a slight time in the microwave to "soften." Also, fresh mushrooms can be "cooked" when microwaved in a small dish of water or diluted marinade.

Eat your leftovers. You can take left-overs from a stir-fry and turn them into a sandwich, or take unused vegetables from another recipe and throw together a quick soup. Waste not, want not...saves time and money.

Beans and Rice Ideas

Bulk beans, grains, and rice are always really cheap. Unfortunately, they often take a while to make. But, fortunately, they also are easy to keep once made. With that in mind, always make yourself a double, triple, or more batch and freeze the rest. In the long run, you'll save lots of money and lots of time.

Vegetarian Baked Beans. Use baked beans that are specifically labeled "vegetarian." Bush's are great. Eat with whole wheat bread, small potato, and side of steamed vegetable.

Vegetarian Chili. Start with canned or pre-cooked beans (experiment with different beans, including kidney beans, black beans, pinto beans, etc.). Things to add: spice (chili powder, cayenne Pepper, etc.), sautéed onions, green pepper, garlic, canned tomatoes or tomato paste, salsa or barbecue sauce, macaroni or other pasta, Bac-O's or other fake bacon/ham bits, crumbled veggie burger (or try veggie ground beef like Ground Meatless from Morningstar)

Refried Beans for Burritos. There are lots of great low/no fat types.

Microwave beans and tortillas separately. Add your favorite veggies, sauces, etc. Chunky salsa is quick when short on time.

Steamed Vegetables or Squash on Rice. Topping ideas: a little grated cheese, lemon pepper, oregano, ground black pepper, salsa and other sauces (For a quicker version than steaming your veggies, you can take refrigerated, pre-cooked rice and microwave frozen veggies on top) Brown rice instead of white will increase the nutrition value of the rice and is just as cheap, but takes a little longer to cook.

Black Beans and Rice. Cheaters version: heat can of beans in a pan, add garlic powder, onion powder, salt and pepper serve over rice. Non-cheaters: Sauté real onions and garlic, then add beans.

Red Beans and Rice. Sauté a can (or two) of red beans in some oil with onions, garlic, and salt add two cups rice 4 cups water and a heaping teaspoon of fake veggie broth powder. Cover and let cook 20 mins. Serve with salsa. (You can add veggies to this too.)

Refried Beans and Rice. Take a can of no-fat refried beans and add an equal amount of salsa. Add a 10 oz. package of frozen peas or fresh veggies. Put in pan and cook until hot. Serve over rice or toast.

Pasta Ideas

"Pre-sauce" pasta will store for a few days in the fridge if you keep it in a closed container. So just like beans, rice, and grains, cook extra pasta and then microwave for a quick pasta meal a few days later.

Spaghetti. Cook frozen mixed veggies and serve them over pasta w/ canned sauce or your own. Note: Traditional Hunt's in a can is always the cheapest and best. Consumer Reports rated it as tasty as sauces costing 2 or 3 times more. No sugar added too!

Mac and Cheese. Topping ideas: broccoli, mushrooms, garlic, oregano, green pepper, cayenne pepper, shreds of veggie meat or veggie bacon bits.

Egg Drop Ramen with Veggies. Boil water, add Ramen, add fresh or frozen veggies (like green onions and frozen peas) and an egg or two. Stir till Ramen is done

Tomatoes and Chiles Pasta. Add a can of tomatoes and chilies to your favorite pasta shape. Possible garnishes/seasonings: salt and pepper, fresh lime juice, coriander leaves, basil leaves, mint leaves, chives, garlic, curry powder (but not much!)

Pizza Ideas

Dough ideas: Store bought pizza crust (readymade), store bought pizza dough (the kind in a tube), French bread, bagel halves, English muffins, tortillas (the kind used for quesadillas), pita bread.

Sauce ideas: If you can't make your own or buy pizza sauce, just use spaghetti sauce (or tomato slices/paste) and spices instead.

Topping Ideas: Mushrooms, garlic, cheeses, bell peppers, onions, veggie meat, veggie bacon bits, sundried tomatoes, spinach, artichoke, eggplant, jalapenos, whatever you can imagine (from pineapples to zucchini)

Salad Ideas

Make salads easy by making them in advance. Pre-cut your lettuce and carefully choose toppings for easy salad making. Cut, wash and dry lettuce on Sunday before the work week. If the lettuce was freshly bought, it should last until Friday. This is where a salad spinner comes in handy. Choose toppings that don't need to be cut or are hardy. Don't pre-dress salads – they will get soggy. Pre-make salad dressing and put into a travel-size bottle. A vinaigrette won't spoil if left on your desk from morning until lunch. Lemon and lime wedges also make a great salad dressings.

Base Ideas: Start with leafy greens, such as lettuce (not Iceberg though!), cabbage, spinach, kale, field greens, etc.

Topping Ideas: Slices or shreds of veggie cheese, feta cheese crumbs, hard-boiled eggs, boiled potato chunks, sliced tomatoes, canned beans, canned or marinated artichoke hearts, pimientos, pepperoncini (and other hot peppers), veggie meat or fake bacon bits, croutons, Chinese noodles, cashews, pecans, walnuts, sunflower seeds, pumpkin seeds, flax seeds, radishes, onions, raisins, cranberries, grapes, cherry tomatoes or grape tomatoes, sundried tomatoes, and any other vegetables you have lying around (like broccoli, carrots, asparagus, green, red, and yellow peppers, cucumbers, etc.)

Sprinkle the whole thing with some dressing or vinaigrette.

Sandwich Ideas

Start with whole grain bread (Try to find "good" heavy bread made from whole grains rather than the super bleached out/processed white flour variety. It's worth it.)

"Meat" Ideas: Sliced mushrooms (dry or marinated), grilled tempeh, veggie patties/veggie burgers (If you're not shopping at a health foods store, veggie burgers are still available in most supermarkets. They are usually found in the frozen food section next to the Egg Beaters, bagels, and waffles), veggie deli meat (also usually available near the produce section), refried beans, veggie chili, marinated/sautéed vegetables.

Other Ingredient Ideas: Lettuce, spinach leaves, other leafy things, jalapeno slices, pickles, sprouts, potato chips, Chinese noodles, hummus, veggie bacon bits, veggie cheese (you really can't taste the difference), garlic powder, cayenne pepper, dill, lemon pepper, tomatoes, mushrooms, onions, pickles, green pepper, barbecue sauce, mustard, ketchup, mayonnaise, salsa.

Stir Fry Ideas

You can stirfry (or sauté) your way into some very easy (and healthy) Asian-inspired dishes. (See "Basic Cooking Techniques") This is a way to get lots of vegetables into your diet.

"Base" ideas: Rice, couscous, lo mein noodles (you can use spaghetti noodles stir-fried with some onion and soy sauce), any starchy product (from bread to pasta)

Topping ideas: Chopped up fresh or frozen veggies (anything you can imagine, depending on the flavor you're going for) veggie meat chunks, eggs (add egg or two, fry rice until egg is done), onions, scallions, mushrooms, soy sauce, hoisin sauce, sesame seeds, teriyaki sauce, salsa, peanut sauce (peanut butter, soy sauce, garlic, and crushed red pepper), peanuts.

Other Ideas

Baked Potatoes (microwaving can work if your time is short). Topping ideas: salsa, barbecue sauce, ketchup, mustard, spaghetti sauce, spice/seasoning (cayenne pepper, garlic powder, black pepper, etc.), broccoli chunks, stir-fried veggies, homemade chili, cheese (colby, swiss, parmesan) or veggie cheese alternative, veggie bacon bits, sour cream and chives, and anything else you can imagine.

Omelets or Hash Browns. Topping ideas: cheese, mushrooms, onions, jalapenos, diced tomatoes, spinach, vegetables.

Quinoa, millet, or other grain with veggies. Sauté grain in oil. Add water, simmer, and add small pieces of veggies. Cook until done

Couscous with veggies or spaghetti sauce. Put couscous in boiling water for 5 min. with a little tamari, salt, onion, and curry.

Soup. Sauté onions, garlic, etc. in oil. Then add canned tomatoes, more water, celery, carrot, basil, bay leaf, other vegetables, dried beans, barley, grains, potato, etc. Throw it all in a pot and cook for 1-3 hours. Not a 15 minute meal, but if you make a bunch, it will pay off.

For more ideas, and over 1,000 of the world's best vegetarian meal and drink recipes, check out *A Taste of Life: 1,000 Vegetarian Recipes from Around the World*, available from Supreme Design Publishing.

DETOX

FASTING AND CLEANSING

Say what you want about 50 Cent's ethics, you can't knock the man's self-discipline. In May of 2010, photos of him hit the web, showing him down from a bulky 214 lbs. to an almost bony (by comparison) 160 lbs. He'd lost over 50 pounds in about two months!

The internet gossipers thought he was smoking crack or had AIDS. That may have been true for ███████████████ and ███████████████, but not Fifty. He did it to star in *Things Fall Apart*, a film he wrote about a football player who gets diagnosed with cancer. I'm not normally a fan of his "act" but can you say anything negative about that? Doesn't matter, because 90% of Curtis Jackson's critics can't do what he does. And I don't mean attending Illuminati meetings and drinking goat's blood, or whatever the latest gossip is. I'm talking about the fact that, **even though he's surrounded by the madness of the music industry, he doesn't smoke, doesn't drink** (Read *How to Hustle and Win* for details), **and can lose 54 pounds when he decides to do so.** And damn, at least it's for a good cause. Most of us want to lose weight just so we can look cute.

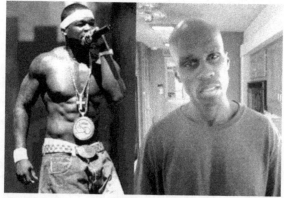

So how did he do it? By going on an all liquid diet and taking daily three-hour walks on a treadmill for nine weeks. That's some serious *drive* and *discipline*. With those two things, anything is possible, whether it's cleansing a toxic system or losing that weight that won't go away. And that type of drive and discipline is not out of your reach. In fact, Fifty ain't the only one in the hip hop world to go on a liquid diet. Trina's done it. Beyonce does it. And plenty of dudes have done it, but probably won't admit it, because fasting and cleansing don't seem like "gangster" things to do. Why not? You really ain't *that* gangster if you start crying and complaining every time you ain't had something to eat. And that's where most of us are at. We can't even imagine going without solid food for a few days, much less nine weeks. Why? We're spoiled. Original people throughout the world survive on less food and drink over a week than what we run through in a day. So it's not impossible. It's just a decision you make.

In *How to Hustle and Win, Part One*, I describe how Buddhist monk Thích Quang Đuc set himself on fire in front of a Cambodian embassy as a political protest...and didn't flinch or scream once as he burned to death. I compare that degree of internal discipline to that of the typical male in America, who can barely control himself once a female touches him the right way...even if it could mean him losing his job, his wife, his freedom, or millions of dollars. I'm sure I don't have to name any examples for those (You may be one of them). Anyway, I use those examples to illustrate how many of us are in serious need of internal discipline. Yet we rarely develop it. **Instead we pursue external discipline, which is when others are responsible for making us do what we should. But external discipline doesn't last. And it's not consistent, like internal discipline, which is when you do what you should even when no one else is watching.**

So how do you start disciplining yourself? As I explain in *How to Hustle and Win*, the way to do that is to deny your "weaker" desires, or those that only satisfy your immediate emotional or physical needs:

So how do you deny yourself? Easy. **You fast.** You're already doing it. Every time you sleep, you're denying yourself of things you do during the day. That's why the first meal of the morning is called breakfast (break "fast"). But to discipline your mind and body, you have to **consciously** deny yourself various things. The following are a few fasts you can take to start developing that Internal Discipline. Man up.

The following are some of the fasts I break down in detail in *How to Hustle and Win, Part One*:

❏ Fasting from Food	❏ Fasting from TV
❏ Juice Fast	❏ Fasting from Talking
❏ Water Fast	❏ Fasting from Sex
❏ Fasting from Meat	❏ Any Vice: (_____)

Pick a fast you plan on doing. How long do you plan on keeping it up? While you're at it, get someone to join you.

21 DAYS

BY SUPREME UNDERSTANDING

ORIGINALLY PUBLISHED IN HOW TO HUSTLE AND WIN, PT. ONE

It takes 21 days to make a habit. Three weeks. **Almost anything you do consistently for that period of time will become habitual.** It's as if you are programming yourself to do something without thinking by doing it over and over again.

I've tried it for myself plenty of times. I've changed the way I walk, the way I get dressed in the morning, how I eat, even how long I watch TV. **People who've read** *How to Hustle and Win* **have told me they've used this advice to do everything from losing weight to quitting smoking.** I even went on a slouching fast that literally made me an inch taller by the 3rd week (You probably slouch more than you know!). **Repetition creates habit.** Why do you think people who have been locked up or in the military act like they are still programmed to make their beds a certain way or hide their toilet paper like an inmate is still going to steal it?

If you part your hair a certain way every day for a period of time, it will eventually start growing out that way until you start brushing it the opposite way. If you start catching yourself every time you say a word like "nigga," in three weeks you won't be saying it by accident any more. It's like a plant being cultivated to grow and produce fruit. You can nurture it with the right elements and bring forth good fruit, or you can water it with poison and produce death.

"Ill habits gather to unseen degrees – As brooks run to rivers, rivers run to seas." – John Dryden (1631-1700)

This information is helpful for two reasons:

First, you can purposefully program yourself to adopt new behaviors in less than a month. If you want to stop wasting money, limit your spending for 21 days and you'll notice your spending habits have changed. The new behavior will now be in place without you having to think about it anymore.

"The unfortunate thing about this world is that the good habits are easier to give up than the bad ones." – W. S. Maugham

Second, you can program yourself without wanting to. If you smoke weed regularly for three weeks, guess what? You've got a weed habit now. I don't care if you never smoked before. In three weeks, you'll have a habit that's hard to shake. You can hang around people with more money than you and overspend for almost a month. After that, you're stuck with spending habits you may not be able to afford. Once the money runs out, you're going into shock. That's when you need another 21 days to reprogram yourself.

Bottom line: Watch your thoughts, they become your actions. Watch your actions, they become your habits. Watch your habits, they become your culture. Watch your culture, it becomes your life. Cultivate yourself or be cultivated. If you can't train yourself, you'll never be in charge.

When you're around others, either you influence them, or they influence you. So, be aware of how you're changing.

DIDDY TAKES A BREAK FROM CHEESECAKE

On March 10, 2009, hip-hop mogul Diddy began a 48 hour juice fast, inspired by producer Jay Electronica. According to Diddy, the "spiritual fast" as he called it, was to help strengthen him in "mind and spirit."

At exactly midnight on the dot, both set out on their journey, writing texts on their official Twitter pages, asking for support and encouragement from their legions of followers.

During the first few hours, the hip-hop mogul joked about smelling some of his favorite foods when there wasn't anything in the room. "I smell fried chicken... even though there's none here... I can still smell it... lol!!!" Diddy wrote.

The next day, there were several times Diddy seemed to almost give in, tweeting, "Man why is everyone eating??? Everywhere I go I see and smell food!!! God help me!" But he managed to "survive" on natural juices for the scheduled two days. Jay Electronica, being a Five Percenter, was more accustomed to fasting (and for much longer). Still, I commend them both. Because the average person can't make it 24 hours without food without losing their mind. Can you? Can you do 3 days?

Things You Should Know about Fasting from Food

On the first day of your fast, you're gonna crave whatever you've been missing…bad. Almost like withdrawal. Especially if you're, say, going from eating a S.A.D. diet to, say, a water fast. Probably not a good idea. You need to move in stages and steps. But even if you transition into a juice fast, and you're already eating light and healthy, it'll still be tough.

You'll probably want to quit, but – unless you're about to pass out – you probably don't need to. You might even feel sick or have a headache, but a lot of that is the toxins leaving you. As a result, your breath will stink too, so brush your teeth often. As Dr. Richard Anderson explains in *Cleanse and Purify Thyself, Book One*:

> It is ironic that, because of cleansing reactions, it sometimes appears that eating fresh raw food makes a person sick, while eating cooked or junk foods makes a person feel temporarily better. All that has really happened in this scenario, however, is that the eating of junk foods has stopped the cleansing process.

Day two will be bad too, because the headaches will really kick in, and you might feel drained, but you'll have less cravings. **By day three, you'll have some incredible mental clarity you didn't have before, your energy will be back, and the headaches will be gone.** This is because your body is making it through a detox cycle successfully.

When you're finally ready to break your fast, it's critical you do it right! Or else you'll actually make yourself sick again! I normally tell people to break fasts with at least one whole day of smoothies, soups, and/or salads only, but other people say you need more time to get the best results. The following guidelines come from *Fasting*, by Tom Coghill (www.fasting.ws):

> For six days, gradually increase the amount of raw fruits and vegetables in your diet. To break a fast and gorge on meat, bread or junk food will be a disaster. Jarring the system this intensely, when the digestive system is re-awakening, can cause stomach cramps, nausea and weakness, negating some of the benefits of a fast.

> First day after the fast: Eat a piece of fruit in the morning and a small bowl of raw vegetable salad for lunch; vegetable broth also is good. Drink freshly made juice for the rest of the day.

> Second day after the fast: Soaked prunes or figs for breakfast. Small bowl of fresh vegetable salad for lunch. Vegetable soup made without salt at dinner. Two apples or a fruit salad eaten between meals. All this in addition to freshly made juices and broths.

> Third day after the fast: Same as the second day, but add a handful of dates or raisins.

Fourth day after the fast: You may return to the diet you have chosen, but it is important to listen to your stomach, eat smaller meals, chew your food and eat according to hunger.

NOTE: When breaking a fast over ten days, a good rule of thumb is that the break-in period should be extended one day for every 4 days of fasting. When breaking from water fasting, go to a juice fast for two days or eat sweet fruits like oranges, mangos or pears.

A fast is like anything that makes you stronger. It's tough in the beginning and toughens you up in the end.

WHY YOU SHOULD FAST
BY YVETTE GZ

To many, fasting is just a remote activity exclusive to religious or spiritual people. Most people associate it with the Muslim Ramadan or the Christian Lent. However, even those folks don't *only* do it for religious purposes. In fact, there's a sh*tload of reasons for one to fast – the 'load of sh*t' in your body being one of the biggest ones.

Why Fasting Works

Iimagine how much power and discipline you would have if you could train your mind to reject the very thing that keeps you alive! This is what fasting primarily teaches you, SELF-CONTROL. **The essential idea is, if you can say no to food, you can say no to anything and everything, even the finest of women/men, the most addicting of drugs, and the most appealing of materials.**

During a fast, you're always aware of your thoughts, behavior, and actions. This is because you've changed an important part of your routine, and you're making a change, consciously.. This awareness gives you more thinking time, and less illogical actions. **In fact, you would most probably reach your highest level of consciousness during a fast.**

Health Reasons

Fasting works wonders on the body. And not just on our bodies but on pretty much every living thing in the animal kingdom, which is why most animals do it when they are sick. Fasting does three main things to the body: cleanses, heals, and rejuvenates.

1. Cleansing: Also known as detoxification, because what you're doing is removing toxins from your body. Too many of them can cause serious chronic illnesses, the worse being cancer. We get toxins in our bodies everyday by drinking unpurified water, eating processed foods or produce that contain traces of pesticides, breathing filthy air, smoking, drinking, taking certain medications, stress and indigestion.

Most of these toxins are stored in your body fat. This is why obese or overweight people have traces of weed/drugs in their system for a longer period than their slimmer counterparts. When you fast, you're cutting off your energy supply (food), which forces your body to go to your stored body fat to produce energy, breaking down fat molecules and releasing toxins and flushing them out. The longer you fast, the more you cleanse your body, and the better you feel.

2. Healing: Your body is smart and usually knows which moves to make whenever changes or incidents happen. When you don't eat, your digestive system works less, which means less energy is being consumed. So instead of that energy just laying around in your body, it goes about to find something else to work on: your immune system. Without food interfering, your body works more efficiently by producing the right amount of hormones and renewing protein and other helpful cells (for example the white blood cells needed to fight bacteria). This is why you lose your appetite when you fall sick. Your body is telling you to take a break from snacking to let it do its job!

The benefit of fasting while healthy is the strengthening of your immune system while it's inactive. With fewer bacteria in your body, it wont need to work twice as hard to keep you healthy. Therefore you don't need to wait until you fall sick before fasting. Preventing the illness in the first place is a smarter move.

3. Rejuvenating: This is pretty much the combination of cleansing and strengthening. As I mentioned previously, fasting helps with the production of cells. You are actually speeding up the rate of which your body renews cells! In fact you're making BETTER cells because you have less toxins from food mixing in your system. And guess what? This will make you look AND feel younger, and possibly increase your lifespan if you keep the habit up!

You don't need money or extra time to fast, since it's free and can be done at any moment. Fasting is one of, if not THE cheapest and most effective way of molding your mind and body into exactly what you want it to be. You get the discipline, high morale, wellbeing, and fresh looking body. Do you need to be any more convinced?

LIVING THE FAST LIFE

BY C'BS ALIFE ALLAH

Western society has numerous holidays that are identified with eating a whole bunch of food (Thanksgiving, Halloween, Christmas) to the point that they have devolved to parodies. They are exercises in gluttony. **In Eastern and Indigenous cultures you have feast days yet they are balanced by times of fasting and reflection.**

One of the biggest myths is of breakfast, lunch and dinner. It is assumed by many that this 'sacred trinity' is the same worldwide. The reality is that most Original cultures don't follow that triad unless they have been influenced by Western society. And even if they do they don't have three BIG meals during the course of the day. That's because most indigenous cultures are aware of the body's cycle which mirrors the sun. **The best time to intake food is when the sun is highest in the sky** (between noon and 6pm). After that point the body goes into digestive mode. The next mode is integration mode (taking those nutrients and putting them to use). The final mode is elimination mode which usually last the whole morning. This is why if you intake anything before noon it should be light like fruit, juices and water.

Agricultural societies didn't just store food in case of famine. They also trained their physical bodies to be prepared for such periods. During my own life on the microscopic level I learned this lesson from my father. There were times when we ate that he didn't eat. It was later on that I learned that there wasn't enough food for the whole family so he made sure that the wife and children were fed. Agricultural societies also fasted in tune with the seasons.

AT LEAST TRY THIS YOU CHUMP

BY SUPREME UNDERSTANDING

So fasting from food altogether is just too hard, huh? C'mon son! When I was first getting Knowledge of Self, I was told by my educator that **"it takes 7 years for the swine to leave your system."** For years, I thought that was just a symbolic way of saying something philosophical, as Five Percenters sometimes appear to do. Turns out there's a lot more science to that statement than I realized (which was true for a lot of the other "outlandish" teachings I questioned at first). You see, that meat sits in your colon for quite a while. And the residues of poor eating stay in your system in other forms for quite some time longer. So while it's metaphorically true that we psychologically have to cleanse ourselves of "swine thinking" for years after quitting the actual diet, the literal meaning of that statement is just as true.

According to Brian Clement, creator of the Hippocrates Health Program:

> Actually, 60 percent of accumulated wastes will be released in the first seven days of your program, but complete healing and restoration of the body takes a number of years and breaks down into stages of 7-year increments. It will take the first seven years to completely rebuild the body in the following phases.
>
> 1 day – 1½ years: Digestive cleansing – major fat deposits and calcifications removed.
>
> 1½ – 2 years: Deep tissue cleansing and joint cleansing.
>
> 2 – 5 years: Bone structure, cartilage, and further joint cleansing.
>
> 5½ – 6¼ years: Organ re-positioning and renewal.
>
> 6¼ – 7 years: Brain tissue and neurological cleansing.
>
> Cleansing reactions may ensue as layer after layer is stripped away. But you will feel better and better as time passes. Due to the body's cellular intelligence, every part is affected by the whole. And, when one part is renewed, this leads to greater and greater integrity and harmony within the whole being.

It's amazing how much our street scholars actually know…

While you will receive great results by your 7th day of fasting, the best results take years. Meaning you will need a healthy lifestyle, not just a fad diet, to get the best out of this.

THE DEF JAM DETOX
BY SUPREME UNDERSTANDING

According to the *New York Post*, when Beyonce gains weight, she turns to the Def Jam Diet. "She has gained a lot of pregnancy weight," a source said. "When she gains weight, she normally does the Def Jam detox, but not now." So what's the Def Jam Detox?

According to Jonny Bowden, PhD, board certified nutritionist and author of *The Most Effective Natural Cures on Earth*, "I'm pretty sure it's a version of the Master Cleanse, which has a lot of traction in the music and acting communities."

"'Def Jam' is just the hip rapper way to say Master Cleanse. We are still talking lemon juice, maple syrup and cayenne. Glad she is not doing the detox if she is pregnant since babies need more balanced nutrition to be healthy," says Dawn Jackson Blatner, RD, Chicago-based dietitian and national media spokesperson for the American Dietetic Association

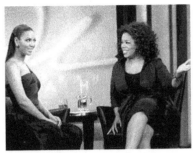

I don't know what all the guessing is about. Beyonce once told Oprah that she did the Master Cleanse for 14 days to prepare for her role in *Dreamgirls*. She lost 22 pounds that time (but she was eating vegetables too). Ashanti did it too (though she ate fruit). Everyone's doing it. And it's not just about losing weight, because it's really a "cleanse" as the name "Def Jam Detox" suggests. This is what Hip Hop's "Baddest Chick," Trina had to say about it:

"It's not that easy to not eat for like three weeks… You're not eating a lot, you're just drinking liquid…[T]hat's all you could do is drink this cleanse. And it's water. All day, any time I had this craving, any urge to eat, I would just drink this water. I did that all day every day for 15 days…You start really wanting food and your body kinda goes into this dysfunctional thing. But if you really want to lose weight and you're trying to get to be a certain size or whatever, it's a good remedy. It's a cleanser, cleans your body out, cleans all the toxins."

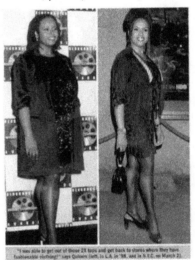

"I was able to get out of those 2X tops and get back to stores where they have fashionable clothing!" says Quivers (left, in L.A in '98, and in N.Y.C. on March 2).

Robin Quivers of the *Howard Stern Show* did it three times and lost 73 pounds. Quivers believes the diet relieved her joint pain and chronic fatigue. Even Denzel Washington and Angelina Jolie have done it. So what *is* the Master Cleanse?

Get the best part from these celebrities. Instead of trying to dress like them, Detox like them.

THE MASTER CLEANSE
BY EBONI JOY ASIATIC

With the changing of every season I endeavor upon a fast of my mind and body. I renew my slacking yoga and meditation routine, and I fast for 10 days with the Master Cleanse "Lemonade Diet."

Cleansing our colon, which in turns clears up our respiratory system due to too much ingestion of dairy and soy products, is a great way to prepare your body to fight off seasonal allergies. My preferred method of cleansing is Stanley Burroughs's *Master Cleanse*. **In his book, Burroughs stated that he invented the Master Cleanse in order to "simplify the cause and correction of all disorders, regardless of the name or names."** His studies taught him that every disease could be corrected by the "same process of cleansing and building positive good health" because dis-ease caused by disease is brought about by our basic habits, improper diet, inadequate exercise, negative mental attitudes and lack of attunement with nature and the universal order of all things, which indicates a lack of self-awareness as well.

So, in order to return my physical to optimal health and proper functioning, I endeavor upon the 10-day Master Cleanse fast from food and beverages; adhering to a strict "lemonade diet" made of:

❏ Organic lemon juice
❏ Genuine maple syrup – preferably Grade B (freshly extracted sugar cane can be used in place of maple syrup)
❏ Cayenne pepper
❏ Water – I prefer distilled because the natural minerals in water are best preserved through this method of purification

Since this is a cleanser and not just a fast, something must also be taken to ensure elimination of waste and clear the intestinal tract. Ideally, you want to have at least two, if not three bowel movements a day (as often as you eat, you should be defecating). Because you are not ingesting food during the fast, you are not producing excess waste that would usually cause you to excrete the waste already in your system. So in order to ensure daily cleansing of the digestive system a person fasting may choose to abide by the book's recommendation, which is to do a "saltwater flush" first thing in the morning before consuming anything. This consists of 1 quart of lukewarm water and 2 teaspoons of unionized sea salt.

You should drink the entire quart in one sitting, lay on the right side of your body for ½ an hour (this enables the saltwater to enter your colon and expedite the elimination), and you will experience a bowel movement typically within one hour. According to Burroughs, this cleans the colon tract like scrubbing a tub, and is often referred to as an "internal saltwater bath," and has no harmful effects like some enemas, nor is it invasive like a colonic.

I, however, have found the saltwater flush harsh on my stomach, so instead I drink an herbal laxative tea to do the elimination job. My herbal tea of choice is Nuevo's Regular Strength Dieters' Nature Slim Tea. The more food you have in your system, the longer it takes to begin working (up to 6 hours), however, once you are on your 3rd or 4th day of the fast it works within an hour, two at the most. You will experience some discomfort due to intestinal cramping, but this is just your body pushing out the waste (much like contractions are your body's natural way of pushing out a baby during labor).

Now, people are often concerned about how they will receive all of their vitamins and minerals while on a Master Cleanse fast. So I've made a list of the benefits of each ingredient used in this "lemonade diet":

Water. Of course, this (along with oxygen and sunlight) is the key to life; it keeps us hydrated, breathing, and the blood pumping through our veins. Nothing could be more basic and absolutely necessary. (See "Water Fasting")

Lemon Juice. It helps balance pH. an acidic pH in women is often associated with yeast infections and bacterial vaginosis; and in men and women it hinders digestion – thus, lemon juice serves to aid digestion by increasing digestive proteins that break down food in the intestines, helping our bowels to move regularly. It has fruit calcium and strengthens teeth, bones and the central nervous system; however, when on the lemonade diet your mouth should be rinsed frequently because lemon juice also eats away at tooth enamel. On an empty stomach, lemon juice eliminates water retention.

Maple Syrup. This is a natural, unrefined sweetener coming directly from tree sap – no artificial anything. It has the minerals manganese and zinc in it as well. (See "The Essential Mineral Guide")

Cayenne Pepper. This increases blood purification and circulation. Like lemon juice, cayenne pepper is also a natural expectorant because it breaks-up, or thins, the mucus built up in your respiratory system.

As you see, your vitamin intake is not diminished with the Master Cleanse, but your waste build-up, excessive mucus and allergy symptoms will be, just as your immune, digestive, respiratory and nervous systems will be strengthened and increase in their functioning.

The master cleanse is an inexpensive way to cleanse the body when compared to how much you'll spend at the doctor and pharmacist.

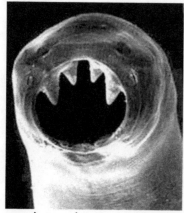

DO YOU HAVE PARASITES?

BY DR. NANCY J. WILLIAMS

The term "parasite" relates to any living thing that lives on or in another living organism. Many parasites interfere with bodily functions, cause irritation, destroy the host's tissues, and release toxins into the bloodstream.

Basically, there are 2 types of parasites: large ones referred to as worms and small ones that require a microscope to see. The large worms, while in an immature form, can travel through your bloodstream and infect any organ, gland or part of the body. Depending on the type of worm, they can grow anywhere from several inches up to many feet in length, and can lay thousands, up to millions, of eggs each day. The eggs stick to the intestinal walls and begin to cause problems. The large worms are called Heminthins or Intestinal Nematodes. Fish tape worm is the largest of the human tapeworms and can reach up to 33 feet in length or more! **Meat eaters, BE AWARE, most meats have some type of parasite in them.**

Parasites can deplete the body of vitamins and minerals and, in some cases, cause anemia from loss of blood. The hookworm, for example, latches onto the human intestine with two sharp hooks, hence its name, takes a mouthful of tissue, dissolves it with enzymes and slurps up blood from ruptured capillaries. In heavy infestation of a hundred or more worm, a person can lose a pint of blood every two days, suffering severe anemia and iron deficiency.

Parasite Symptoms May Include:

- inability to gain or lose weight
- chronic candida
- yeast infections
- chronic sinus or ear infections
- urinary tract infections
- itchy ears or nose
- anal itching
- especially at night
- digestive problems
- gas and bloating
- diarrhea
- mucusy stools
- hemorrhoids
- constipation
- irritable bowel syndrome
- grinding teeth while sleeping
- heart pain
- pain in the navel
- arthritic pains
- burning in the stomach
- bed wetting
- drooling while sleeping

- cysts and fibroids
- eating more and still being hungry
- all skin problems
- depression
- chronic fatigue

- prostate problems and sexual dysfunction in men
- water retention (mostly from tapeworms)
- crawling feeling under the skin
- liver/gallbladder trouble
- and more

Sources of parasites may include food and drink, that romantic kiss, the barbecue next door and the swim you took in the lake two years ago when you accidentally swallowed a little bit of water and have had diarrhea off and on ever since. Yes, they live in us, around us and among us – but they can be properly diagnosed, dealt with and eliminated!

Parasites are among us, so detoxing regularly is so important to a healthy lifestyle. **I always start my clients off with a total body detox.** This includes detoxing the large and small intestine, all the organs, and purifying the blood. **We typically rid the body of over 100 parasites and their eggs.** The results are astonishing, and include more energy, better circulation, mental clarity, weight loss, clearer skin, better digestion and much more.

There are many methods of removing parasites from the body. Some of the ones that I use to keep my clients parasite-free are herbal remedies, colonics and detox foot baths. If you've never done a parasite cleanse, now is a good time to get started on a good detox program. For example, I give a free 20 minute consultation to those who know that they need to get started, but do not know where to begin. Also, keep in mind detoxing is a complete personal journey – it does not look the same for everyone. Getting help is important, so that you don't waste your time and money.

> Did You Know?
> It is estimated that more than 80% of people in the western world have some parasitic or semi-parasitic animal living inside their body. According to a *Scientific American* titled "Worms N Us," over 3 billion people worldwide are infected with at least one of the three worms forming what Columbia University parasitologist Dickson Despommier calls the "unholy trinity" – large roundworm, hookworm and whipworm. Everyone is a potential host for parasites, so I recommend that everyone do a regular detox program to rid their body of the intrusive organisms.

There are parasites within and without the body. Many things can suck the life out of you, eliminate them all.

YOU FLUSH THE TOILET RIGHT?

WELL, IF YOU DON'T, YOU A NASTY MOFO

BY C'BS ALIFE ALLAH

How to Flush Each of your Internal Organs

In addition to periodic fasting and a once a year detox a one year cyclical flushing of each organ should take place. **This means that you should flush out each organ in the body during the course of a year.** This will keep your whole physical in good shape. What follows is a list of the internal organs and simple flushes that one can do for each one. There are natural products you can buy that promise to get the same results (with various degrees of success), but I'm gonna show you how to do it all without spending any real money.

Lungs

The lungs are the largest detox organ in the body. Each exhale dispels cellular waste out of the body. Due to poor eating habits (hella dairy), vices (smoking) and general ignorance (shallow breathing) most peoples' breathing in the Western world isn't at the optimum level. People ain't taking out the trash the way they should be, in other words. Taking any form of Yoga or Chi Gung/Qigong (or any of the internal martial arts) teaches one to breathe deeply. The simple way to do this is to lie on your back and fill your lungs until your stomach is rising and falling in a rhythmic pattern. This means the lower parts of your lungs are being filled up. To do a detox, along with deep breathing, utilize the herbs loelia, mullein, mugwort, sage, or ma huang. Also for general upkeep trying singing or chanting. This will allow you to find new areas of the lungs that you might not have been familiar with.

Lymph Nodes

Toxins from your blood filter first through your lymph nodes before they are flushed out through your urine, sweat or skin. If your lymph nodes get clogged up toxins will start to collect. The fluid in the lymph nodes react to gravity. The way to detox them is simply to be inverted like in a handstand. Another way is by getting a slant board or table. This is a board that is set at an angle of 45 degrees. You can make a simple one by having a table that has two legs on one side removed. The same effect can also be achieved with gravity boots. Invert for approximately 15 minutes.

Blood

Blood is composed of plasma, hemoglobin, vitamins, minerals, sugar, oxygen and white blood cells. The way to rejuvenate the blood is by diluting the blood plasma with a parallel plasma substitute. One of the best substances for this is coconut water. It's the most natural analog to human blood in existence. In the Pacific during World War II loss blood was replaced with coconut water. To flush the blood drink a quart of coconut water in the morning and then one pint every hour for 1-4 hours. You should be pissing like crazy at this point. At this point keep drinking approximately a pint an hour yet add some spirulina. You're basically doing a one day water fast.

Stomach

To clean out your stomach drink a whole gang of water. Eat a whole bunch of straight alkaline raw foods like green papaya and pineapple. Another thing that you can do is a salt water flush where you drink about one liter of water mixed with 2 teaspoons of sea salt. You have to chug it though and gravity will do the rest. Before you do this though make sure you have eaten light foods the day before. Don't go from eating some fried chicken to immediately doing a salt flush or you will be sorry. Another recipe for a stomach flush is 1+ cup of distilled water, 1 cup cabbage juice, ½ cup raw white potato juice, ½ tsp. cascara sagrada powder, 1 tsp. comfrey powder, 1 tsp. horseradish root powder, 1/8 tsp. (a pinch) cayenne

Kidney

The kidney filters the blood and handles the salt balance in the body. It's like a battery, when you take good care of it you'll be able to have more energy. Fasting on organic water (from fruits and veggies) flushes it out. A good flush recipe is ½ cup fresh lemon juice, ½ cup fresh grapefruit juice, 1 garlic clove or 1 tsp. garlic powder, 1 tsp. ginger root powder, 1/8 tsp. cayenne

Liver

The liver handles filtering your blood and your glycogen sugar conversions for later use. To start off, overconsumption of fried foods, cooked oils, and high glycemic starches like potatoes, wheat, corn and rice will jack it up, along with smoking and alcohol. To flush it out, you can drink some beet juice or chlorophyll water, eat watermelon (with the rind), and a salad of dandelion greens with parsley. Try fasting on just that for one day to induce a flush.

Gallbladder

The gallbladder handles bile. People pass about 100 gallbladder stones a year naturally. They're basically composed of rancid fats, oils and calcified minerals. Yet there's a way to dissolve them internally so they won't later come back to kick your ass (literally). It involves a 3-5 day flush. You start off drinking apple juice and eating low glycemic index soups. The acid in the apple starts to wear away the outsides of the stones. When you are ready to flush (about the 4-5 day) drink an 8 oz. of lemonade and 12 oz of olive oil at once. The best way to do it is to drink shots of olive oil followed by lemon juice chasers. Try doing it at noon (to pass at around dinner time) or at 11 pm (to pass in the morning). Lay on your left side and have some hot water bottles available. Massaging helps. They'll be either greenish yellow or orange brown when they pass.

Spleen/Pancreas

For a flush do a day of drinking panini juice while eating a salad of green leafy greens with sunchokes (Jerusalem artichokes). Take in some pure licorice which will restore sugar balance in those organs while things that are bitter, like a tea or coffee, will assist in a flush.

Bladder

You know how it is when you have a bladder infection. Though it may burn like hell the best thing to do is to keep pissing. This is where the water is removed from the body. To flush it the same thing that is good for an infection is good for flushing, cranberry juice. Take one day and drink only cranberry juice NOT one of those sugar laden cranberry cocktails that you can find anywhere. I'm talking about that bitter stuff that makes you curl up your face. You can also add veggies heavy in organic sodium like celery, cucumber, and seaweed to your flush.

Colon

One of the best ways to clean out the colon is to do a colonic. This is not something that should be done annually though. In fact, unless you have an unusual medical disorder you should only do it a couple of times. It cleans out the whole lower intestine by irrigating it with water via the anus. When you irrigate the lower intestines you are getting rid of bad AND good flora/bacteria (this is what antibiotics do which is why you shouldn't depend on them they don't choose what to kill in the body). This is why after you have a colonic you need to restore the good bacteria/flora (acidophilus) by eating bifudus rich foods like cabbage, kim chi, sauerkraut, seed cheese, rejuvelak, miso, amazake, and yogurt. You can also take probiotics which are basically anti-antibiotics. In terms of a yearly flushing of the colon you can take chompers. Chompers are basically items that naturally scrub the walls of the the colon by either expanding with water or scrubbing against the wall (which is why you need to get a lot of natural fiber this scrubs your interior). Some well-known chompers are psyllim husk and cassia pods. Senna is a well-known natural laxative that can be found in herbal laxative teas. Also, to get rid of various parasites that may be inhabiting your intestine you can ground up walnuts and make a paste with water that is almost liquid. Walnuts have been shown to remove worms from the body.

Holistic health means to take care of every component. Cleanse an organ a month; it's a days' work that can add years of health.

MAGIC POTIONS

TONICS AND TEAS FOR THE ORIGINAL MAN
BY C'BS ALIFE ALLAH

A tonic is a drink that is restorative, invigorates, and strengthens. It works best if your system is cleaned out. Yet even with a messed up system you can still get a few of the benefits. Many of the tonics are fermented so they'll give you a slight buzz. Now these tonics got to me via urban Orientalism. **Urban Orientalism**, as defined by I majestic Allah, is the connection and relationship between Black, Brown, and Yellow communities in the Wilderness of North America and filaments of Asian culture. **It's how aspects of Asian culture have integrated itself into the urban environment.** I learned of the following two tonics from the Gods, some of who learned about it from Black Muslims and others who learned of them through their experience with Asian Martial Arts.

Many of these tonics are *aperitifs* and *digestifs*. That's fancy French talk. An *aperitif* is a drink that is taken before a meal (many times in the past it was a liquor used to conceal medicinal herbs) and a *digestif* is a drink taken after a meal often times to assist in digestion. You will find a lot of these types of drinks in Original cultures, especially in ancient Egypt, India, China and Japan, where digestion and metabolism were a big deal.

"You got that Chih"

Shou Wu Chih is my tonic of choice. I keep about three bottles of it in stock at all times. It's an acquired taste. It's sweet bitter. It warms the blood and increases your energy level. It tones up the liver and kidney. Since these are also waste elimination areas the side effect is that your vision is clearer and if you have grey hairs coming in, that vitality will be turning them black again. Taken regularly it is said to improve bones and tendons. I do knowledge that it does ease sleep. You can mix it with just about anything yet I like to just hit it by itself.

"I got that Chiew"

Baji Chiew is my second tonic that I keep on my shelves. It goes down smoother than Shou Wu Chih (no this is not a malt liquor commercial) and is a little sweeter. It focuses on that same area; kidney, lower back, prostate, etc. In terms of stamina vs. sexual dysfunction you should be hitting both of these tonics on the regular. To make sure you aren't harboring internal anger, slow thoughts, and crystallized emotions make sure this is on your routine.

Tiger Bone

Now the last two tonics work as relaxants. They balance you out and take some of the stress out of your life. Tiger Bone is the shot of life. It's the "get up and go" tonic. It ups one's blood circulation, nerve stimulation and glandular activity. Some of the active ingredients in there are ginseng, saw palmetto, astragalus, and guarana seed. Kinda tastes like Hennessey. Get you a shot of this and you're good to go.

Baba Roots

If the Rastas roll deep in your hood, then you know about Baba Roots. There are several Jamaican roots drinks yet this one is probably the most well-known. **This is that energy drink that will bring you up yet not drop you from a mountain top when it's done with you.** It does other things also like builds the blood foundation and circulation. On the low it also works to detoxify several internal organs like the liver. Get hip to it.

"Let me hit this Ginseng Tea"

I start my mornings with a shot of either tonic and a cup of ginseng tea. Now I know in the hood you are used to seeing those little finger length bottles of colored ginseng shots or the 'honey water' bottle with a ginseng root. You may also see that prepackaged ginseng. First off if you see something with 'Siberian ginseng' on it, pass. There ain't no such thing as Siberian ginseng. It's just a marketing ploy.

The best way to rock a ginseng tea is to just steep a sliver of ginseng root in hot water and make a raw tea. You can also steep the root with another bag of tea to give it some additional flavor. Let it tumble down your throat. Ginseng is an adaptagen; it helps your body fight stress and ups your immune system. It also hits your central nervous system and taps the gonads, so yes, it's an Asiatic aphrodisiac. When you get more in tune with your body you can definitely detect that natural ginseng high that enables you to maneuver with clarity through your environment.

Wait! Where Can I Find This Stuff?

Shoh Wu Chih and Baji Chiew can be found in any Chinese/Asian grocer or emporium (hit up the Asian neighborhood in your town and you'll find one...because they do for self) or you can order them online. Baba Roots can be found in health food stores, Jamaican food spots or online. Ginger root can be found just about anywhere. And while these are great for improving vitality among men, there is a whole host of different tonics for women. That would require a whole separate article, so look out for that at www.HoodHealthHandbook.com

---

If you can buy a six pack of beer or take shots of liquor, you can afford and like this stuff. Replace a can of soda, with a shot of tonic.

PASSING THE DRUG TEST

BY SUPREME UNDERSTANDING

Of course, the smartest (and safest) way to pass any drug test is simple: Don't do drugs. Beyond that, drinking vinegar, lemon juice, and/or bleach – while commonly recommended – are still not your best bets. Apple Cider Vinegar is probably the safest and most effective out of the approaches I listed above (though it does cause some burning in your stomach and sometimes diarrhea), but it's only going to reduce levels of THC (and some other substances) somewhat, possibly enough to pass if your test is a few days away, but not enough if it's tomorrow. Not only that, but if they send the sample off for further testing, known as "specimen integrity tests," the lab will detect the presence of whatever chemicals you thought you masked because of altered pH, specific gravity or creatinine level. Drinking other commonly recommended liquids like green tea, coffee, cranberry juice, grape juice, beer, iced tea etc. will help even less because these products neither mask THC in the urine nor eliminate it from fat cells. Taking Niacin (as a supplement) works, but you have to take it for several days and at least 750 mg a day, which will cause itching and burning. So if your test is coming up real soon, you've got only a few options. You can secure someone else's urine (but then the tricky part is how to reheat it, and not OVERHEAT it). And this only works if you're not being closely monitored. So the other option is choosing an effective, research-based, and often expensive detox drink. Ideally, you want a product that promises to:

❏ Contain ingredients like papain which destroy THC in the urine
❏ Contain herbs which act as soft diuretics that help your body flush out marijuana metabolites from your urine without drinking large quantities of water
❏ Provide fiber to absorb excess water and marijuana metabolites as well as other pollutants and impurities from the digestive system
❏ Provide vitamins and minerals to replace whatever gets depleted, especially B-group vitamins (Thiamin, Riboflavin etc) which color your urine bright yellow so it doesn't look like water
❏ Contain the creatine monohydrate, which your body is using to produce creatinine in the metabolite process

Finally, you want all this to be scientifically studied, and preferably with some sort of guarantee. And if it's effective, it's gonna cost you. You can find these kinds of products at smoke shops, sex shops (yup), and just about any shops that sell "water pipes" (bongs) or other creative smoking devices. You can also probably get a kit to test yourself at home before the real test. (you can find them at Amazon.com for less than $8). Hope that helps.

---

if you're on probation or working a job that requires sobriety...stay sober! If you still can't stay sober, you may have an addiction and need further help.

Notes:

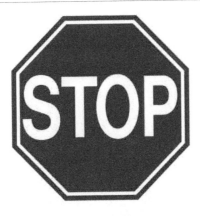

Take a break.
Put this book down for a minute.

Do NOT go back to reading this book until you do one (or more) of the following things:

- ☐ Call somebody who is going through some rough sh*t and make sure they are okay.
- ☐ Eat something that your body is telling you it needs, or drink some water.
- ☐ Wrestle, spar, or slapbox someone to make sure you "still got it."
- ☐ Take a walk through your neighborhood and see if somebody needs help with something.
- ☐ Clean up a part of your house, or organize some f*cked up part of your life.
- ☐ Tell somebody about this book and what you're learning. Invite them to come read it.
- ☐ Give this book away to somebody who needs it and get another copy for yourself.
- ☐ Cook something good, and make enough to share. Invite people.
- ☐ Check yourself out in the mirror and pick something to improve.
- ☐ Identify ten positive things about your life and stop forgetting them when you're stressed.
- ☐ Tell somebody you love them, cause it might be your last chance.

This has been a PSA from 360 and SDP.
Once you're done, carry on.

WE THE ILLEST

Asthma. Bronchitis. Cancer. Diabetes. Eczema. Fibroids. Gallstones. Heart Disease. We could literally go through the entire alphabet, naming diseases and conditions that affect Original people at higher rates than whites, that strike the poor harder than the rich, and that kill more Black people than anyone else in this country. Matter fact, we've got enough of those to run through the ABCs 3 times over. If you don't believe us, you'll see the statistics throughout this book, but you see our list of documented health disparities at www.HoodHealthHandbook.com

Why are Black and brown people so sick? There are some people who will argue that it's yet another symptom of our incompetence and inability to take care of ourselves, but there's no scientific evidence for that, no matter how many stupid people you know personally. **What countless studies have shown us is that there are *systemic* factors in place – which have been in place since the founding of this country (and before) – that have set the stage for what Dr. Vernellia Randall calls a "Slave Health Deficit."** And very little of that has changed today. If anything, the society and system had more to gain if Blacks lived longer during slavery than they did afterwards. In effect, Original people are more expendable now than ever. Only thing saving us might be how much money we spend with them.

"One-quarter of what you eat keeps you alive. The other three-quarters keeps your doctor alive." – Hieroglyph found in an ancient Egyptian tomb

And those sicknesses? It wouldn't make any sense to actually CURE you, would it? Where would be the profitability in that? **Western medicine is a BUSINESS. These hospitals ain't nonprofits! These drug companies ain't gonna stay paid without repeat customers!**

"And we have made of ourselves living cesspools, and driven doctors to invent names for our diseases." – Plato

So doctors tell us the name of our disease or condition, and we say "okay." Then they tell us about a drug that will make it "better" (but not fix it), and we say "okay." Everybody gets rich. And we stay sick and die quick. A doctor in Costa Rica (who understandably wanted to remain anonymous) once said:

> The word incurable is modern…The word incurable is not found in any indigenous language. Translated it means: I do not know how to cure you. But instead of taking the responsibility to tell you that, or refer you to someone who might be able to help with your cure, I will instead guilt trip you and blame YOU for being incurable and ruining my day.

> *"I find medicine is the best of all trades because whether you do any good or not you still get your money." – Moliere, "A Physician in Spite of Himself," 1664*

So this chapter exists to describe and discuss all that ails us in this society. Our goal isn't to just make us aware of the problem, but to take things a step further than others, and actually provide solutions. We'll cover all the conditions that disparately affect Original people in America, the signs and symptoms of conditions you may not know you have, the reason why these illnesses aren't actually treated, and solutions for our struggle against sickness.

When there is an everyday system to keep you sick, you need to be on your job as much as them to be healthy. This means 24/7.

DIET VS. DRUGS: WHAT CURES DISEASE?
BY KING G DELGADILLO

Is there a cure for cancer? Diabetes? Heart disease? It depends on who you ask. Most doctors and pharmacists will tell you no. Although alternative medicine practitioners have been saying for years that there *are* cures for all these diseases (even cancer), many of us are skeptical (and with good reason) because there are so many nut-jobs, idiots, and pretentious people on the Internet and elsewhere, speaking on things they genuinely know nothing about…and a doctor just makes things sound a lot more sensible…even if it's untrue.

> *"The carpenter desires timber, the physician disease." – Rig Veda IX. 7.9*

Back in the late 1920s, there was a German physician named Dr. Max Gerson who documented the effects of diet on eliminating disease from the human body. Dr. Gerson discovered that the human body, when polluted with contaminants and unhealthy foods, combined with a deficiency in proper nutrition, could create numerous unhealthy circumstances to the body, depending on what was consumed and what was lacking. He theorized that if the opposite was done that the body could reverse effects and illnesses.

Dr. Gerson then experimented with 450 patients who all suffered from various ailments such as chronic headaches and different variants of tuberculosis. **Much to his disappointment, he noticed no improvement in any of the patients' health...until he discovered that a nurse was sneaking pastries, sausages, and beer to the patients.** Once his approved diet was properly enforced and adhered to, 446 of his 450 patients recovered from their conditions. And Dr. Gerson's diet therapy wasn't just good for healing headaches and tuberculosis. **He found that he was able to effectively reverse cancer and cure diabetes by simply modifying his patients' diets.**

> Did You Know?
> A scientist named Royall Raymond Rife also came up with a cure for cancer in the 1920s, but the American medical industry saw it as a threat to all the money they were making off a sickness that 'couldn't be cured.' Rife was killed, all of his work was destroyed or 'lost', and everyone who supported him was threatened into denying any knowledge of his cure. Even now, it has become increasingly hard to find information on Rife.

After publishing his book, *A Cancer Therapy: Results of 50 Cases*, Dr. Gerson was criticized by the American scientific and medical community, most notably by Dr. Morris Fishbaine, editor of the Journal of the American Medical Association, who said Gerson was "Treating cancer patients with diet and warning them about cigarettes." Dr. Gerson had also warned patients about the risk of tobacco and openly expressed his opinions about tobacco industry advertising, where doctors recommended smoking a particular brand of cigarette because of how it improved one's lifestyle. During the 1940s-1950s, Phillip Morris was one of the bigger tobacco companies in the United States and was the biggest source of advertisement for the Journal of the American Medical Association, a big reason for the journal's criticism of Dr. Gerson and his work. Ridicule followed Dr. Gerson for most of his career, along with constant attempts to suppress his findings.

In July of 1946, Senator Claude Pepper held a series of Senate subcommittee hearings over Dr. Gerson's cancer therapy. News commentator Raymond Swing reported the testimony on ABC Radio. The public reaction was overwhelming positive, yet Raymond Swing was fired within a couple of weeks, due to pressure from the American pharmaceutical and medical industries. **Despite the effectiveness of Gerson's therapy on diseases such as cancer, muscular dystrophy, diabetes, and even in healing heart arteries, Gerson's work remained unpopular among his peers.** Why? Because his practices challenged the need for pharmaceutical drugs and the established (yet flawed) practices that generated high revenue for the American medical establishment. Despite the overwhelming evidence that supported his practice, Gerson's alternative diet therapy was largely forgotten and overlooked.

More proof that diet affects your health came from Dr. Weston A. Price. In the 1930s, Price travelled around the globe to study native cultures who had rarely (or never) been exposed to modern civilization's diet of processed white flour. As a result, these cultures averaged less than 1% tooth decay. What was also surprising was that many of these native cultures also never practiced any form of dental hygiene yet had better dental health than many people in western civilization (At the time, 30% of adults in the US age 45 and older were beyond tooth decay, they were literally toothless). **He noted that once processed food was introduced to the native people, disease followed soon after.** Dr. Price also studied how diet played a large role in birth defects in animals and humans, especially in skull formation. However, like Dr. Gerson, Dr. Price's research was later ignored because it interfered with the sales of chemicals like fluoride which were purported to help improve dental hygiene, even though diet clearly played a larger role in dental hygiene. Fluoride has been shown to only be effective when applied topically, rather than drinking it through the water supply. The toxicity (not health benefit) of fluoride has been increasingly well-known for quite some time. In fact, it was rumored that, during World War II, Hitler would have sodium fluoride poured into the water because it would result in sterilization.

So why are we being sold lies? Simple, it keeps the people in power PAID. If people knew that we could find simple cures for our health problems simply by changing our diets, there'd be no need for the sale of prescription drugs, organizations like the FDA, and the many pharmaceutical companies they supposedly monitor (when they actually work together). (See "I'll Be Your Pusher"). So don't be surprised if this book ends up being criticized heavily (or worse). Just keep in mind that we personally have nothing to gain from teaching you how to save yourself…and our opponents have everything to lose if we succeed.

You're paying for what you don't know. They hide the facts so you can depend on them. But you know better now. Don't be exploited.

DIABETES

BY SUPREME UNDERSTANDING

"Seventeen, tryin to man up/ Feed the fam boy, I put that on these canned goods/ All I got was diabetes and a damn hug" – Rick Ross, "Usual Suspects"

What do Shawty Lo, Dame Dash, Phife Dawg, Lil Boosie, and Ghostface Killah have in common?

Same disease my mother's got…same disease that a LOT of people in our families and communities got. And yet…we still don't talk much about it, still don't know much about it, and definitely ain't doin much about it. **Diabetes currently affects about 285 million people worldwide.** With the steadily rising numbers of overweight people in the world, it's expected to hit over 400 million in the next 20 years. **And like damn near every other illness, it hits Black and brown people the hardest.** Over 3.2 million Black people in America have diabetes, and ONE-FOURTH of all Black women over 55 have Type 2 Diabetes.

And for most people, having diabetes is a death sentence. More than one-third of all Type 1 diabetics die before the age of fifty, and more than 70% of Type 2 diabetics die of heart attacks and strokes (and way before people without diabetes). And like every other disease, we also get the worst treatment. Often, doctors will amputate the feet or lower legs of diabetics with infected feet (its common). Guess who's feet they cut off the most? Black people. Since the days of Kunta Kinte, ain't much changed. **The rates of Blacks undergoing amputation and suffering from blindness and kidney failure from this disease are skyrocketing, and at rates exceeding those of any other racial groups.** But those premature deaths and complications don't have to happen. **The most common form of diabetes, Type 2, is nutritionally related, and is both preventable and reversible through a change in diet and regular exercise.** Which means, if you don't want to die early, or lose your feet, you need to stop eating that bullsh*t and get your ass up offa that couch or Walmart scooter.

How Diabetes Occurs – Warning: Science Content!

Diabetes occurs when the body is not able to regulate levels of sugar in the blood, resulting in too much sugar in the blood. Your pancreas monitors sugar levels in the body. When the sugar level gets too high, the pancreas kicks into action and releases a hormone called insulin. The body needs insulin to regulate sugar in the body. Insulin sends a hormonal message out to the liver and muscles telling them to absorb the excess sugar so the body can remain balanced. The heavier you are, the greater the risk you will develop Type 2 Diabetes. This is because when you have more fat in your body, you need more insulin to get the sugar to your cells, because the fat around your cells makes it difficult for the insulin to do its job. **Just 20 pounds of extra fat and your pancreas is forced to produce twice as much insulin.** Imagine how overworked your pancreas would be if you were fifty pounds overweight for twenty years. Then what happens? It quits. And now you're a diabetic.

Signs and Symptoms of Diabetes

There are two main types of diabetes. High sugar levels in Type I are due to a lack of insulin because the insulin producing cells have been destroyed. Type II diabetes occurs when the body's cells become resistant to insulin that the pancreas produces. I think Lil Boosie explains it simpler when he says, "I have type one, which happens, in general in younger patients. [Type one diabetics] don't make insulin, which helps bring down your blood sugar. Older people in general get type two diabetes; they make insulin but the body can't use it properly." In any type, your blood has too much sugar in it and your cells aren't getting the sugar that they need. As a result, your body's alarms go off by giving you these signs and symptoms listed below.

> **Did You Know?**
> Blacks are 1.8 times more likely than whites to have diabetes. Latinos are 1.7 times more likely to have diabetes than whites. And because of the crappy food provided to Native Americans on reservations, they are 3.2 times more likely than whites to have diabetes.

- ❐ Frequent trips to the bathroom
- ❐ Unquenchable Thirst
- ❐ Losing Weight Without Trying
- ❐ Weakness and Fatigue
- ❐ Tingling or Numbness in Your Hands, Legs or Feet
- ❐ Other Signs and Symptoms That Can Occur: Blurred vision, skin that is dry or itchy, frequent infections or cuts and bruises that take a long time to heal are also signs that something is amiss.

If you notice any of the above signs, schedule an appointment with a trusted medical professional. They will be able to tell you if you have reason to be concerned about a diagnosis of diabetes or not.

Discovering Diabetes

Discovering you have diabetes can be rough. Often, people don't have a clue until the doctor breaks the tragic news. Ghostface Killah, in the 2007 song "Trials of Life" (featuring Prodigy), raps about how he thought he had an STD until he got the diabetes diagnosis. And check out the following story from Shawty Lo:

It was crazy when I first found out. I was doing a lot of urinating, having to go to the bathroom like every 20 minutes. I remember one night lying in bed and it was like I was having an out of body experience; I could see myself sleeping. When I first went to the hospital, the doctors said I could have been, was supposed to be like in a coma because my blood sugar was so high – over 1600. They couldn't believe it was that high, saying most people would either be dead or in a coma. It seemed like I could barely walk, like I weighed 300 pounds. All this had gone on for about a week before I went to the hospital. When they checked me in, that's when they found out, I was diabetic. I didn't take it seriously at first. It took me having to go to the hospital 2 or 3 times before it really sunk in. I was in denial. I just didn't want to accept that I had diabetes, but my family really clamped down on me. If you've ever seen the movie Soul Food, that's how my family is. We're real tough and we were raised to be that way and take care of each other. When my grandmamma died, our family came together; my mama, my aunties, all my family. It took all their help to make me do right and realize that I had to make some changes and how serious diabetes was and that it could take my life. And ever since then, I've been pretty good.

Lil Boosie had a similar experience when he found out, admitting, "The first two years, it was real hard. I was in and out of the hospital, and I didn't wanna take my medicine. I didn't wanna accept that I had Diabetes." I can understand, considering that Boosie and Shawty Lo were neither elderly or obese – the typical characteristics we associate with diabetes. But in Shawty Lo's case, it was a combination of lifestyle (the crap you eat when you go from "the trap" to being on the road touring) and genetics. In Boosie's case, he says himself that he feels his success in hiphop is what brought Diabetes into his life. All this just goes to say, don't think it can't happen to you. And if it does, be prepared to do what's right.

As Boosie explained to the HipHop Doc, Dr. Rani Whitfield:

I been diagnosed with type one diabetes four and a half years now; I got diagnosed when I was 20, and you know it's been a struggle for me. As the years go on though, I learn more about the disease and I get better with it, you know...Now I'm taking a pill called Actos and I'm on that 70/30 [insulin] also...Have to give myself shots at least twice a day and check my sugar as well...It gets old, but I know the importance of taking care of myself. You know really I just

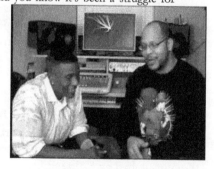

keep fresh alcohol pads and I have to alternate spots on my body where I give myself insulin injections. I use to get knots under my skin that were painful, so now I go to my arm one day, stomach the next...

As you can tell, managing can be tough, especially if you live a hectic lifestyle, celebrity or not. Boosie continues:

[Dr. Whitfield: So, do you ever have days where you say, I'm tired of this, I'm not dealing with this, I'm not going to eat right or exercise?] Yeah man, I have days when it's like all falling down on me. If I like go two to three weeks of taking care of myself, that one day I slip, I might get sick. You know I have to really be on it and the lifestyle I have – this lifestyle I'm surrounded by, you know, I feel like I need more people around to help me with this. It's hard Doc. You know those couple of nights I had to call you when I'm on the road feeling bad; sh*t man, I was down. But it's all good when I take care of myself.

Shawty Lo, who recently started a health foundation called L.O.L.O. (Loving Our Little Ones), struggled as well, but also came up with a game plan to do better:

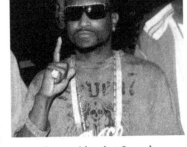

I try to exercise, drink plenty of water and take vitamins but lately I've been so busy on the road that I don't do all that stuff as often as I'd like; but I do the best that I can. My work schedule affects my diabetes a little bit because when you're traveling as much as I do, there's not too many places to stop off and get a good wholesome meal and sometimes I end up just eating what's convenient. But I'm about to put in my rider that I need to have special meals prepared for me when I do shows cause I can't be eating crazy.

Both rappers expressed hope about their conditions:

Shawty Lo: Diabetes is not the end of the world, but it is a lifestyle change and that's hard because you've been stuck in your own ways for so long, eating and doing whatever. It's hard to change that up. When you first find out, it's hard, but in time, you learn to accept change and just take one day at a time; small steps. I think once you start eating right and get into a workout habit and stay focused and believe in yourself, you'll get through it. Staying as healthy as I can is a priority. It's about longevity and having a quality life because you can lose limbs or even go blind from diabetes. That's something people don't really know; you can lose legs, toes, feet, have kidney problems and heart problems. Anything I can do to help raise awareness about diabetes, I will be there, not only because I have it, but because it's a disease that affects millions of people. Everybody knows at least one person that has diabetes, so it's like when we participate in events, walks and things of that nature, we're really helping somebody we care about and ourselves because you never know when it can affect you.

Lil Boosie: At first it was like, how am I going to accept it? But now I talk about the disease and motivate other diabetics to take care of themselves and prolong their lives. It's like a blessing; at first it felt like a curse, but now, to me it's like a blessing. It's millions of people with this disease and I'm a big influence to a lot of people. So, if I can help people to live longer by talking about it, then I'm going to keep doing it…I know this, diabetes is not HIV; it's not AIDS. Take care of yourself, keep your sugar under control and you can live better and longer. Keep your head up and take pride in yourself. Don't feel like you are alone with diabetes.

Diabetes will be a growing problem until you inform yourself, friends, and family. Setup a weight loss challenge to motivate everyone.

PREVENTING TYPE 2 DIABETES
BY KING DIVINE ALLAH

Recent studies by Harvard researchers have concluded that moderate exercise and a healthy diet can prevent most cases of Type-2 Diabetes. **The study overwhelmingly indicated that by making appropriate lifestyle changes, diabetes can be prevented over 90% of the time.** The study also concluded that lifestyle changes significantly reduced the risk of getting the disease by 58% among people who already showed signs of developing diabetes.

Diabetes is one disease in which genes play an important part. If you have these genes and are at risk of developing diabetes, you lifestyle decisions very well determine whether these genes become active or remain dormant.

Being overweight is the number one reason people contract diabetes; 61% percent of all cases are attributed to obesity and weight problems. Overweight women cut their risk by 24% simply by walking regularly. The more exercise, the less likely you are to have any instances with the disease. **Those who did 7 or more hours a week of exercise had a 29% lower risk than those who did not exercise or exercised less than 30 minutes per week.** Eating a diet that is high in fiber, low in fat and low in partially hydrogenated oils also significantly decreases your risk. So it's crucial to read labels. (See "Reading and Understanding Food Labels")

Foods that Help Beat Diabetes
There are foods that you can add to your diet that can help manage and in some cases reverse the symptoms of diabetes or eliminate the

disease all together. These foods provide powerhouse nutrients like fiber, vitamins and minerals and these foods are also low in fat. Making these foods part of a comprehensive diabetes diet can make a real difference in managing diabetes.

Beans. A wonderful food for managing sugar levels in the blood, giving the body nutrients to slowly digest and process.

Fish: Many fish are high in omega 3 fatty acids and have been shown to be heart-healthy. This doesn't mean that your fish fries are a healthy solution. **Some studies show that eating two servings of baked or broiled fish may protect people with diabetes from kidney problems.**

Nuts. Some nuts and seeds like walnuts and flaxseeds contain omega-3 fatty acids. Nuts also deliver healthy doses of fiber and magnesium.

Berries. Compared to other fruits they are relatively lower in calories and carbohydrates considering their serving size.

Broccoli. Another low-carbohydrate, low-calorie, high-fiber food that has antioxidant and anti-cancer properties. Broccoli also fills you up which are a plus for people that want to lose weight.

Sweet Potatoes. I know potatoes are good but they contain high levels of starch that can be harmful for individuals with Type 2 Diabetes. A healthier alternative is sweet potatoes. They are high in fiber and vitamins A and C.

Dark, leafy green vegetables. Spinach, collard greens, and kale pack high levels of nutrients like vitamins A and C and calcium, as well as being low in calories and carbohydrates. Other great choices in this group include Bok Choy and mustard greens. Please leave the fat back and neck bones out, because that would totally defeat the purpose.

Whole Grains. The germ and bran contained in whole grains have large amounts of nutrients like magnesium, chromium, omega-3 fatty acids, and folate; these nutrients are stripped out of the grains when they are processed into white flour products.

Tomatoes. Here's another colorful vegetable that contains large amounts of nutrients like iron and vitamins C and E. Tomatoes are very versatile and can be used in many different recipes. Cooked tomato products like stewed tomatoes and ketchup also deliver the important nutrient lycopene.

Get the nutritional content and further benefits of these foods in our "Healing and Treatment" chapter.

Adjust your diet to what you need to be healthy.

HEART HEALTH

BY QUEEN RIGHTEOUSLY REFINED

Despite losing both of his parents to heart attacks, rapper turned actor Ice-T didn't know that he was at high risk for heart disease. In fact, like many of us, he only found out after going to the doctor for an unrelated problem:

> After I learned I have high blood pressure, I had to slow down. I don't drink, I don't smoke. I was just overworking myself and pushing myself too hard and letting myself get frustrated," he says. "Finally, the doctor basically told me, 'You can die from this.' That's when I really had to shape up...The truth is that anyone who has a history of heart disease in their family should be having regular check-ups. You need to have check-ups continuously to be safe...The trouble with high blood pressure is that you may not know you have it. It absolutely can go undetected. It's not something that you feel, it's not a normal sickness, it's not an ache, it's not a pain. You just have high blood pressure and it can kill you.

High Blood Pressure

Hypertension a.k.a High Blood Pressure is one of the top "silent killers" in African American communities. **High blood pressure is a leading cause of heart attack, stroke, heart failure and kidney disease.** HBP also increases the odds in the favor of you developing cardiovascular disease, commonly referred to as heart disease. HBP basically works your heart like a slave in the field just to pump enough blood and oxygen to your organs. It can cause the heart to enlarge and weaken, and can cause major damage to your artery walls.

Studies have shown that Black people are about 40% more likely than Whites to develop high blood pressure. According to the American Heart Association, in 2006 the death rates per 100,000 people from high blood pressure were 15.6 for white males, and 14.3 for white females, versus 51.1 for Black males, and 37.7 for Black females! And guess who's got it even worse? **Puerto Ricans actually have a higher death rate linked to high blood pressure than blacks, whites or other Latinos.** Health officials don't know why, but one expert said it could be related to health care, diet or genetics.

There are many contributing factors to this gap in numbers, such as environment, diet, economics, psychological facts and other differences.

The first and foremost thing in preventing and treating any condition is to be in the know. Those that are reading this book are on the right track by seeking out information. Getting regular check-ups are important things that many of us in the Black community avoid because of lack of time, money, lack of insurance or just a fear of medical institutions altogether.

There major risk factors for HBP are:

- ☐ Poor diet.
- ☐ Being overweight.
- ☐ Drinking too much alcohol and caffeine.
- ☐ Smoking.
- ☐ Stress.

Coronary Heart Disease

I have heard that the heart of a man is the most important part. So it is crucial for this area of your body to be in healthy operating order. Coronary Heart Disease is exactly what it says. It is a disease that affects the coronary arteries that route blood to the heart to be pumped back out through other arteries. Again, this is another area where Black people are affected much worse than their white peers. **What's ironic is that studies have found that Black people actually have a natural genetic PROTECTION against heart disease** (one that scientists are studying to develop new medicines), **which makes this huge disparity especially sad**.

If so much fat builds up in your "blood pipes" that the proper amount of blood can't get to and from your heart, then you may experience some serious chest pains that is 20 times worse than your worst gas pain ever, called angina.

Over time pieces of that fat may bust loose from the walls it was attached to and a blood clot might form. This could totally block blood flow to that part of the heart and that part of the heart will start to die. This is called a heart attack.

Heart Attacks

DJ Unk, (best known the hit single "Walk it Out") was rushed to the hospital in August of 2009, after he complained he was having trouble breathing. Doctors examined him and told the Atlanta rapper that he'd suffered a mild heart attack. He was only 26 years old.

During the experience, Unk posted

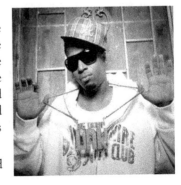

updates on his Twitter. Of course, people speculated that it was caused by drug use, but he shut that down quickly, blaming it on the same factors that are causing more and more young Black men and women to have heart problems: a bad diet.

"Never...wanna go through that again," he wrote. "Got to change my diet and slow down! Scared the sh** out of my family and friends. Luv life." he tweeted. He told his followers that he was "still walkin it out," but called the heart attack a "wake up call" that had given him immediate motivation to adopt a healthier lifestyle:

> No more Kush, Purp, Piff, Haze, Sour diesel for me! No more drinks! Got to do this for my health...No more hot wings, no fried food, no more seafood! Dam what must I eat? (air) and (water) lol... What's sum good healthy food anybody?

Would you know if you were having a heart attack? Do you know how to prevent yourself from ever having one?

Over a million people in the U.S. alone have heart attacks every year. Half of that million die from it. Some of the symptoms of an attack are...

❏ Having a feeling of a lot of pressure, squeezing, or pain in the center of the chest that lasts more than a few minutes. This can go away and come back.

❏ Having shortness of breath along with or without chest pain or pressure

❏ Breaking out in cold sweats, feeling sick to the stomach or lightheaded.

❏ Having pain or pressure in one or both arms, the back, neck, jaw or stomach

❏ A sore jaw, when combined with chest pain, can signal a heart attack – especially among women

According to the American Heart Association (www.heart.org), the most common heart attack symptom is chest pain or discomfort for both men and women. But women are somewhat more likely than men to have some of the other common symptoms, particularly shortness of breath, nausea/vomiting, and back or jaw pain. If you experience these symptoms, you know you're at risk. Get to the hospital right away!! The sooner you get there, the greater the chance to save your heart.

Healing and Prevention

These are some things you can do to prevent heart disease and rehabilitate your heart after damage has already been done:

❑ Reach a Desirable Blood Pressure by limiting salt intake to slightly more than 1 teaspoon a day and if you drink, limit alcohol to no more than 1 drink per day

❑ Limit Trans fatty and processed foods, saturated fats like butter, and eat more whole grains and unsaturated fats from vegetables, fish, and nuts; The fiber from these sources are very important.

❑ Get down to a healthy body weight by healthy dieting and proper exercise.

❑ QUIT SMOKING!!!! Smoking is one of the most important preventable causes of premature death in the US. Each year 430,700 deaths are reported due to smoking. Cigarette Smoking is the most important risk factor for coronary artery disease that you can change. When you smoke it decreases HDL (good cholesterol) and increases LDL (bad cholesterol)..

❑ Reduce your stress and anxiety. Studies that examined what victims of a heart attack were doing and feeling in the hours preceding the event found acute emotional stress to be a common trigger.

Learn the symptoms of a heart attack, if not for your own good, do it for your family. Follow the above steps to keep your heart healthy.

STROKES

BY YVETTE GZ

In 2008, Nate Dogg suffered from his second stroke in less than a year's time. The first stroke had left him partially paralyzed and confined to a wheelchair. The second stroke put him on life support. "He has suffered another stroke from his bad eating habits and unhealthy lifestyle," said old

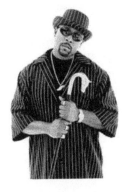

friend Lil Half Dead, "All we can do now is pray for him." Fortunately, he made it off life support, but as of 2010 was still in recovery. "He's in therapy getting himself together, that's all I can tell people," Warren G said in a recent interview. "I see him any and every time I want to. It's hard when you have somebody that got two strokes, usually the person don't make it. But he's strong. He's getting good therapy and he's pulling out of it." Currently relearning basic movements and functions, Nate Dogg is finally able to lift his head, but still can't communicate verbally. "It's hard when you first have a stroke, you got to learn everything over again," Warren G continued. "It's like you're a baby again. You gotta learn everything."

What is a Stroke?

The simplest way to describe a stroke is a brain attack. It's what happens when the blood flow and oxygen to the brain gets cut off or when a blood vessel in the brain gets ruptured and leads to a deadly hemorrhage. During a stroke, about 2 million brain cells die every minute, resulting in brain damage or death. There are many reasons why a stroke occurs, and unless you're very healthy, it can happen anytime to anyone.

☐ Arteries or small blood vessels that carry blood and oxygen to the brain can be blocked by blood clots, plaque build-up, cancer cells, or deposits of fat in the bloodstream.

☐ Sickle cell anemia can cause blood cells to clump up and block vessels.

☐ Head injuries that damage tissue and big or small important blood vessels can cause strokes by compressing the brain or leaking blood into it (hemorrhage).

☐ High blood pressure increases the risk of a hemorrhage when an injury occurs.

☐ Extremely low blood pressure can also cause a stroke since it reduces the blood flow in parts of the body, which is also what a cardiac arrest (heart attack) does.

☐ Smoking increases the risk of stroke.

How it Affects Us

It is claimed that African Americans have twice the risk of stroke compared to whites, but that really goes for anyone who maintains the same lifestyle since the risk of stroke is linked to sickle cell anemia, diabetes, high blood pressure, obesity, and a high sodium diet. Unfortunately, Black people have the highest rate of diabetes, sickle cell anemia and obesity in the country, so stroke should be a big concern in the community and measures should be taken to avoid it.

Signs and Symptoms

Strokes happen quickly. Once the brain is deprived of blood and oxygen, it only takes a minute for the body to shut down. The immediate signs of stroke are:

- ❑ Sudden numbness or weakness in facial and limb muscles
- ❑ Trouble walking or standing up
- ❑ Confusion or difficulty making simple sentences
- ❑ Headaches, dizziness, and trouble focusing
- ❑ Droopy face

Recommendations

The only thing you can do when you see symptoms of a stroke is call the ambulance. There's no point trying to figure out what you can do. The more you wait, the more brain damage will ensue. **What you CAN do is take precautions to prevent a stroke.** You can do that by dealing with the root causes of stroke. Get your blood pressure checked to make sure it's not too high or too low. Eat a healthy low sodium and low sugar diet; it helps regulate your blood pressure and keep your cholesterol and diabetes in check, especially raw fruits and vegetables. Visit a doctor every now and then to check your heart condition. Last but not least, cut down on smoking and drinking and exercise more often. A fast walk 20-30 minutes every day can do miracles for your heart.

More Tips on Stroke Identification

STROKE: Remember the 1st Four Letters…S.T.R.O.

SMILE: Ask the individual to SMILE.

TALK: Ask the person to TALK or SPEAK A SIMPLE SENTENCE coherently. (i.e. It is sunny out today.)

RAISE: Ask him or her to RAISE BOTH ARMS.

OPEN: Ask the person to OPEN their mouth, just enough to stick out the tongue. If the tongue is 'crooked', that is, if it goes to one side or the other, that is also an indication of a stroke.

If he or she has trouble with ANY ONE of these tasks, call emergency number immediately and describe the symptoms to the dispatcher.

The best approach is prevention. If someone's having a stroke quickly call 911. Learn the signs and symptoms to get help faster.

CANCER IN THE BLACK COMMUNITY

BY EARTH EM'MAYA JEWEL

Loyola University researchers conducted 35 clinical trials in which they followed nearly 20,000 adult cancer patients for 10 years after treatment. The study revealed that African Americans, which made up 12% of the patients, were more likely to die from breast, ovarian and prostate cancers. **Experts think there are genetic and hormonal factors that make the diseases more deadly for people of color.**

Black men living in America have the highest rate of occurrence of prostate cancer, about 60% higher than that of whites. When famed singer Charlie Wilson, former front man for the Gap Band, learned he had prostate cancer in the early part of 2000, he was devastated. He felt like he was too young to be getting a cancer like that. The singer said he was astounded to learn that African American men are 1.6 times more likely than others to be diagnosed with prostate cancer. But he was lucky. The doctors caught the cancer early enough to be able to completely get rid of it. Today a healthy and touring Wilson urges African American men to get tested.

Early detection is critical in successful treatment, but many people of color won't go to the doctor for the most severe ailment or chronic condition. These can often be signs and symptoms of pre-cancerous conditions that can be stopped with early detection and proper treatment.

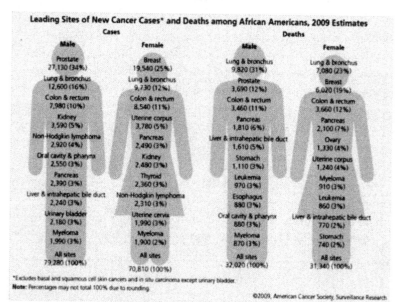

Leading Sites of New Cancer Cases* and Deaths among African Americans, 2009 Estimates

Cases		Deaths	
Male	**Female**	**Male**	**Female**
Prostate 27,130 (34%)	Breast 19,540 (25%)	Lung & bronchus 9,820 (31%)	Lung & bronchus 7,080 (23%)
Lung & bronchus 12,600 (16%)	Lung & bronchus 9,730 (12%)	Prostate 3,690 (12%)	Breast 6,020 (19%)
Colon & rectum 7,980 (10%)	Colon & rectum 8,540 (11%)	Colon & rectum 3,460 (11%)	Colon & rectum 3,660 (12%)
Kidney 3,590 (5%)	Uterine corpus 3,780 (5%)	Pancreas 1,810 (6%)	Pancreas 2,100 (7%)
Non-Hodgkin lymphoma 2,920 (4%)	Pancreas 2,490 (3%)	Liver & intrahepatic bile duct 1,610 (5%)	Ovary 1,330 (4%)
Oral cavity & pharynx 2,550 (3%)	Kidney 2,480 (3%)	Stomach 1,110 (3%)	Uterine corpus 1,240 (4%)
Pancreas 2,390 (3%)	Thyroid 2,360 (3%)	Leukemia 970 (3%)	Myeloma 910 (3%)
Liver & intrahepatic bile duct 2,240 (3%)	Non-Hodgkin lymphoma 2,310 (3%)	Esophagus 880 (3%)	Leukemia 860 (3%)
Urinary bladder 2,180 (3%)	Uterine cervix 1,990 (3%)	Oral cavity & pharynx 880 (3%)	Liver & intrahepatic bile duct 770 (2%)
Myeloma 1,990 (3%)	Myeloma 1,900 (2%)	Myeloma 870 (3%)	Stomach 740 (2%)
All sites 79,280 (100%)	All sites 70,810 (100%)	All sites 32,020 (100%)	All sites 31,340 (100%)

*Excludes basal and squamous cell skin cancers and in situ carcinoma except urinary bladder.
Note: Percentages may not total 100% due to rounding.

©2009, American Cancer Society, Surveillance Research

Another reason why Black people are likely to die from the disease may have something to do with a lack of bone marrow donors within the African Diaspora. (See "Leukemia")

What Causes Cancer?

"It is time to lay to rest the notion that germs jump into people and cause diseases." – Emanuel Cheraskin, M.D

Contrary to popular belief, cancer doesn't just "happen" to people. It's not a mysterious plague. **It's VERY clear and well-known what kinds of things contribute to causing cancer.** And most of them are avoidable. But because people are making billions of dollars selling those same things, don't expect to hear much about it. Case in point: Using tobacco is the easiest (and most preventable) way to serve yourself some cancer. Not just lung cancer, but any of the 100+ types of cancer that can occur anywhere in the body. But how long did it take for that information to come out and become public knowledge? For decades, doctors and the American medical industry were some of the biggest supporters of the tobacco industry!

The cells in your body are set up a certain way to make sure that you get what you need as far as vitamins, oxygen, and whatever chemicals you need to produce at any given time. **Your job is to feed your body the right foods, give it enough exercise and rest so that the cells can do their jobs and take you into old age.** If you feed your body the wrong foods, don't exercise and smoke cigarettes your cells become weak and damaged and are not able to do their jobs right. They start to change as they multiply and eventually, they send the body into a sort of self-destruct mode (also called auto immune disease). And this is what causes cancer.

When mutated cells begin to multiply too fast, they form tumors or masses. These abnormal growths can be harmless (benign) or deadly (malignant) depending on the factors involved in their creation. **Carcinogens can boost the rapid growth of abnormal cells causing them to take over healthy cells and tissues in the body, causing the cancer to spread.** Carcinogens are just substances that can get into the blood stream and activate a sort of self-destruct mechanism in cells that turn them cancerous.

There are many risk factors involved in the development of cancerous cells within the body. Many of them are preventable (eating right and exercising), or avoidable (staying away from tobacco smoke). Some of the most common risk factors for cancer are aging, smoking, not being physically active, alcohol, certain hormones, sunlight, certain chemicals, family history and poor diet. **It is unlikely for cancer to 'run' in families, but some genetic mutations are passed from** parent to child, causing every cell to carry the mutation and leave the child at an increased risk. Melanoma (skin cancer), breast cancer, and cancers of the colon, ovaries and prostate can occur more often in some families. More often they are the habits and traditions that we pass on to our children, such as what we teach our children to eat (by example) or when they inhale our secondhand smoke, only to eventually smoke on their own.

Warning Signs of Cancer

One thing you have to understand about cancer is that it is not just "a" disease. **Cancer is actually a group of diseases that can cause different signs and symptoms depending on where it is, how big it is and how long it's been there.** As cancer grows within the body, it can put pressure on blood vessels, nerves and organs causing noticeable reactions or changes. In some of the more sensitive areas of the body like the heart or brain, even the smallest growth can bring on symptoms. Oftentimes people will ignore these symptoms, writing them off as stress or "growing pains" and there are those who just don't know or think their symptoms are anything serious. Some may just be afraid to seek medical advice, fearing the diagnosis and what it may mean for their finances, their families and their futures. But cancer is best beaten the earlier it is found. The earlier cancer is detected, the less likely it has time to "metastasize" or spread, which means treatment can be direct and quick.

> **Did You Know?**
> Our oldest description of cancer (although the word cancer was not used) was discovered in ancient Egypt and dates back to about 1600 B.C. It is called the Edwin Smith Papyrus, and is based on an even older Egyptian textbook on trauma surgery, possibly dating back to 3000 B.C. and the teachings of the Egyptian father of medicine, Imhotep. It describes eight cases of tumors or ulcers of the breast that were treated by cauterization with a tool called the fire drill. There is also evidence that they were able to tell the difference between malignant and benign tumors. Inscriptions suggest that surface tumors were surgically removed in a similar manner as they are removed today.
> At the same time, a recent study by Michael Zimmerman has revealed that cancer doesn't go much further back than this era: 'The virtual absence of malignancies in mummies must be interpreted as indicating their rarity in antiquity, indicating that cancer-causing factors are limited to societies affected by modern industrialization.'
> Colleague Rosalie David added, "There is nothing in the natural environment that can cause cancer. So it has to be a man-made disease, down to pollution and changes to our diet and lifestyle."

The following are some of the most common warning signs of developing or existing cancer. All should be addressed by a doctor for diagnosis.

Lumps: Unexplained or new knots, tough spots or sensitive bumps on your glands or lymph nodes, breasts or testicles may be cancerous.

Persistent cough: A cough or a hoarse throat that does not go away; ever, may be an indication of lung cancer or cancers of the throat.

Sores that won't heal: A sore in the mouth that doesn't heal could be an oral cancer; especially white patches inside the mouth or on the tongue. This can be a precancerous condition caused by smoking or alcohol consumption. Sores on the penis or vagina may either be signs of infection or an early cancer and should not be overlooked.

Unusual bleeding or discharge: Abnormal vaginal bleeding can be a sign of cervical cancer or cancer of the uterus. A bloody discharge from the nipple can signal breast cancer. Blood in the toilet can be a symptom of colon cancer. And coughing up blood can signal lung cancer.

Pain: A headache that never goes away, even with treatment can be a sign of brain cancer. Chronic pain in the back, groin or hips can signal cancers of the colon, rectum or ovaries. Pain when urinating, especially when blood is present may be bladder or prostate cancer.

Unexplained weight loss: Sudden and unexplained weight loss of 10 pounds or more can be the first sign of stomach cancer, lung cancer and cancers of the throat or pancreas.

Skin changes: Abnormal and excessive hair growth, persistent or extreme itching, any change in warts, moles or skin color are all indications of cancer of the skin or melanoma.

Extreme fatigue: When rest does not alleviate the feeling of extreme tiredness, it's called fatigue. Chronic or extreme fatigue could be due to blood loss which is common in stomach or pancreatic cancers. Rapid spread of cancer can also cause chronic fatigue.

Look out for any abnormal marks or feelings. Get checked out if you find anything. The earlier you get help, the better your chances.

THE OUTRIGHT FRAUD OF FINDING A CURE FOR CANCER

BY DR. SCOTT WHITAKER, CO-AUTHOR OF MEDISIN

Most cancer organizations including the pink ribbon cancer non-profit groups are a total fraud. They refuse to teach women about the basics of cancer prevention. They won't teach anyone about vitamin D or the anti-cancer properties of fresh produce. **Their focus in October is to trap women in a system of cancer screening that actually causes cancer: Mammography!** They irradiate the breast and heart. If you get enough mammograms, you'll eventually get breast cancer. (See "The Importance of Pap Smears and Mammograms"). Once you're given a cancer diagnosis, they've got you trapped in a system of dangerous chemotherapy treatments that will absolutely destroy your health.

It's quite a racket. An incredible scam, but hey, if you believe that buying "pink" candy or buckets of KFC made with cancer-causing chemicals is a great way to support cancer "research" (whatever that means), then go ahead! Buy all the pink crap you can find in the stores! Just don't kid yourself into thinking you're helping find a cure for cancer. **The truth is; they're not looking for a cure.** They're just looking to make a quick buck by selling you false hope... the hope that by buying more junk, you will be part of finding a "solution" for cancer.

Well, the solution already exists, people. It's found in anti-cancer foods, herbs and supplements. It's found in the sunshine over your head, in pure & clean water, in the super foods & nutrients like Wheatgrass, Goji berries, Flax seed oil and Selenium. The solution to cancer has already been found. It just can't be patented. It's not a drug. So the cancer industry has zero interest in actual cancer solutions that really work, and they keep selling the lie that they're "looking" for a cure.

> Did you Know?
> There is a well-known link between obesity and cancer. In fact, according to an American Cancer Society study, as many as 90,000 cancer deaths each year could be prevented if Americans could only maintain a normal., healthy body weight. It's believed that one of the important ways obesity increases your risk for cancer is by causing the body to produce more of the right circumstances, these hormones are critical for our health. But when someone is obese and these hormones are too high, they can actually stimulate the growth of cancer. The good news is that, to some degree, we can control many of our risk factors for these cancers by good eating habits and exercising. Achieving and maintaining a healthy weight is not just about what you look like in the mirror or the number that registers on a scale.

At the same time, they are doing their very best to try to scare people away from nutritional supplements that actually protect healthy cells: Pau d' Arco, chlorella, Vitamin B17, Magnesium, Resveratrol and so on.

That's the sad (but true) state of our modern cancer industry. It's a racket run by deceptive, dishonorable people who are far more interested in making a quick buck than solving the world's cancer problems. Their jobs, after all, depend on cancer. (See "Diet Vs. Drugs: What Cures Disease?").

Don't fall for propaganda from "non-profit" cancer organizations. Instead of reading into their message, make healthy life changes.

SKIN CANCER IS **NOT** PREJUDICED

BY EARTH EM'MAYA JEWEL

"The Black man is the original man of this Earth/ We can live under the sun, it give us strength/ The white man gets sunburn, and cancer of the skin" – Prodigy, "My World is Empty Without You"

If you are of African descent; Latino, or Asian don't be fooled into thinking that you can't get skin cancer. Most people link skin cancer to white people due to too much direct sunlight or tanning. As it turns out, it doesn't matter what color you are; sunburns and tanning beds instantly increase your risk for getting a cancer of the skin. People of color may have an advantage, but we do not have a "skip" card when it comes to skin cancer. As a matter of fact, **even though we are less likely to get a cancer of the skin, we are nearly twice as likely to die from it.**

The most common types of skin cancer are basal cell carcinoma (BCC), squamous cell carcinoma (SCC) and melanoma. All of these are caused by chronic or even occasional over-exposure to sunlight. Now, keeping in mind that ultra violet (UV) rays in sunlight cause the skin to produce vitamin D (which is good for us), so you shouldn't be "scared" of sunlight. But too much of anything is never a good thing, so also keep in mind that there are different types of UV rays coming from the sun that can also do damage to our skin cells. UV rays are what cause you to burn when you spend too much time in direct sunlight. **Without good sunscreen or sense enough to cover your skin if you have to be in it for long periods, you put yourself at risk for sunburns. And it only takes one burn to put you at risk for skin cancer.** People of color who live in places like Arizona and New Mexico are especially prone to burns and cancers because of the sunnier weather. Here are some ways to avoid getting burned:

- ❏ Once you've gotten your daily dose of Vitamin D (sunlight), there's no need to overdose. Seek shade if you are outside for longer than 4 hours between 10 in the morning and 4 in the afternoon.
- ❏ Avoid UV tanning booths.
- ❏ If you live in a scorching hot area, use a sunscreen with an SPF of 15 or higher every day.
- ❏ Know how much sun your own complexion can take. Whether you are dark or light skinned, your skin may be more or less sensitive to direct sunlight.
- ❏ Wear clothes when you are out and about in the hot sun! No amount of naked will keep you cool and only make you more prone to burns all over.
- ❏ Keep newborns out of the sun. They also need sunscreen and clothing to protect their delicate new skin from the dangerous UV rays.

Melanoma is the deadliest and most common skin cancer of all and it's caused by too much sun/UV rays and heredity in white people, but nobody knows for sure how it develops in people of color. Earlier I stated that people of color are more likely to die from skin cancer than whites. Why? Because many cases of melanoma in this group go undetected and without treatment until it's too late. The tumors are big, the spots have been there for years, and now the cancer is deep and spreading. Once a cancer has begun to spread, it is harder to stop and remove. It starts as a tiny spot on the palm of your hand and 5 years later, you're dying and a doctor gives you 3 months to say your goodbyes.

Familiarize yourself with your body from head to toe and check yourself out for any new spots, moles, discolorations or lumps. Don't get too much sun.

LEUKEMIA
BY YVETTE GZ AND C'BS ALIFE ALLAH

My mother's sunrise was January in the year of 1935 and her sunset was in October of 2001. My mother grew up in Arizona picking cotton and went on to become an elementary school teacher. My grandmother picked cotton in the same fields that they use to spray with DDT. She died of cancer before I was even born and later on in my life it came down to us that my mother had leukemia. – C'BS Alife Allah

What is Leukemia?

Leukemia is one of the top 10 most frequently occurring cancers in all races or ethnicities. Leukemia is cancer of the blood and/or bone marrow. To keep it simple, leukemia develops when there's an unusual increase of bad blood cells. A dysfunctional cell (usually a white blood cell) is formed in the bone marrow and survives then multiplies and crowds other cells over time. They reproduce at a much higher rate than healthy cells, and that's damaging to the body because those cells don't work like normal cells and prevent the healthy ones from growing. If those cells spill to the bloodstream, they can slowly or rapidly spread throughout the body and destroy vital organs. Also, the lack of healthy white blood cells means a weaker immune system and inability to fight off infections, and that can lead to serious illnesses and death. Leukemia also changes the blood cells count in your body, creating an imbalance between white blood cells, red blood cells and platelets. Since a cell is the basic unit of the body, when one goes wrong, it can affect the function and condition of your tissues, organs, and overall system.

How It Affects Us

Leukemia can affect anyone at any age. Even though it's more common in people over 60, young children can get it too. All it takes is a bad cell to survive and reproduce. That usually results from genetic mutations or viruses. Usually those mutations are a direct result of exposure to radiation and carcinogens from smoking and chemicals (hair dyes, relaxers, ammonia, etc...) and Black women are especially known to relax their hair or visit nail salons and breathe in toxic chemicals. Children with Down syndrome also have a risk of developing leukemia since they have a defect in their DNA.

Signs and Symptoms

Since leukemia makes the body weaker, you'd be more prone to infections, diseases and fatigue if you had it. Look for tiredness, night sweats and fever, slow healing of small cuts, random bruises from nowhere, bone and joint aches and weight loss.

Recommendations

"You cannot poison your body into health with drugs, chemo or radiation.
'Health' can only be achieved with healthful living." – T.C. Fry

Again, you would have to do a physical check-up to determine whether you have leukemia or not. Most forms of are treatable with medication or chemotherapy, but pills and radiation usually cause more complications and aren't completely healthy. In some cases, a bone marrow transplant may be needed.

The best way to protect your body is through a healthy diet.

How you can Help Someone with Leukemia

When my mother was getting sick and we were contemplating a bone marrow transplant, her Japanese doctor told me that Original people were the "superset" in terms of bone transplants. This means that (as long as other factors are met) **Original people's bone marrow is useful for transplanting into the bodies of all Original people AND white people** (sometimes known as a "universal donor"), **while white people's marrow, generally, is only geared toward the bodies of other white people.** Now, if Original People aren't entering into the database to be a possible bone marrow donor, what do you think is going to happen to all of those Original people who become afflicted with leukemia? That was actually a rhetorical question. To find out more about how to save someone's life by becoming a possible donor, keep reading.

50 Cent is a Bone Marrow Donor

WHY AREN'T YOU?

BY SUPREME UNDERSTANDING

Feel how you want about his public image, but don't talk bad if you're not doing better. I'm talking about 50 Cent, who recently registered as possible bone marrow donors in an effort to help save the life of 11-year-old Broadway star Shannon Tavarez, who was recently diagnosed with leukemia.

Fifty, right-hand man Tony Yayo and G-Unit artist Young Hot Rod got swabbed at DKMS America, the world's largest non-profit marrow donor center, which they documented in a viral clip for his official website. Considering that rappers are now making viral videos of themselves snorting cocaine, this is definitely a promo plug I can support. 50 explained:

> My son is just a couple years older than Shannon and I can't imagine if his life was needlessly cut short when there is someone out there that could save him. Shannon's chances of finding a matching donor are slim because she's African American and Dominican and minorities are underrepresented in the national registry. Everyone, regardless of their race or ethnicity, deserves a fair chance at life. Registering to become a bone marrow donor starts with a cheek swab, but it's more than that. It's a commitment to save a life.

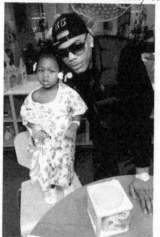

50's not the first celebrity to push for more bone marrow donation in the Black community. Earlier in 2010, retired NBA great, Kareem Abdul-Jabbar, revealed that he'd been diagnosed with a rare form of leukemia and was being treated. Abdul-Jabbar told *CNN* that he's going public now to educate people about this disease:

> My grandfather died from colorectal cancer, my uncle died from colorectal cancer and my father almost died from colorectal cancer...I think it's possible for someone in my position to help save lives.

But before 50 and Abdul-Jabbar, Nelly was pushing the issue. In early 2003, Nelly and his sister Jackie started the "Jes Us 4 Jackie" campaign after Jackie was diagnosed with leukemia on March 29, 2001. The cancer was in remission for nearly two years before she suffered a relapse, prompting Nelly to arrange a number of bone marrow drives in search of a match. Nelly, identifying with the Five Percenters' concept of "self-savior" used "Jes Us (Just Us) instead of "Jesus" to signify the need for us to proactively create the solutions needed in our communities, without waiting passively on divine intervention. The campaign's goal was to educate Blacks and other minorities about the need for bone marrow transplants, and to register more donors. Nelly planned on kicking off the campaign with a huge bone marrow drive to be held at Spelman College in Atlanta in April of 2004, but found himself stuck in a controversy. Because of his "Tip Drill" video, particularly the scene where he swipes a credit card down a stripper's butt crack, Nelly had become the new whipping-boy for male misogyny and female objectification in hip hop. Nelly certainly didn't create the culture, but he had become its new poster boy. As a result, Spelman women protested his appearance there and demanded he agree to a panel discussion on women and hiphop, or not come at all. Of course, not all the students agreed with the approach. "I didn't agree with it since he wasn't coming to promote himself," Nzinga Fielder, a Spelman sophomore told The Final Call. "He wanted to get bone marrow donors for his sister. I didn't think it was proper to protest this; she didn't make the video…People could have benefited from the event. I agree with them totally about his lyrics and the video. I just don't think this was the appropriate time to do this."

Nelly never came to Spelman. The Spelman students never followed through with their promises of holding their "own" bone marrow drive. And Jackie lost her battle with leukemia less than a year later on March 24, 2005, almost two years after the campaign began and no match had been found. In 2006, Nelly talked about the events:

> I come down there to teach people about leukemia and help benefit and try to help save lives and try to find a donor for my sister…Instead of doing that and helping and teaching our community about a bigger issue as far as healthcare, you want to have a three hour conversation about a f*cking video. Now, where are our priorities in it?… Why didn't you take that same three hours and educate brothers and sisters up on leukemia and what I came down there for? Now the same fight you are fighting in 2005, are you fighting that today? Because I don't have my sister today! No, I don't have her today!

Regardless of how you feel about what happened,[24] I hope you get the

---

[24] I agree that the portrayal of women in such videos is often tasteless, and leads to a variety of issues among both the girls and boys who grow up watching them. However, I think it's actually demeaning to women to claim that they are being "objectified" by Black men, as that idea takes away all "agency" from Black women, who have the ability to make their

MAIN point at hand, which is the immediate need for more Black and Latino men and women to AT LEAST become registered as POTENTIAL bone marrow donors. And bone marrow donation isn't just for people with Leukemia. It's probably the best way to address Sickle Cell Anemia as well. And considering how easy it is to get registered (just a cheek swab), you've really got no excuse to let anyone else die unnecessarily.

For more information, check out www.marrow.org or join the registry at www.getswabbed.org

---

Register to become a possible bone marrow donor. You don't have to do it alone, do it with a group of friends, it'll strengthen the bond.

IS IT A TUMOR?

BY YVETTE GZ

West Coast rapper Saafir found out he had one in his spine. T-Boz of TLC found out there was one in her brain. Actor Michael Douglas discovered one in his throat. Beastie Boys member MCA had one in his salivary gland. Tumors are real, and they're not so rare that you'll never find one in you. But because we don't know what to look for, we usually don't find out until it's too late.

What is a Tumor?

A tumor is a swelling or abnormal growth of cells and body tissue. They can be cancerous or noncancerous. A tumor occurs when there's an imbalance in cell division and you're creating more new cells than you can kill. The noncancerous ones are usually not dangerous depending on their location, size and cause. Sometimes genetic mutations can cause the swelling of body tissue in harmless areas. **The real problem is when they occur in important organs like the brain, lungs, colon, breast, or cervix.** When that happens, they can create blockades due to excessive tissue and interfere with body functions. They become cancerous when they help cancer cells grow and spread. That's when they become real uncomfortable and fatal.

How It Affects Us

Although a tumor is not always synonymous with cancer, it's still not healthy, and not pretty to look at either. And when it IS cancerous, it speeds up the growing process. **Cancer and cancerous tumors are very common in smokers, alcohol abusers, obese and inactive**

---

own decisions based on costs vs. benefits. After all, the dancer in the credit card shot actually CHOSE to be in that scene. Not to mention that the industry is not really driven by the Black men in the spotlight, but by the white men in the shadows people, as well as people exposed to toxins, radiation, and harmful chemicals. Toxic waste is dumped near a lot of Black communities, and breast cancer risk is very high in Black women. Look out for symptoms of a tumor so that you can get it treated as fast as possible.

Signs and Symptoms

These depend on the location of the tumor. A brain tumor can cause severe and painful headaches while a lung tumor will make you cough and have difficulty breathing. A tumor in the colon can make you randomly lose weight or give you diarrhea, constipation, anemia, or bloody feces.

Recommendations

Because these symptoms are not unique to tumors, it's best to check with a doctor to perform scans to locate tumors and determine whether they are cancerous or not. Once they are found, they can be removed by surgery or chemotherapy, but that depends on the stage of the tumor. Some can't be treated if they've spread to vital organs or blood vessels. However you can reduce your risk of getting a cancerous tumor, like many other conditions, if you exercise often, eat a healthy diet, reduce smoking and chewing tobacco, drinking alcohol, and keep a good weight.

What you allow to grow around/in you can strengthen or ruin you. Whether cancer, bad people or habits. Build or Destroy accordingly.

THIS ISN'T WORKING FOR ME
BY YOUR LIVER

Hello. You might not even know me, but you should. I'm your liver. Let me tell you how much I do for you.

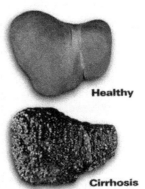

Healthy

I store the iron reserves you need, as well as a lot of vitamins and other minerals.

I make bile to help digest your food.

I manufacture new proteins that your body needs to stay healthy and grow properly.

Cirrhosis

I store energy, like a battery, by stockpiling sugar (carbohydrates, glucose and fat) until you need it.

I make the blood that got your system going even before you were born.

247

I detoxify poisonous chemicals you put in your system, including alcohol, tobacco, and other drugs (prescribed, over-the-counter, and illegal).

I also remove poisons from the air, like exhaust smoke and other chemicals you breathe.

I make clotting factors that stop the bleeding when you're hurt.

I help defend you against the germs going into your body all the time. I can't always kill them, but I help weaken them.

That's how much I love you! Without me, you wouldn't have the strength to carry on! Without me, there'd be no point to eating, you'd have no energy and fall into a coma. Without me to save you, your "bad" habits would destroy you. You wouldn't even be here! Without me, you'd die from poisoning just by breathing, you'd never recover from a wound and you'd be a dead man walking, a target for every bad guy out there. But do you love me? Here are some ways to show me you do.

- ❑ Don't drown me in alcohol! Even one drink can be too much and could scar me for life. I scar easily and those scars, called "cirrhosis" are permanent.
- ❑ Leave the drugs alone! ALL drugs are chemicals, and some can damage me badly. Sure, medicine is sometimes necessary, *but taking pills when they aren't needed is a bad and dangerous habit.*
- ❑ You've gotta be careful about what you are breathing. Aerosol sprays, including cleaners, bug sprays, mildew sprays, paint sprays and all those other chemical sprays you use can hurt me because I have to detoxify what you breathe in. So when you are cleaning with aerosol cleaners, make sure the room is well ventilated, or wear a mask.
- ❑ Stop putting crap on your skin! All those chemicals you put on your body or touch with your hands eventually get through to me and destroy my cells.
- ❑ Stop overeating and feeding me garbage! I can't process all that junk. What's even worse is that the "food" you eat is already processed, so I don't even know what to do with it sometimes!
- ❑ Give me a break sometimes. Try drinking only water for a day or two (I like a little lemon in the water). See. "You Flush The Toilet, Right?"
- ❑ A *blood screening test* can identify some trouble. If your doctor suspects trouble, an ULTRASOUND and CT scans can look into it. If I'm soft and smooth, that's good. If I'm hard and bumpy, that could mean trouble.
- ❑ Remember: I don't complain. I won't tell you I'm in trouble...until it's too late. So, this may be the only warning you will ever get!

Now you know how much I care for you. Please take care of me like I take care of you. My life, and yours, depends on it.

Your silent partner, Liver.

P.S. Heart, colon, lungs, kidneys, and the intestines also want to talk with you. And prostate said "What's good?" He said you'll know what he means.

It's better to take care of your liver than get a transplant! Don't neglect what has been with you thru your most F*up moments.

KIDNEY DISEASE

KIDNEYS ON $OME $HIT
BY ANGET MARCUS PANAG

Most people might not have heard of the rapper **Bo$$** (or 'Bitch On Some Sh*t'). Known for her tracks **"Recipe of a Hoe"** and **"Mai Sista Izza Bitch,"** she was the first female gangsta rapper out there and even landed herself a spot with Def Jam Records in '93. Her first and only album *Born Gangstaz* managed to push half a million sales, but unlike a rapper pushin a Beamer, Benz or Bentley, she literally needed the cash to survive. It turned out she wasn't even from the hood. And she certainly wasn't no gangsta, but she disappeared from the public because she was fighting another battle; she was fighting to live.

Like so many people in our community Bo$$ was suffering from **kidney failure.** She spent a lot of time in the hospital or on daily doses of medicine.

Yet another boss, who goes by Young Boss (no relation), an up and coming artist who already worked with the likes of Trina and Pitbull, known for his "fat boy fresh" image is suffering the same. The 25 year old hustla has been grinding his way into the scene for the past 5 years and has finally landed a record deal.

However, behind all the glamour of gettin big, Young Boss is still struggling medically, with kidney disease. Often kidney disease affects both of your kidneys, so the only real cure would be replacing them. Problem is that ain't so easy considering the average wait time for a person Boss' or Bo$$' age (18-34) was 1557 days way back in 2000. In 2004 that number had risen to 1782 days, about 5 years. **Even though that seems like a long time, the wait time is even longer in communities of color...especially for Black folk.** When the doctors do a kidney transplant, they have to be sure that the donor has the same genes as you or the body could reject the kidney and it'd be of no use. So they try lookin at family first and then check people from the same racial culture (we all family) but if there are only 20 kidneys available and they need 100, you can imagine that the wait is gonna be much longer.

Young Boss sat down for an interview with Allhiphop.com talking a little about his condition:

AllHipHop.com: What were some of your symptoms?

Young Boss: Swelling in the legs, in the hands and in the face, from the fluid not being kicked out by the kidneys. No energy, I would be at my sister's house laying on the couch talking to her and then I would just fall asleep. Bleeding from the nose, just a whole bunch of random stuff that you would never think, you know.

AllHipHop.com: Are you on any medications?

Young Boss: Yeah, I take 13 pills a day. For example, I take pills to limit my phosphorus, pills for energy. I'm going to need my energy and it's kind of hard to have a lot of energy when you rip and run as much as we do in the industry.

AllHipHop.com: Now, is there anything in your life that you could have been doing differently that may have prevented this?

Young Boss: Been skinny probably. [laughs] Nah, size, and when you're young you just eat. You don't really watch what you eat, you're just out there. I was good in high school because of football, so I was alright and it wasn't as bad as it is now. But of course you get older you start doing less, you start driving instead of walking, so I just gained weight – but I think it could happen to anyone. It just kind of happened to me. I'm still young and I was told that I only had a year if I didn't get dialysis or a transplant.

AllHipHop.com: So what are you doing different? Are you eating different or exercising?

Young Boss: I still eat, but I do it differently, I don't eat as much as I used to. Before my mom would cook and I would eat two, three, four plates, but now I just eat a plate or sometimes I don't eat at all. But now I eat differently, what I eat, the amount of what I eat, and I eat more meals, [smaller] portions.

AllHipHop.com: Are you on a waiting list for a kidney transplant?

Young Boss: After I drop 30 to 40 more pounds, then I can get on the waiting list because I don't meet the numbers. Your body has to match a certain number, so it has to do with your weight and your body levels, your blood count. It's so much of your life on a piece of paper when it comes to this. Hopefully when I get my kidney, my brother Dwayne and I match blood types.

So what is kidney disease?

Chronic kidney disease is when you have some type of kidney abnormality and decreased kidney function for three months or longer. Normally, this is because you've abused your kidneys (overworked them), or they've been affected by another disease like diabetes (the leading cause) or high blood pressure, which also results from constantly putting garbage in your body.

Some kidney conditions are *inherited* (run in families) or *congenital* (produced by a birth defect), but these aren't nearly as common as the above causes. If your family has a history of diabetes (high blood sugar) or high blood pressure, you are much more likely to suffer from kidney disease. Drugs and other toxins can also cause kidney problems. **Using large numbers of over-the-counter pain relievers for a long time may be harmful to the kidneys** (which is ironic, since that's what most doctors will prescribe once you have kidney disease!). **Certain other medications, toxins, pesticides and "street" drugs such as heroin and crack can also cause kidney damage.**

What Are the *Warning Signs* of Kidney Disease?

Many forms of kidney disease don't show any symptoms until late in the course of the disease. However, here are six common indicators:

☐ High blood pressure.

☐ Blood and/or protein in the urine.

☐ A blood test that shows your *creatinine* and *Blood Urea Nitrogen (BUN)* levels outside the normal range. BUN and creatinine are wastes that build up in your blood when your kidney function is reduced.

☐ A *glomerular filtration rate (GFR)* less than 60. GFR is a measure of kidney function, and can also be calculated from a blood test.

☐ More frequent urination, particularly at night; difficult or painful urination.

☐ Puffiness around eyes, swelling of hands and feet.

And finally, for the record, kidney disease ain't always caused by not eatin or drinkin right. You are also at increased risk for kidney disease if you:

☐ are older

☐ have a family member who has chronic kidney disease

☐ are Black, Latino, Asian/Pacific Islander or Native American (basically anyone "not white" but ESPECIALLY so if you are Black)

If you are in one of these groups, have any of the common indicators, or think you may have an increased risk for kidney disease, ask your doctor about getting tested...immediately

---

If you're in one of these groups, have common indicators, or think you may have an increased risk for kidney disease. Talk to a doctor.

WHAT IS LUPUS?

What could artists as different as Trick Daddy and J-Dilla have in common? Lupus. In an interview on *The Rickey Smiley Morning Show*, Miami rapper Trick Daddy talked about his personal experience with the disease:

I went to the doctor like 12 years ago. He took all kinds of tests, because I was trying to get rid of what we call dry skin. She did biopsies and blood tests and swab tests. She told me I have lupus. I am allergic highly to the sun, that's my worst enemy. It's like an AK-47 with a double clip on it. I could jeopardize kidney and liver failure from the treatment and the medication.

But Trick also explained that he refused to let the disease dictate his life:

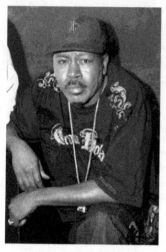

A lot of people try to cover it up with regular make up. It makes your skin pigmented. You can go from dark to light and not light to dark. You have to cover it up and conceal it...[But] my mama had 11 children from 10 different men. If she can live with that, I know I can live with this.

Unfortunately, living is not a guarantee. Lupus took the life of legendary hip-hop producer J. Dilla in February 2006, just three days after his 32nd birthday. This was a reminder that Lupus is NOT a "white folks" disease, nor is it something to ignore: In fact, just the opposite.

So...what IS Lupus?

Lupus is an incurable, life-threatening, autoimmune condition affecting the skin, joints, heart, and several other organs in the body. **And in case you didn't know, lupus afflicts people of African and Asian descent at higher rates than Caucasians.** Why? It appears that a gene that prevents malaria, common among many Blacks and Asians, also raises the risk of lupus. Lupus is incurable, but it is treatable once detected.

Keep in mind that no two cases of lupus are alike, and lupus symptoms can develop slowly or suddenly. **People with lupus often experience episodes known as flares, which can then improve or disappear, causing more confusion.** Lupus signs and symptoms depend on which body systems are affected by the disease, but may include:

- ❏ Fatigue
- ❏ Fever
- ❏ Weight loss or gain
- ❏ Joint pain, stiffness and swelling
- ❏ Butterfly-shaped rash on the face that covers the cheeks and the bridge of the nose
- ❏ Skin lesions that appear or worsen with sun exposure
- ❏ Mouth sores
- ❏ Hair loss (alopecia)
- ❏ Fingers and toes that turn pale when exposed to cold or during stress
- ❏ Shortness of breath
- ❏ Chest pain

| □ Dry eyes | □ Anxiety | □ Memory loss |
| □ Easy bruising | □ Depression | |

Recommendations

Here are a few pointers to increase the possibility of obtaining remission or improvement with autoimmune diseases, such as lupus:

- □ A nutritious, plant-based diet, without flour and baked goods, is usually necessary; a lower protein diet is helpful.
- □ Making sure you have a healthy fatty acid balance in your system. Fish oil and/or flaxseed oil can help.
- □ Fasting can be an extremely effective way to regulate your autoimmune response and reset the hyperactive immune system to a more normal (lower) level of activity. (But don't fast without talking to your doctor, especially if you are on medication. This is critical if you are on immunosuppressive drugs, such as Methotrexate and Immuran).
- □ Get on a food elimination diet to uncover hidden food sensitivities and allergies. The offending foods are most typically animal products, wheat and dairy; but you may find other foods can worsen your condition as well.

Follow the above recommendations if you have an autoimmune disorder. Do all you can to remain or go into remission.

MAKING SENSE OF HIV AND AIDS

BY ADRIAN BLACK

What is HIV?

HIV is a "REAL" diagnosable and observable virus which CAN be treated and conquered. However, HIV can also sit practically dormant (but not completely) in the body and can do so for the rest of your life. Truth be told, the problems usually begin when a person (A) does not have access to adequate nutrition in their daily diet; (B) is stuck with poor/unsanitary sources of food/water and/or living conditions; and (C) is regularly exposed to pathogens (bacteria and viruses).

This is because, like most viruses, HIV tends to temporarily (sometimes permanently) lower the T-cell count in your body (CD4+ T-cells are the cells that help your immune system function adequately). After this happens, the body has lowered its defenses to combat the virus thus leaving it slightly more vulnerable to any other invading viruses or bacteria. If a person is poorly nourished or has lived in unsanitary or toxic conditions, then their T-cell levels would have ALREADY been lowered. Thus, if a person living under these conditions contracts HIV, the effects will "most definitely" be more drastic than if contracted by the average "fairly" healthy human being because their body's defense mechanisms are preoccupied, combating other threats. In such situations, HIV can actually be a significant factor in someone's death. Otherwise, it's unlikely.

What is AIDS?

A lot of people get caught up in the hype of the "incurable disease" but don't understand the medical definition of AIDS. **Acquired immune deficiency (AIDS) is an umbrella term for any or all of some twenty-eight previously known diseases and symptoms.** When a person has any of these diseases or infections and also tests positive for antibodies to HIV, an AIDS diagnosis is given.) I often hear a lot of people still talking about a "Cure for AIDS." The problem is, AIDS is not as simple as it sounds, and in my personal opinion, the word should not exist because there is no "distinct" condition called AIDS. **In reality, the common diagnosis of AIDS is based on common factors/characteristics/symptoms but no "set" catalyst** (or we wouldn't be able to have HIV negative AIDS patients…more on that in a bit).

In places such as the rural parts of Africa, based on the current medical protocol, "ANY" physical condition you have, which could cause you to physically deteriorate, could have you diagnosed with AIDS (even without HIV!). This is one of the biggest factors behind how the phenomenon of the "AIDS pandemic" came about. **The standard diagnosis for AIDS in Africa is this simple: If your T-cell count falls below 200 cells per cubic millimeter of blood** (about a drop)**, you have AIDS.** No virus required.

The Diagnosis Flaw

The problem with this diagnosis is that MANY factors (other than HIV/ AIDS) **can cause an individual's T-cells to drop well below 200.** This is why there is a common pattern with "large findings of AIDS" around the world: the locations are usually extremely poor, the locals often drink from poor water sources, the kids are malnourished and diseases such as Malaria, Cholera and parasitic infections are commonplace (hence the stereotype of AIDS making you skinny when, in fact, an immune deficiency would not necessarily affect a person's metabolism). Each of these factors can lower an individual's T-cells.

"AIDS is a multi-factorial and conductive disease caused by simultaneous tensions over the immune system, like drugs, diseases of sexual transmission and multiple viral infections." – Dr. Gordon Stewart, Professor of Public Health at the University of Glasgow

Now in the case of many Black, South American and South Asian people where "AIDS" is documented at fairly high rates, these characteristics (mass poverty/poor living standards and a lack of medical resources) are nearly parallel, and based on Western standards a diagnosis of AIDS is performed nearly the same way.

"The dogma that HIV causes AIDS is the biggest and perhaps morally the most destructive fraud ever perpetrated in the western world." – Dr. Charles Thomas, Professor of Biochemistry at Harvard and John Hopkins Universities

Many people from scientific and medical backgrounds have voiced similar concerns about flaws in the modern diagnosis of HIV, particularly in 3rd world countries. For starters, in places such as Africa, India or Brazil, people's bodies often produce high levels of antibodies to fight off bacteria or foreign proteins. These same antibodies can cause you to show up as positive on a HIV test. In fact, many pathogens, such as Hepatitis viruses, Herpes viruses including Cytomegalovirus, Herpes simplex, Treponema pallidum, the cause of Syphilis, Epstein-Barr Virus, Mycobacteria, and others, are just as prevalent in AIDS-patients as is HIV.

"There are too many deficiencies in the theory about HIV as the cause of all the signs related to AIDS"– Dr. Luc Montagnier, Virologist and alleged discoverer of the supposed HIV at the Pasteur Institute in Paris

If you have pneumonia with 600 T-cells, you just have pneumonia. If you have pneumonia with 100 T-cells, you have AIDS. Don't expect many specifics beyond that. **Nobody can tell you how HIV is supposed to cause the loss of T-cells, even though that's the whole basis of the HIV=AIDS argument.** You mean to tell me after TRILLIONS of dollars spent (more than on any other illness EVER found on the planet) we can't even get a simple answer as to HOW HIV causes AIDS? Think about it. Have you ever heard that connection explained?

"We couldn't find any good reason for which most people on Earth believe AIDS is a disease caused by a virus called HIV. Simply there is no scientific evidence somewhere that demonstrates that this is true." – Dr. Kary B. Mullis, Chemistry Nobel Prize in 1993 for inventing the PCR technique

Better yet, I'd like someone to explain how does a person WITHOUT HIV contract AIDS? The logic is pretty basic – if HIV causes AIDS, why are 2-10% of AIDS patients HIV negative? The math just doesn't add up. If the equation is "HIV + Human = AIDS" how do you get AIDS without the key ingredient? Can you make Chicken Soup without chicken? Does 1 + 0 = 2?

Distortion of Statistics

There's also an ongoing outrage within the global community related to inaccurate, practically made-up, statistics being distributed about HIV/AIDS. **For example, in November 1997, the World Health Organization made a famous blunder when it announced that, since its previous report in July 1996, there had been a further 4.5 million AIDS cases in Africa. In this period, however, only**

120,000 AIDS sufferers were actually registered.

So my question is: How did the remaining 4.4 million AIDS cases become "Official Statistics" for the globe to absorb as factual? Perhaps it's the way the "estimates" are made. The current UNAIDS figures state that there are approximately 30 million people worldwide, currently suffering from AIDS, mainly in Africa, South Asia and South America – the only locations on earth where people of color are the majority. **What we are not told about this "official figure" is that it is not actually based on any physical data but merely a computer generated estimate formulated via a Simulation program called Epimodel.**

Been Diagnosed with AIDS?

In ALL cases of people diagnosed with AIDS/HIV the most important thing anyone can do is seek a second, third and fourth opinion from specialists. As Queen Zafirah Aqueous writes in "WTH.I.V.?":

> If you are faced with a positive HIV diagnosis, be sure that all the tests have been taken: ELISA, Western Blot, and even PCR. Discuss with a doctor, preferably your own, factors that may cause a false positive. Keep on top of your t-cell count and t4 cell to t8 cell ratio. Get the test repeated even after a positive diagnosis.[25]

It's up to you whether you notify the lab of your status when seeking a second opinion, because you may not want them to misdiagnosis based on the last diagnosis. And go for as MANY professional opinions as possible, as misdiagnosis is a very common practice in Western Medicine. What one doctor may overlook, another doctor may pay closer attention to. So do NOT give up on yourself. Being told you have AIDS merely means you have a physical condition in which your immune system is weak or deteriorating. But, in reality, this provides no "reason" as to why, or what is causing the condition. The blame will often be placed on HIV, and in "some" cases HIV can/may be the cause of the defective immune system, but that's not the case every time, nor does such a diagnosis mean the battle/war is over.

---

[25] Her article (which you can find online at www.HoodHealthHandbook.com) offers another perspective on HIV/AIDS, as well as some details on the actual origins of HIV and AIDS.

What Can I Do for my Health?

If you're diagnosed as having a low T-cell count, it's important to try and stay clean and exercise and be very careful regarding what foods you consume. Animals such as pigs (pork) carry a lot more bacteria and parasites than most other meats, which can lead to problems your immune system can't handle, also avoid processed foods, caffeine, and alcohol.

Also, be sure to prepare fruit and vegetables very carefully. Raw vegetables, while richer in nutrition, often carry a lot more bacteria. Some fruits and vegetables to be especially careful about include broccoli, cauliflower, cabbage, Brussels sprouts, kale and collards. It's also a massive bonus in nutrition to eat fermented vegetables, but if not "properly" fermented, there is a risk of botulism, so choose wisely.

In terms of vitamins and nutrients, it's important to have a solid balance of Vitamin C, Vitamin E, Beta carotene, Bio-Flavonoids, Zinc, Magnesium, Selenium, Cysteine, Glutamine, and Tryptophan. (**Many of these,** particularly Selenium, **are highly effective in improving immunodeficiency disorders – and strongly connected to death when they are deficient.**) Also, onions and garlic (cooked) – as a side or seasoning – are beneficial because of their anti-bacterial and antibiotic properties: **Have your diet consist of the appropriate foods from our "Healing and Treatment" chapter.**

It's also extremely important to stay active (but don't overstrain yourself or "burn out." Exercise lightly and build up over time as exhaustion can also affect your health. **Be sure to get 8 hours of sleep a day, as rest allows the body to fight infections/viruses more effectively, as does making sure you spend enough time getting sunlight** (and thus Vitamin D).

Don't give in to depression. While its normal to experience some degree of low feelings, deep depression can actually weaken your immune system and negatively affect your internal health.

Finally, while it's important to do research and look up as many sources on treating the virus as possible, BEWARE that there are many con-artists with monetary interests "hustling" people into paying for bogus treatments. Look for proof, and we don't mean "personal testimonials." Ask to see "before and after" blood work and to talk to some references. It's also important to be aware that most known HIV treatments merely slow the process of the virus but do not destroy it. Therefore, it's very important to maintain a healthy lifestyle comprised of (1) Exercise, (2) Good Diet, and (3) Enjoying yourself rather than recessing into depression.

A PERSPECTIVE ON ANEMIA

BY CY

The very first time I was diagnosed with anemia, I took it upon myself to learn what that meant. Anemia is basically a deficiency in your blood, typically a decreased number of healthy red blood cells. These cells are the main transporters of oxygen to the organs. If red blood cells are deficient in hemoglobin, then your body doesn't get enough oxygen. That's why people get fatigued and sometimes pass out if they are anemic. **Anemia is the most common blood condition in the U.S. And, like everything else, it affects Blacks and Latinos more than whites** (Iron-deficiency anemia affects 3.3% of whites compared with 24.4% of Blacks and 8.7% of Mexican Americans).

It also turns out that there are different perspectives on whether or not anemia is an actual disease or merely a genetic trait of certain individuals. The standard for "normal" does not take into account gender, weight or other individual factors. **Women, in particular, experience a higher degree of variation due to menstrual blood loss, pregnancy and childbirth.** Some argue that some forms of anemia may be genetic adaptations, particularly in those with African heritage.

As a woman dealing with anemia I learned to observe my menstrual cycles as a basic indicator of overall health. When I was younger, still subjecting myself to processed junk foods, I had very painful and immobilizing periods. As I have adapted my lifestyle to include life enhancing fresh and natural foods, my cycle feels more like the cleansing process that it is. I feel no pain, have no need for medication and have observed less bleeding.

If you decide to treat your anemia through diet, it is important to debunk a few myths. One is that vegetarians/vegans are more susceptible to iron deficiency. Not true. Lentils, lima beans, dark leafy greens and even prunes are great sources of iron and easy to add to your diet. Eating raw steak will probably make you too sick to fulfill your daily need for iron. You'll throw up any beneficial vitamins and a layer of your stomach. Another myth goes back to standardizing anemia levels for everyone and universally labeling it as a disease. A better approach is to treat it on an individual basis. If you have been diagnosed as anemic, assess how you feel. Look at your diet. Ask yourself if you have any symptoms of the disease, especially persistent fatigue. If you need to increase your iron intake, focus on whole foods which help the body to absorb beneficial vitamins like iron.

> **Get enough iron in your diet. Vegetables, fruits, and nuts/seeds are great sources. Check the appendix of this book for specific sources.**

SICKLE CELL ANEMIA
BY DIERDRA BAPTISTE

On Prodigy's "You Can Never Feel My Pain" he raps about the disease that has consumed most of his life. His words are jarring and harsh, but they convey a sense of pain that few of us can understand:

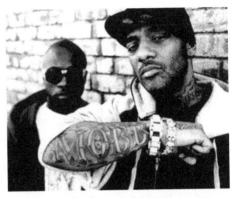

> 1974 motherf*cker, I was born with pain/ My moms and my pops pass it down to me/ So don't talk to me about, can I feel yours?/ Cause I ain't feelin you at all, your pain is impure/ You cryin cause you grew up in the projects/ That's not pain, that's emotions, you a bitch/ I'm talkin bout permanent, physical suffering/ You know nothin about that

What is Sickle Cell Anemia? The term "Anemia" is typically used to describe a blood deficiency (See "A Perspective on Anemia"). In the case of Sickle Cell Anemia, the red blood cells are shaped like a "C" or a sickle, caused by an abnormality in the cell's hemoglobin.

What is Hemoglobin? This is an iron-rich protein that gives blood its red color and disc shape, which allows it to move freely through your blood vessels. This is particularly important for carrying oxygen-rich blood from the lungs throughout the rest of the body. But sickle-shaped cells are stiff and clump easily, blocking vital passageways in the body. This blockage results in infection, pain and damage to organs.

How does this Happen?
Red blood cells are formed in your bone marrow, the spongy stuff inside of your large bones. This is a constant process performed by your body daily so that new red blood cells can replace the old ones which only last approximately 120 days. However, the life span of a sickle cell is typically 10-20 days and the body can't replace them at the rate of loss. This is what also accounts for the anemia or lower than

normal red blood cells needed for healthy performance of the body.

Who has Sickle Cell and Why?

This disease affects mainly people and/or descendants of those from tropical or sub-tropical regions, with over one-third of the Sub-Saharan African people as carriers of the gene. It remains most prevalent in regions where malaria was/is common. This includes parts of Southern Europe (especially Spain and Italy), the Middle East, and India. This is because in areas where malaria is common, there is a survival value in carrying only a single sickle cell gene (sickle cell trait). That is, if the person has the trait and not the disease, they are less likely to develop a significant infection from malaria. Yet those who have the disease (sickle cell anemia) have a high mortality rate from malaria and even if they survive, are severely weakened.

Is it Contagious?

No. Sickle cell anemia is inherited; it's passed down from parents like blood type, eye color, or hair color. A person who has inherited a normal gene from one parent and a sickle cell gene from the other will have sickle cell trait but not sickle cell disease. However, a person who has inherited the sickle cell gene from both parents can be born with sickle cell anemia. Two parents with the sickle cell trait have a 1 in 4 chance of producing offspring with sickle cell anemia, meaning, out of four children, two will likely have the trait, one will likely be genetically normal and the other will likely have the anemia.

> **Did You Know?**
> Books like *The African Exchange: Toward a Biological History of Black People* by Kenneth F. Kiple and *Black Superman: A Cultural and Biological History of the People Who Became the World's Greatest Athletes* by Patrick Desmond Cooper actually explain how diseases like malaria actually strengthened West African populations and paved the way for Black physical dominance in the Western world.

Symptoms

It's not a death sentence but the life expectancy is currently listed at 48 years for women and 42 years for men. It can lead to acute and chronic complications, some of which can be deadly. Symptoms are not limited to but include the following:

❏ Fatigue	❏ Jaundice	❏ Skin ulcers
❏ Paleness	❏ Bone pain	❏ Breathlessness
❏ Rapid Heartbeat	❏ Chest pain	❏ Excessive Thirst
❏ Delayed Growth	❏ Frequent urination	❏ Stroke

Sickle Cell Crisis

These are acute, severe episodes that usually last between five to seven days.

Aplastic Crisis (a worsening of the anemia), Vaso-Occlusive Crisis (obstruction of the capillaries by sickle cells), and Splenic Sequestrian Crisis (large amounts of blood are sequestered in the spleen). **The one thing all these conditions have in common is PAIN. You may have no idea what it feels like to have your blood get stuck somewhere in your body, but just imagine it hurting like hell...sometimes for days at a time.**

There are various other crises, including Acute Chest Syndrome, which produces similar symptoms to pneumonia, and is therefore hard to diagnosis. There is also Dactylitis, which is inflammation and swelling of an entire finger; it can be seen as early as six months of age and in those with just the sickle cell trait. Additionally, there is hemolytic crisis, which is an increased or accelerated drop in the blood's hemoglobin and break down of the red blood cells and most often requires treatment with blood transfusions.

Complications

Complications from the crisis stage and infections are severe and can be fatal, depending on the type of complication.

Eyes: Hemorrhage and retinal detachment can occur, causing blindness

Penis: Infarction (tissue death) or Priapism, a very painful state in which the penis does not lose its erect state. These episodes can last anywhere from several hours to even days. It's a significant problem for young males because it usually begins while sleeping and then the erection lasts for up to two hours. Besides the pain, an erection over four hours can result in impotence.

Stroke: Due to lack of oxygen to the brain caused by narrowed blood vessels from the blockage. Cerebral hemorrhage or infarction can occur.

Gallbladder: Gallstones and inflammation of the gallbladder (cholecystitis) from overproduction of the bilirubin during increased breakdown periods of the red blood cells

Bones: Increase in susceptibility to Salmonella and Staph infections; avascular necrosis, mainly of hip and other joints. The bone cell/tissue death occurs due to loss or interruption in the blood supply.

Kidneys: Necrosis (death) of tissue and papillary (ducts). This leads to renal failure, requiring dialysis, the need for transplant and can lead to death.

Heart: Pulmonary hypertension and heart failure

Limbs: Skin ulcers due to lack of blood supply

Complications in **pregnancy** include spontaneous abortion (miscarriage), pre-eclampsia (pregnancy induced hypertension) and intrauterine growth retardation.

Immune System: Those with the disease suffer from what's known as OPSI or Overwhelming Post-Autosplenectomy Infection. The spleen is usually completely dead or auto, .i.e. self-removed by the effects of the disease during childhood. This leaves the door wide open for infections like Staph, Strep and Flu and can overwhelm the immune system.

Alloimmunization is another problem that occurs with patients who frequently require transfusions. **African Americans make up a substantially smaller portion of blood donors than their white counterparts.** Therefore, most transfusions received by African Americans are from European Americans. **There are minor differences in the blood's antigens between those of African descent and European descent, and after a while, antibodies are built up against them.**

Treatment

While there is no cure other than bone marrow transplant for Sickle Cell Anemia, various treatments are used to combat and/or relieve the symptoms and complications.

Bone Marrow Transplants: Although not a common procedure for Sickle Cell Disease, it's been proven effective in children. However, the risks are great including transferred disease from the donor, rejection of the marrow from the donor and infection. (See "50 Cent Is A Bone Marrow Doner")These risks are cited as the reason bone marrow transplants for Sickle Cell are rarely done in the U.S., even though it's proven to be a cure.

Nutritional Supplements: Folic Acid or Iron is usually taken daily at a dosage of 1 mg from childhood throughout life whether in crisis stage or not. But other nutrients have been found to help, such as zinc, which studies have found to improve overall health among people with Sickle Cell Anemia, and Vitamin E, which several studies have found to significantly reduce "irreversible" sickling.

Herbal/Holistic Approaches: Maureen Henry, founder of the African Children's Holistic Health Foundation, described her search for a "natural treatment" for her son's Sickle Cell Anemia, noting that she'd heard about Africans returning to their village to obtain a traditional herbal remedy which they'd bring back to the U.S. At her site, she **lists several findings, most notably the use of prickly ash and gingko biloba, a treatment also used by the**

Nigerian Health Services, which is said to reduce the number of crises by 75 percent. She tells the following story:

> Since we have started treating my son naturally, we see a noticeable difference in him. His appetite has increased and when I recently took him to the children's hospital he had gained three and a half pounds in one month. His eyes were once yellow and now they are completely clear; he has much more energy and he doesn't cry and cling to me as much. Before we started working with the homeopath, I thought the hospital wouldn't allow me to treat him holistically but I was wrong. They are not pleased with it because they have seen many children suffering without their treatment but they understand our position.

Penicillin: Usually given from birth to five years because of childhood illnesses to which those with the disease are more susceptible. Hence why some parents supplement their children's diets with immune-boosting foods and supplements.

Anti-microbial ointment: Usually the only thing topically that can be used for the skin ulcers. Skin grafts are not performed due to low blood supply to the region.

Drug Rehab: Pain medication, as noted, is often required to ease symptoms and after back to back episodes of crises, some may become addicted to these drugs and seek them even when the pain is not severe. Prodigy continues:

> You just complain cause you stressed/ Nigga, my pain's in the flesh/ And through the years that pain became my friend; sedated/ with Morphine as a little kid/ I built a tolerance for drugs, addicted to the medicine/ Now hospital emergency treat me like a fiend/ I'd rather die sometimes, I wish a nigga'd OD/ Beggin God for help, only to find/ that I'm all by my goddamn self

Counseling: For psychological effects the disease has on the person and possibly family members and mates. Prodigy continues:

> When I speak, sit up in your seat/ Pay attention to the words, cause the story is deep/ In and out of crisis, since before I could walk/ It gave me strength, though nowadays I hardly talk/ It made me cold-hearted, anti-[social], I won't play sports/ I barely joke or play games, take it how you want/ My handicap took its toll on my sanity/ My mom's got me at the shrink at like 13/ And doctors called the cops on me/ Cause I be throwin IV poles when they ignore me/ I gotta try to calm down and breathe/ I can only hold it but for so long; put me to sleep/ Do I sound insane? If I do/ Then this here was written for you/ Cause you could never feel my pain nigga

There's a huge stigma attached to Sickle Cell Anemia. It's called the Black disease and often the men with it are portrayed falsely as weak. Most notably is when Prodigy was called out by Tupac on Hit 'Em Up, saying "Don't one of you niggas got sickle cell or somethin'?/You f*ck around and have a seizure or a heart attack." This was said as though his sickle cell held him back from carrying his own weight. Not true. **With the right treatments, healthy living adjustments, counseling, and a good support system and attitude, people (and children) with Sickle Cell can manage their condition very well.** In fact, the frequent pain crises Prodigy rapped about on "You Can Never Feel My Pain" are what led him to finally stop smoking, drinking, and eating meat.

After the change, Prodigy's health (and general well-being) improved immensely. Other famous folks who have sickle cell and are doing their thang include Larenz Tate, T-boz, Tiki Barber, and Miles Davis.

> **Did You Know?**
> The "reading in the dark is bad your eyes" scare is just a myth. Although reading in dim light is unwise because it may cause your eyes to feel tired or uncomfortable, it can't hurt your eyes. There really is very little you can do that will permanently damage your eyes. Similarly, reading small print or reading extensively cannot cause damage to the eyes. This is true even for people who already have poor vision. Although using computers will not damage your eyes, fatigue, eye strain or dry eye may occur with prolonged use. The eyes are meant to be used!

GLAUCOMA AND VISION LOSS
BY PATRA AFRIKA

Unbeknownst to my mother, I would deliberately break every pair of glasses she bought me when I was a child. I hated the way they looked and I especially hated getting teased by other kids. My mom used all sorts of scare tactics just for me to wear them. When she told me I'd go blind and could forget about playing and having fun with my friends, I used to walk around in the dark or with my eyes closed to pretend I was blind to see what it felt like and whether or not I could manage to get around. I must have broken at least a dozen pair of glasses. I never gave any thought to the possibility that it could really happen to any of us, especially not my mom who always boasted about having 20/20 vision.

Wouldn't you know it, when my mom was in her mid-50s, she woke up one morning and went to reach for the light but couldn't find the switch. When she tried to focus, all she could see were colored halos around the light bulb and a fogged vision everywhere else. And there was tremendous pain around her eyes and forehead. After being admitted into the hospital, that same day she was diagnosed with *acute closed angle glaucoma*.

I didn't think it could happen to me until I saw it happen to my mother with my own eyes. As conscientious as my mother had been about her health, she had developed glaucoma and nearly lost her sight. But as a result, she began to find ways to incorporate a better diet, nutrition and exercise into her daily routine. And fortunately she recovered by undergoing eye surgery. **My mom remains a powerful** example to me, on many levels. One level of which is because I share her genetics. Yes, glaucoma is hereditary which means I'm at risk. **Having a family history like mine is a good reason to have your eyes carefully examined at least once every year.** (See "Knowing Your Family's Health History")

What is Glaucoma?

Glaucoma is a group of diseases that can steal sight without warning or symptoms. **Over three million Americans have it. Only half know.** The two main types of glaucoma are primary open angle glaucoma (POAG), and angle closure glaucoma. These are marked by an increase of intraocular pressure (IOP), or pressure inside the eye. When optic nerve damage has occurred despite a normal IOP, this is called normal tension glaucoma. Secondary glaucoma refers to any case in which another disease causes or contributes to increased eye pressure, resulting in optic nerve damage and vision loss. Glaucoma can cause headaches where fluid in the eye does not drain properly, or there is over-production of fluid, which causes increased pressure within the eye. Prolonged increased pressure can lead to vision loss if not corrected.

Who's at Risk for Glaucoma?

Though everyone is at risk for glaucoma, certain cultures are at higher risk than others. **People at high risk for glaucoma should get a complete eye exam, including eye dilation, every one or two years.** The following are groups at higher risk for developing glaucoma.

People Over 60. Glaucoma is much more common among elders who are six times more likely to get glaucoma than a younger person.

Family Members with Glaucoma. Family history increases risk of glaucoma four to nine times. The most common type of glaucoma, primary open angle glaucoma, is hereditary.

Hispanics in Older Age Groups. Recent studies indicate that the risk for Hispanic populations is greater than those of predominantly European ancestry, and that the risk increases among Hispanics over age 60.

Asians. People of Asian descent appear to be at some risk for angle closure glaucoma. Angle closure glaucoma accounts for less than 10% of all diagnosed cases of glaucoma. Otherwise there is no known increased risk.

African-Americans. Glaucoma is the leading cause of blindness among African-Americans. It is six to eight times more common in

African-Americans than in Caucasians. Primary open-angle glaucoma (referred to as glaucoma going forward) affects people of all ages and ethnicities.

While glaucoma symptoms vary among Black populations in different international regions, it clearly affects those of African heritage more.

Six Ways to Prevent Glaucoma and Improve Your Vision Naturally

Exercise. I don't mean to sound like a guru, but I can't stress enough how important diet and exercise are in maintaining eye health and glaucoma prevention. **It keeps our weight down and increases the blood flow to our major organs, our eyes being one of them.** Increased weight means increased disease risk and poor blood flow cause hardening of the arteries and of course there are veins and arteries in and near the eyes.

Quit Smoking. Cigarette smoking and secondhand smoke can damage your eyes and your eyesight as fast as it can damage any other part of your body.

Keep allergies under control. Allergies can cause us to rub our eyes sometimes to the point of corneal injury.

> **Did You Know?**
> Contrary to popular notions, a headache is a valuable tool; an indicator that some kind of imbalance is present and needs immediate attention. Unconscious consumption of foods and other substances can cause headaches which medications only mask. Assessing ones dietary habits and environmental surroundings can lead to insights that can resolve the problem permanently. A headache can also indicate the need for the body to recover from a lack of sleep, stress or other physical or chemical factors. Relieving stress through healthful practices, light physical activity, sleep, relaxation techniques and healthy lifestyle changes can assist with internal sources of the headache. Avoiding harsh chemicals and ensuring time and space to breathe in clean air with live plants if possible, is key if complete relocation is not an option. Some natural forms of headache relief include applying pressure to the soft spot at the back-center of the head (where the cranium makes way for the neck) or applying peppermint leaves or oil to the temples.

Keep diabetes under control. Diabetes is the number one contributor to eye disease. Preventing it by eating a proper diet without a lot of sugar is the preferred way to deal with it. If you can't prevent it, then keeping it under strict control is the next best option.

Have regular eye checkups. Every one to two years is good and will help guard against developing glaucoma.

Nutrition and Healthy Eating Habits. If you knew that eating junk food all the time would cause you to go blind, and healthy would keep you from developing glaucoma and saving your eyesight, which would you choose? Not such a hard choice anymore, is it?

Treating Vision Issues with Nutrition

Here are 14 vitamins, minerals, and herbal supplements that medical research has shown to support your vision and improve or maintain eye health. Many of them are found in fruits and vegetables, while others require a trip to wherever you can buy herbs or supplements. You can check the extended version of this article at www.HoodHealthHandbook.com for details:

- ❐ Alpha-Lipoic Acid **(nutrient)**
- ❐ Bilberry (fruit)
- ❐ Bioflavonoids (nutrient in food)
- ❐ Copper Gluconate (mineral)
- ❐ Eyebright (herb)
- ❐ Ginkgo Biloba (herb)
- ❐ Glutathione (nutrient in food)
- ❐ Lutein/Zeaxanthin (nutrient)
- ❐ Rutin (nutrient in food)
- ❐ Selenium (mineral)
- ❐ **Vitamin A**/Beta Carotene
- ❐ Vitamin B12
- ❐ Vitamin C
- ❐ Vitamin E
- ❐ Zinc (mineral)

Protecting your vision is about more than just wearing glasses.

ALLERGIES
BY GENIALLY GREEN UNIQUE EARTH

Allergies occur when the body's immune system overreacts to normally harmless substances. Doctors call these substances "allergens." Almost anything can be an allergen to any given person. **Food allergies are triggered by your body's intolerance to the chemicals in** (or on) **foods.** An allergic reaction to food is an immunological reaction to food proteins. Remember your last doctor's visit when your doctor asked, "Are you allergic to any medicines?" Doctors ask this because there are some non-protein allergens that exist in medicine, like penicillin. And for other allergens think of the springtime when every other person has itchy eyes and is sneezing all over the place. These are also non-protein allergens. They must bind to a protein within the body before they can cause an allergic reaction. It all boils down to external agents upsetting the proteins in your body. Listed below are common allergens, in two categories, environmental and food:

ENVIRONMENTAL ALLERGENS	FOOD ALLERGENS
Pollen from trees and grasses	Medicines
House dust mites	Nuts and Seeds
Mold spores	Starch
Animal dander	Dairy: eggs, cheese, and yogurt
Wasps and bees	Shellfish

Industrial/household chemicals	Wheat
Latex	Pitted fruit
Feather pillows	Chocolate
Poison Ivy	Pork/Bacon
Poison Oak	Artificial coloring

Someone who suffers from allergies is really experiencing a war inside their body. Their immune system believes the allergens to be a threat and accordingly attacks them. As in any war there are styles of warfare. The body uses chemical warfare; what's the chemical of choice? Histamine, which unfortunately, causes the allergic reactions in you. The most common allergy symptoms are:

- ❑ Sneezing
- ❑ Hives or skin rash
- ❑ Runny nose
- ❑ Itchy eyes and ears
- ❑ Severe wheezing
- ❑ Coughing
- ❑ Shortness of breath
- ❑ Sinus problems
- ❑ Sore or closed throat
- ❑ Eczema
- ❑ Hyperactivity in children
- ❑ Nausea, vomiting, diarrhea

I'm sure you know all symptoms mentioned here can be caused by other factors besides allergies, but we can say for sure allergies do cause the above symptoms.

To treat an environmental allergy, you will have to systematically remove the things that may be causing it. You can do this by removing EVERYTHING that could be causing a reaction, then gradually reintroduce things one at a time to measure your reaction. For beginners, try removing pets (cats are particularly troublesome because they wash their fur and emit 'dander' that even sticks to the wallpaper, and comes off as you walk), synthetic detergents, synthetic soaps and lotions, and even old sheets, pillows and carpets.

To treat food allergies, first and foremost cut out all unnatural and processed foods or drinks. If you have the willpower (which you should if your allergies are persistent) you should fast. Make the proper preparations, take a week to plan, and fast. I don't mean "water only" fast, but a fast from all meat, processed foods, unnatural foods, dairy, nuts and of course any particular foods that you know may trigger your allergy. (See "Why You Should Fast")

After you complete your fast begin to re-introduce one excluded food at a time to your diet. Try a small dose, wait two hours and then if no reaction, complete the portion. Wait a couple of days between each new food before you introduce another. NO meat, seafood, dairy, grains or potato. Leave those till last because they are the most likely culprits of all.

Keep in mind not all food intolerances are related to meat and dairy products, but it can be said that vegetarians, and particularly vegans, will suffer less from food intolerance because they already eliminate the most common causes of allergic reactions.[26]

Remove anything you may be allergic to and reintroduce it once it's been "cleared." Do this for all that troubles you, especially people.

I CAN'T BREATH! ASTHMA AND WAYS TO COUNTER IT
BY C'BS ALIFE ALLAH.

I've had asthma practically since birth. It took me out of the running for playing team sports and though I was generally active I had longed to play things like football. I was guaranteed to get asthma attacks at the drop of a dime. In the Spring and Fall, due to certain types of plants pollinating, I would get attacks. During the Summer time if the humidity was high I would get an asthma attack. If I was in a panic or had anxiety from school work I would get an attack. I would lose out on many days of school and general fun plus my parents would have to figure out whose turn it was to stay home with me.

I would have to drink this pink stuff that would practically make me throw up. I had to take two little white pills that were supposed to do something. I graduated up to various types of inhalers. One type that was supposed to prevent attacks and another type that was in case of an attack. I even had to get a steroid shot at one point when I had a pretty vicious attack.

Now the first thing you need to know about asthma is it feels like someone is literally lifting you from the planet Earth's atmosphere into outer space. You start to cough, wheeze, your chest tightens and finally it feels as though someone is vacuuming all of the air out of your lungs. That windpipe of yours is getting smaller and smaller. You start to panic. And because you start to

[26] For more on allergies, particularly as they affect children, see "Why do Black Children have the Most Food Allergies?" in the chapter of this book dealing with Raising Healthy Children.

panic your breath quickens. Your asthma attack now goes into overdrive.

Asthma claims approximately 5,000 lives annually in the United States. And deaths from complications related to asthma have increased significantly during the past two decades. From the 80s to the mid-90s the death rate for asthmatic children ages 5 to 14 doubled. From the Mid 90s to the late 90s it roughly doubled again. Blacks are 4 to 6 more likely than whites to die from asthma. One thing we do know is if you are of color and live in the inner city the rate of having asthma goes up tremendously.

In fact Bronx County has one of the highest rates of asthma in the world. This is due to it being a junction for 18 wheelers and travel. The hospitalization rate is 5 times higher. In some neighborhoods 20% of the children have asthma. Why do we get hit hard in the hood?

- ❏ Many of our family members and caretakers smoke. It's not just being around active smokers that aggravates asthma, either. The presence of tobacco smoke in clothing and furniture acts as an allergen.
- ❏ Rodents and cockroaches carry allergens. The level of infestation in the hood doesn't even need to be written about.
- ❏ Nitrogen Dioxide, another allergen/irritant, covers the dwellings in the hood due to inadequately vented stoves and heating appliances
- ❏ Air pollution. Everything from the buses, cars and trucks to trash incinerators (trash burners are usually placed in the hood). That toxic smoke binds with pollen and jacks people up.
- ❏ The presence of one or more of these triggers in early childhood makes it more likely that a child will develop asthma. And growing up in this environment makes less likely that a child will grow out of it.

So as you can see a lot of what causes asthma are environmental factors. Also asthma is hard to 'cure,' yet there are a number of things you can do to lessen the intensity of an attack and/or prevent attacks:

- ❏ Cut the dairy out of your diet. It forms mucus in your body (which is basically what milk is, a form of mucus). That clogs up the lungs and attaches itself to all of those allergens.
- ❏ Eat hot peppers during attacks. Hot peppers cause blood to rush to the windpipe and lungs. During an asthma attack, they close up. When you ingest those hot peppers they start to expand.
- ❏ Take a shot of coffee. Coffee as a stimulant causes the heart to beat a little faster and moves blood to the lung and throat.
- ❏ Get the carpet out of your house. Go for hardwood floors. Carpets are breeding grounds for allergens. Vacuuming takes up surface dirt yet you would have to deep clean your carpet at least once a week

to get out the microscopic allergens. Keep your house as clean as possible.

☐ Do mild exercise to build up your lung capacity.

☐ Practice some form of meditation. This teaches awareness of your breathing so you can slow it down during times of anxiety before a full blown attack develops.

☐ Get a neti pot, a small ceramic pot that looks like a small tea pot. They use it in the East. By mixing up a solution of salt water you basically irrigate your nasal cavity. This cleans out all of those allergens and stuff that get caught up there. Done on the daily as a preventative, it helps not just with asthma, but with allergies and colds in general.

☐ Take hot showers. It cleans out the pores and the steam cleans out the nasal passageways. It gets allergens off of your body.

☐ Eat locally-made honey. It has to be locally made. It works to inoculate you against the pollen in your area so that you won't be allergic to it.

☐ Take trips to areas that are devoid of pollution. If you are going on nature walks try to choose days where the pollen index (they usually give this on the news when they give the weather report) is low. Going near water (beach, lake, running water) is great because the ions in the water attract the allergens giving you some clean air.

☐ Invest in an air filter that ionizes the air taking out pollution and allergens in your house. If you have an air conditioner make sure that you clean the filters regularly.

☐ With all of the above being said, go to the doctor to get a proper view of how severe your asthma is. Move from there.

Avoid anything that can clog up your airways. Practice mindful breathing, breathing slow will decrease the anxiety of an attack.

THE CURE FOR THE COMMON COLD

BY SUPREME UNDERSTANDING AND DIVINEGOD B ALLAH

Your immune system is your body's armor when it comes to harmful germs and bacteria. The best way to prevent catching a cold is to have a healthy immune system. Here's a few easy ways to do that:

☐ Get regular exercise, followed by good rest.

☐ Drink plenty of fluids, especially water.

☐ Wash your hands regularly.

☐ Get as much fresh air as you can steal.

☐ Minimize your stress. Yoga and Tai Chi are two great forms of relaxation on an ongoing basis.

Once you've got a cold, there's not much you can do but fortify your immunities to fight it off. Here's some advice on that:

- ❏ Ever heard the saying "Feed a fever and starve a cold"? old wives' tale, right? Well, research by Dutch scientists suggests that eating boosts the type of immune response needed to fight off the common cold virus, while fasting from food promotes a different type of immune reaction necessary to overcome the bacterial infections that trigger most fevers. So it seems like they just had it backwards. You should feed a cold, and starve a fever. No matter what you do, the key is WHAT you eat and drink.

- ❏ When you're sick, drink plenty of liquids (especially those high in Vitamin C) and eat fresh fruits and vegetables, especially the colorful ones that are high in Vitamins A and C.

- ❏ If you want to starve that fever by only having soup, I recommend a spicy, garlicky vegetable broth over chicken and noodles. Unless the soup is full of garlic, ginger, hot pepper, and vegetables the chicken and noodles isn't what's helping anyway!

- ❏ Take some herbs, like those listed below (see *Herbs = Medicine by Supreme Understanding*). Garlic, ginger, and cayenne make a very effective tea.

- ❏ At the supermarket, you can also find a natural cold and flu remedy known as Airborne. You drop it in some water and it makes an orangey drink that helps quickly boost your immune system.

If you can't make it to the health food store or even the supermarket, here's a ghetto remedy: A 99 cent bag of Lay's Flaming Hot chips (the hot pepper opens up the sinuses) and a 20 oz. bottle of 100% orange juice (boosts the immune system).

I can't promise you any results, but it works for me.

Herbs that Help Fight Colds and Flu Symptoms

Astragalus	German	Licorice root	Siberian
Celery seed	Chamomile	Peppermint	Ginseng
Eucalyptus	Goldenseal		Wild yam

Colds generally go away in about 7 to 10 days. Many holistic practitioners see the symptoms of a cold as the body's natural way of eliminating a virus. However, if you have an underlying lung condition, like asthma or emphysema, and you see your conditions going from bad to worse...it's time to see a doctor. (See "Healing and Treatment")

Take the above measures to eliminate or prevent a cold. If your coughing and sneezing everywhere, get some fresh air and sun.

Healing and Treatment

Elder Wisdom

BY KING DIVINE ALLAH

I often hear people say, "My grandma lived to be 100 years old and she ate the same thing I'm feeding you." This is a large misconception. For example, I have a great grandmother who lived to be 106 years old. When I started changing my diet, that's all I heard my parents say. They failed to realize that they were feeding me store-bought foods, while the foods my great grandmother ate came from her farm or her garden. She was not exposed to all the processed, cloned, and grafted foods that we are subjected to today. My grandmother lived a long life and one of the lessons that I took from her is that it's best to live off your own land and grow your own food.

One thing every hood needs is a community garden. We sometimes have rose gardens or flower gardens but what about planting fruits and vegetables? Agriculture is one of the areas that we need to move forward in as a people. **One way to produce plenty of fruit, vegetables, and flowers at one time would be to invest in a "square foot garden."** Square foot gardening is the practice of planning small, but intensively planted, gardens. The practice combines concepts from other organic gardening methods, including a strong focus on compost, closely planted raised beds, while attention is focused on small clearly defined areas. **Proponents claim that the method is particularly well-suited for areas with poor soil, beginning gardeners or as adaptive recreation for those with disabilities.** This is ideal for any area where it's difficult to grow plants, making it easier for us to grow our own food in the hood. An even MORE resourceful way of gardening with even LESS space is known as "container gardening."

More "elder wisdom" that we should never forget is all the home remedies that they use to cure common ailments. We have ancestors' that lived to be 100+ using these methods of survival during the harshest of times, yet today we are dying at the average age of 63.

Learn some gardening techniques. Not only will you be able to produce your own food but it's a great workout as well.

TRADITIONAL MEDICINE VS. THEY MEDICINE
BY SUPREME UNDERSTANDING

People of color have used holistic approaches (like the ones in this book) to heal their ailments for hundreds of thousands of years. And not just bug bites and stomach aches, either. **I can show you records of Black and brown people doing brain surgery 6,000 years ago.** Don't believe me? As always, you can look it up (but we'll go into full details in *The Science of Self*).

But I've gotta give you both sides of the story. Even with our incredible collective knowledge of traditional healing, I wouldn't advise you to go see the roots man when you've got a bullet wound or a serious life-threatening condition that requires immediate attention. Why? The following excerpt from *The Sacred Formulas of the Cherokees* by James Mooney (available for free download on www.SupremeDesignOnline.com) illustrates an important reality:

SHAMANS AND WHITE PHYSICIANS

Of late years, especially since the establishment of schools among them, the Cherokees are gradually beginning to lose confidence in the abilities of their own doctors and are becoming more disposed to accept treatment from white physicians. The shamans are naturally jealous of this infringement upon their authority and endeavor to prevent the spread of the heresy by asserting the convenient doctrine that the white man's medicine is inevitably fatal to an Indian unless eradicated from the system by a continuous course of treatment for four years under the hands of a skillful shaman. The officers of the training school established by the Government a few years ago met with considerable difficulty on this account for some time, as the parents insisted on removing the children at the first appearance of illness in order that they might be treated by the shamans, until convinced by experience that the children received better attention at the school than could possibly be had in their own homes. In one instance, where a woman was attacked by a pulmonary complaint akin to consumption, her husband, a man of rather more than the usual amount of intelligence, was persuaded to call in the services of a competent white physician, who diagnosed the case and left a prescription. On a second visit, a few days later, he found that the family, dreading the consequences of this departure from old customs, had employed a shaman, who asserted that the trouble was caused by a sharpened stick which some enemy had caused to be imbedded in the woman's side. He accordingly began a series of conjurations for the removal of the stick, while the white physician and his medicine were disregarded, and in due time the woman died. Two children soon followed her to the grave, from the contagion or the inherited seeds of the same disease, but here also the sharpened sticks were held responsible, and, notwithstanding the three deaths under such treatment, the husband and father, who was at one time a preacher still has faith in the assertions of the shaman. The appointment of a competent physician to look after the health of the Indians would go far to eradicate these false ideas and prevent much sickness and suffering; but, as the Government has made no such provision, the Indians, both on and off the reservation, excepting the children in the home school, are entirely without medical care.

This book was written in 1891, and Native Americans are still underserved by American healthcare. Not to mention that they're still dying at record numbers. In fact, healthcare is so lacking in Native American, Black, and Hispanic communities in America to the point where we might as well be living in a third-world country (yet we never stop bragging about this golden land we live in, huh?).

But let's talk about the story above. What went wrong? Was the shaman clueless? A stick in her side? Sounds stupid right? Not really. You see, "consumption" was an old word for the disease we now call tuberculosis, which got its name from tubercles bacillus, a stick-shaped bacterial microorganism that attacks the lungs, the kidneys and other organs on the side of the human body. Chew on that for a minute. So what this says to me is that our traditional healers have some incredible knowledge from a remote past when we understood way more than we do now, especially considering that Europeans named tuberculosis "consumption" because they believed "something" was eating people up from the inside. Before that, they called it "King's Evil" because they believed it could be cured by the touch of a king.

But let's be real. This knowledge we "once" had, we don't all have it anymore. Some of these traditional healers are just traditional crooks. They make their living selling hope to people who are willing to believe them, and unwilling to consider a second opinion. Some of them haven't been properly trained by anybody, and don't have a medical degree, a naturopathy degree, or even a high school degree. But they're getting paid. Some of these folks have even killed their "patients" through their bad advice, while some of us have killed ourselves trying to treat infectious diseases with roots and candles.

I understand the fear many of us have about going in for a routine physical and then being told we have HIV (See "False Positives in HIV Testing"). But Western medical science has made a lot of progress in terms of diagnosis. **And if you can find a doctor you trust, preferably one who is also familiar with traditional medicine, that's a lot better than choosing someone who doesn't**

have a proven track record of success with traditional healing. The key is finding someone with expertise in their field, who values your approach to health. If you're trying to avoid pills and prescriptions, find a doctor who understands that and who can suggest alternatives. If you're using a healthcare provider directory, I suggest checking out people who have Asian or African names. But just be warned. A so-called holistic doctor nearly killed my wife with her backwards approach to her hyperemesis gravidarum. (See "I'm Not a Doctor") Again, the key is expertise. This lady was clueless. We saw it in our first conversation with her, but we weren't smart enough to run when we should have. Now, our family's approach to medicine and healing looks like the following:

Whenever we aren't super-sick, we strive to heal ourselves through our diet. Either we fast, eat foods that have the appropriate healing properties (See "The Health Benefits of Fruits and Vegetables), or we take the appropriate herbs (See "Herbs = Medicine").

In more serious cases, we consult with someone we know who is very knowledgeable in treating such cases holistically. If we decide that we most likely need an antibiotic, we go to the CVS Minute Clinic (it's quicker and often cheaper than waiting for a doctor's appointment) for a prescription.

In the most serious cases, particularly when there is significant pain or need for immediate attention, we go see our doctors, who are all familiar with our family's approach to health (meaning they're not going to prescribe any medicines that aren't absolutely necessary).

In closing, there are traditional methods to cure just about anything. There are even traditional methods to treat bullet wounds. But, unfortunately, the roots man down the street probably doesn't know how to do it right. So, don't be dumb about your well-being – go to a doctor when you need to. On the other hand, if you don't believe that traditional medicine – when done correctly – is all you really need, check out the following story about rapper MCA from the Beastie Boys, who was diagnosed with cancer in 2009, but beat it after going to India and following a traditional Tibetan approach:

> MCA (Adam Yauch), 45, now says that he is on the road to recovery and getting healthier and stronger daily...He reportedly feels that he is hopeful that he has beaten the cancer after undergoing successful surgery and visiting Tibetan doctors in Dharamsala (India). He has been reportedly taking medicine recommended by these practitioners of Tibetan medicine and eating a vegan/organic diet, which he said was helping...Welcoming Yauch's interest in India and its institutions, acclaimed Hindu statesman Rajan Zed has wished him a speedy recovery. According to Zed, Tibetan medicine is an art, philosophy, and science combined, which provides a holistic approach to

health maintenance, and it includes the key Buddhist principles of karma, ethics, and altruism. According to Tibetan medical theory, all things in the world are made up of the five proto-elements: chu (water), me (fire), nammkha (space), rlung (wind), sa (earth). Changing a patient's lifestyle and/or diet is the first form of treatment in Tibetan medicine. Medicines are considered only if lifestyle-diet change fails to cure an ailment…Zed, who is president of the Universal Society of Hinduism, says that India also offers another herbal-based health care system known as ayurveda (life-knowledge) whose thesis is that disease is due to imbalance of three bodily humours – pitta (bile), kapha (phlegm) and vata (wind) – and balance can be recreated by changing person's diet, thoughts and habits. Ayurveda covered complete wellbeing of the person – mental, physical, and spiritual.

See the common denominators here? Among Original people (not just those in the East), we have traditionally recognized that health and illness prevention are accomplished through a healthy diet, a healthy mind, and a healthy lifestyle, even down to how we treat other people. This is why you hear about those "medicine men" in different societies telling people they need to "appease the gods" before they can get well. That's just a corrupted form of the original science of "making yourself right with the universe" and "cleansing your mind and body." Doing these things won't cost any money on their own, but if the medicine man or healer tells you that you need "special" items, which only he can provide (and bless appropriately), then you've gotta spend money with him to get better. Hence, even the first instances of medical corruption (putting profit before the patient's health) can be found amongst us. That should be expected, considering that we've been on the planet for millions of years, which is plenty of time for some of us to start becoming selfish. But this type of behavior isn't a characteristic of the ENTIRE system, as you'll find with Western medicine, which is almost entirely built on staying in business by keeping people sick and in need of more medicine and more diagnosis. Instead, you can still find plenty of examples of traditional healers who will teach you how to get your body (and mind) so 'right' that you'll never have to visit them again. And ain't that the kind of doctor you'd want to see?

Always check credentials and background.

DRUGS ARE BAD

BY C'BS ALIFE ALLAH

"One of the biggest tragedies of human civilization is the precedents of chemical therapy over nutrition. It's a substitution of artificial therapy over nature, of poisons over food, in which we are feeding people poisons trying to correct the reactions of starvation (malnutrition)." – Dr. Royal Lee, 1951

If you're familiar with the Iphone, you've heard the running joke,

"They've got an app for that." In the United States the mantra might as well be, "They've got a pill for that." **The United States is the pill-popping capital of the world.** This is based on the medical profession's tendency to (A) treat everything as an illness, and (B) manage symptoms through pillage (pun intended), rather than getting to the root of a disease.

Prescriptions run the whole field of drugs, everything from non-steroidal anti-inflammatory to cholesterol-lowering drugs. In the medical industry, prescription drugs are the fastest growing expenditure, rising at least 15% every year since 1998. **Every year, over 125,000 people DIE because of drugs prescribed by their doctors.** Why isn't this being addressed? Because pharmaceutical companies like Pfizer make billions of dollars off each new drug they introduce to the market. And *they stay rich as long as you stay sick.* So you can guess how dedicated they are to "curing" you.

The majority of pill prescribed within what is called "drug therapy" have nothing to do with curing the cause of your symptoms. It's like when you take Tylenol for a bruised hip you got playing football. Tylenol doesn't heal your bruised hip. It just relieves you of some pain. When you have a larger issue in your body, taking pills ends up covering the real issue, which gets worse when not addressed, and then you end up consuming even more pills.

"If we doctors threw all our medicines into the sea, it would be that much better for our patients and that much worse for the fishes." – Supreme Court Justice Oliver Wendel Holmes, MD

Drugs often help with one symptom, while messing with your body in other ways. How often have you been prescribed a drug for one issue, yet prescribed ANOTHER drug to help with the symptoms from the first pill? Most medication is registered by the body as poison. They are eventually filtered through the liver and kidney. They increase the toxicity of the body. Just read the small print of your medication. They talk about how they will mess up your inner organs. The suggestion to drink a lot of water with the pills is not just to help swallow it. It is to flush the residue out of your body.

Did You Know?
Current statistics show that half of all Americans are taking at least one prescription drug. Going further, one in six is taking three or more medications regularly. And pill popping is on the rise within all age groups. When you get to the 65+ age range, we're talking five out of six people are taking at least one type of medication. That means only one out of six people can function without some chemical cocktail. Does that sound right? Does that sound like the pills make us better?

To NOT be a pill popper, it's important to get yourself on the road to nutritional wellness, utilizing holistic interventions and really getting to the root cause of your body's sickness. As Dr. Joe

Fuhrman has written:

> The answer to a long, disease free life will not come from a pharmacy company or from your typical doctor. It will come from an understanding that when you supply the body with the prerequisites of optimal health (superior nutrition, avoidance of excesses, elimination of deficiencies, exercise, satisfying relationships and adequate light), and remove the stressors that cause disease, the miraculous self-healing properties of the body will be given free reign and you will be able to sustain excellent health into your later years.

Some pharmaceutical drugs are anti-healing

"All drugs are poisons. The benefit depends on the dosage." – Philippus Theophrastrus

Yes, some pharmaceutical drugs help save lives. We're not denying that fact. However, every drug has a side effect. These side effects range from nausea to death. Yes, *death*. That's ON the label. This is because (A) most pharmaceutical drugs are chemically-altered and unnatural versions of the "natural" remedies originally used by indigenous people, and (B) many pharmaceutical drugs are focused on dealing with a symptom, rather than the root cause. **This narrow focus causes the drug to interfere with the body's natural path of healing.** For instance, a fever is the result of your immune system going into overdrive, working to prevent or resist something bad from happening. A rise in temperature of just one degree signals that your immune cell travel time has doubled to get to the site of the bacterial infection. When you take Aspirin, Ibuprofen, or Acetaminophen, you are effectively shutting down your body's immune system. So unless you have an abnormally high fever, you should literally just sweat it out. Also you can just take a cold shower. Similarly, arthritis medications weaken the intestinal walls which allow undigested food proteins into the bloodstream, which is bad for arthritis. Also, excessive or unnecessary use of antibiotics destroys good bacteria along with the bad, plus they have no real effects on viral infections. But this is because prescription drugs are big business in the United States (See "I'll be Your Pusher"). The real drug kingpins dress up in suits and go to board meetings in skyscrapers.

> **Did You Know?**
> Recently, the government was trying to get at Toyota for all the cars they had to recall. But the amount of people who die from a car flaw is minuscule, compared to the number of people who die from prescription drugs! We're talking at least 98,550 people per year! This is not even counting those who have severe reactions. ONE type of drug alone, (a non-steroidal, anti-inflammatory drug) causes 76,000 hospitalizations a year. Imagine what all of these over-the-counter/prescription drugs are doing. This still doesn't take into account damages done by long-term use of prescription drugs, which may make people susceptible to other types of diseases and disorders.

Okay, now that you've scared me to death, what can I do?

Well, in reality, drugs are drugs, whether

they are pharmaceutical or illegal. You follow the same process in dealing with relieving yourself of them. Some drugs, like weed, you can go cold turkey on. Other drugs, like heroin, you need a straight up plan to get off of. It's the same with pharmaceutical drugs.

"The doctor of the future will no longer treat the human frame with drugs, but rather will cure and prevent disease with nutrition." – Thomas Edison

So here are some ways that you can work to be free from the pillage.

☐ Find someone who has knowledge on holistic medicines or find a book on herbal remedies. Read and research to find out how to replace the pharmaceuticals you are taking (which are only suppressing symptoms) with natural remedies which will address the symptoms AND the root cause.

☐ Monitor your body. Even when taking a natural cure, you need to be on watch to see if you have any negative reactions.

☐ Surgery may be necessary for some of your issues. Be prepared to deal with that fact. It is good to know, however, that a lot of things don't require surgery (a lot of things that people end up having surgery for).

☐ When dealing with serious issues get more than one reference and weigh all your options. In the end, seek out ways to promote your body's own ability to heal itself.

☐ Remember that the goal is for long term health, not a quick fix. Taking 5x the recommended amount of an herb will not cure you overnight and may jack you up in other ways. After all, what is bothering you didn't happen overnight so don't expect it to just go away.

If you ARE going to use prescription drugs, ask questions and educate yourself. Here are some questions you should ask your doctors, nurses, and/or pharmacists:

☐ What are your meds made of?
☐ Who makes and distributes the meds?
☐ What will the meds chemically and physically do to me?
☐ Where are the meds made?
☐ What is the goal of the manufacturers of the meds?
☐ What are the side effects?
☐ What are the most dangerous side effects of the meds?[27]

Know about your medication. Have a discussion with your doctor or pharmacist about side effects and research alternatives.

---

[27] From "Medication Education" by Lee Williams, CPS. Williams adds, "When seeking answers about your meds, remember that you deserve to know anything that you seek to learn about what is going into your body. Besides, the more you know, the better your recovery process will be."

HERBS = MEDICINE

BY SUPREME UNDERSTANDING

On January 18, 2008, the Botanic Gardens Conservation International (representing botanic gardens in 120 countries) found that five billion people rely upon traditional plant-based medicine for health care.

And it's not just Chinese herbs like ginseng and gotu kola, either. While Traditional Chinese Medicine has preserved the ancient practices of using thousands of local herbs, thousands of indigenous societies throughout the world have been using these methods as well, only with less recognition from the rest of the world. **Only recently, Western scientists have begun studying the many plants used by so-called "primitive" groups like the Bushmen** (or San people) **of South Africa, such as** *Boophone*, **used for the treatment of mental illness and depression,** and *Hoodia*, **used for appetite suppression.** Their studies found such strong results that these drugs are now being worked into the modern pharmaceutical industry. Although the San were worked into the profit-sharing agreement for the use of Hoodia, they have yet to profit from this agreement. Surprised? That's nothing new, considering that so many pharmaceutical

> **Did You Know?**
> The word drug comes from the Old Dutch word drogge, meaning, "to dry," because traditional healers, and later doctors, dried plants to use as medicine.

drugs are based on traditional plants. Over 120 of the most commonly used modern drugs contain at least one active ingredient derived from plants. The rest are chemically synthesized. For example:

- ❏ Sudafed: Ephedrine (Ephedra)
- ❏ Birth Control: Dioscegenin (Wild Yam Root)
- ❏ Morphine (plus Oxycodone, Hydrocodone, etc.): Poppy
- ❏ Aspirin: (Willow Bark and Meadowsweet)
- ❏ Ex-Lax: Senna
- ❏ Valium: Valerian Root
- ❏ Atropine: Nightshade (cardiac sedative, pupilary dilator)
- ❏ Quinine: Magnolia, Dogwood, Cinchona
- ❏ Codeine: Wild Cherry Bark, Poppy

And that's just to name a few. Even Menthol is based on extracts from peppermint, eucalyptus, wintergreen, and/or spearmint; plants we traditionally chewed in our homelands (which may answer Dave Chappelle's question about why Black people crave cigarettes with menthol).

Anyway, these plants had much fewer side effects, but they also weren't making the drug companies any money, so you know how that story went. And now it's becoming more and more difficult to legally pursue or promote alternative healing methods. **This type of "monopoly" on medicine was predicted by some of the country's founders, who saw clearly the European tendency to "take over" and take total control of all human activity.** Benjamin Rush, MD., a signer of the Declaration of Independence and personal physician to George Washington, once noted:

> Unless we put medical freedom into the Constitution, the time will come when medicine will organize into an undercover dictatorship to restrict the art of healing to one class of men and deny equal privileges to others; [thus] the Constitution of the Republic should make a Special privilege for medical freedoms as well as religious freedom.

And in 1903, Dr. J.N. McCormack, of the American Medical Association confessed: "We must admit that we have never fought the homeopath on matters of principle. We fought them because they came into our community and got the business."

Fortunately, herbal medicine hasn't been outlawed...yet. So here's an abridged list of herbs you can find: (A) in your kitchen cabinet; (B) at most health food stores, or (C) in your own garden if you grow them yourself, followed by their traditional uses. In many cases, there's also information from "scientific" studies on whether they work or not. For more, you can also see the section titled "Healing Fruits and Vegetables."

In your Kitchen Cabinet

"Let food be thy medicine, and let thy medicine be food." – Hippocrates

You may already have plenty of these "medicinal herbs" in your kitchen cabinet. You may not know it, **but even hot sauce, mustard, and ketchup can be good for your health!** It's important that I mention that commercial spices and herbs (from regular stores) are usually very old which means you won't get the full health benefits from them. **You** (ideally) **want non-irradiated spices and herbs, which are available at many health food stores. Fresh spices should smell fragrant, not like powdered dirt.** You can get them pretty cheap if you buy them in bulk at a farmer's market, or – better yet – get them whole and grind just before use. It's actually easier than it sounds, and the difference in taste is obvious. You know what I mean if you've ever compared the taste of garlic powder to fresh garlic. **Here are some of the health benefits of common spices we use in cooking.**

Allspice: Great at relieving flatulence, nervous exhaustion, and diarrhea.

Basil: Basil tea lowers blood sugar levels, blood pressure, relieves cold symptoms, indigestion, headaches, cramps, nausea, and constipation, and is anti-inflammatory, a slight sedative, and can be applied to insect bites.

Bay Leaf: It supports the nervous system and stomach, helps dispel gas, stimulates menstrual flow, stimulates appetite, promotes digestion, and relieves colic. Externally used for dandruff, boosting hair growth, rheumatism, sprains, scabies, and bruises. Also can be applied as a poultice.

Black pepper: Helps prevent constipation. It is considered useful for asthma, boils, colic, cough, diarrhea, fever, gas, hemorrhoids, indigestion, chronic rheumatism, sinus congestion, skin diseases, sore throat, and worms. More significantly, it guards against cancer.

Cardamom: Cardamom is often used to treat indigestion and gas. It warms the body and is good for diarrhea, colic and headaches.

Cayenne: Cayenne is an excellent "activator herb," amplifying the benefits of other herbs you take. For any sudden gash, nick, or serious cut, just apply enough cayenne pepper to the injury until the bleeding stops. Both cayenne pepper and products made from it (like hot sauce) are known to increase metabolism and fat-burning ability.

Chili Powder: A blend of spices including chili peppers, cumin, oregano, paprika, salt, and garlic powder. The health benefits of chili powder are derived mostly from the capsaicin in the red pepper which is used in skin creams to reduce pain, including that of osteoarthritis. It also has antioxidant and blood-thinning qualities.

Chives: A member of the same family as garlic, chives contain cholesterol-lowering organosulfides.

Cilantro: Used for digestive and gastric complaints and for coughs, chest pains, bladder complaints, fever, headaches, and removing toxins from your body. Can be applied externally for rheumatism and painful joints.

Cinnamon: Recent research found that ¼ tsp to 1 tsp of cinnamon daily improves insulin function and, in turn, blood-sugar control. Helpful for digestive problems especially when accompanied by gas and cramping, diarrhea, vomiting. Also used to treat colds, flu, arthritis and rheumatism. Cinnamon is also astringent, anti-bacterial, and anti-microbial.

Cloves: an anesthetic, works well for toothaches (chewed, or a drop of the oil on the sore tooth) and as a sore throat gargle. Internally cloves help to relieve pain, nausea, vomiting, and digestive problems. Cloves kill intestinal parasites and act as an anti-microbial agent against fungi and bacteria. Externally it is good for insect bites and rheumatism.

Coriander Seed: Steeped in tea, 2 teaspoons of crushed seeds is useful in relieving fevers (black pepper may be added to stimulate its action). Before toothpaste, coriander seeds were chewed to clean teeth and freshen breath.

Cumin: Aids digestion and helps flush toxins out of the body.

Curry: A blend of ginger, turmeric, cardamom and other spices that have been shown to increase metabolism, help breathing, and reduce cholesterol. Research has shown that saffron, which gives curry its yellow color, helps keep vision sharp and can prevent blindness.

Fennel: Naturally sweet fennel helps stabilize blood-sugar levels and curbs the appetite. The herb relaxes the smooth muscles of the digestive tract, which helps with flatulence and indigestion. Fennel will also ease throat tension and coughs as well as bring up phlegm from the lungs.

Garlic: Contains cholesterol-fighting organosulfur compounds. Garlic helps many illnesses, because it stimulates your immune response, and promotes sweating. It also helps prevent heart disease by lowering cholesterol levels. It also boosts levels of T-cells, a critical component of the immune system. Destroys cancer cells and may disrupt the metabolism of tumor cells. Studies suggest that one or two cloves weekly provide cancer-protective benefits. Let fresh garlic sit for 10 to 15 minutes after chopping and before cooking so the active form of the protective phytochemicals develops. Studies have shown that garlic also relieves arthritis.

Ginger: Prevents nausea (including morning sickness), motion sickness and can stimulate the appetite. Ginger may also relieve pain and inflammation associated with arthritis. A quarter-size piece of fresh root contains about 1,000 mg of powdered ginger. More than 6,000 mg can cause stomach irritation. For more, see "Add a Little Spice to Your Life!"

Horseradish: Whether it's fresh, jarred or in the sharp green wasabi served with sushi, horseradish can help you fight cancer. Compounds in the roots and leaves of the horseradish plant, can increase your liver's ability to detoxify carcinogens and may suppress the growth of existing tumors, says a study in the Journal of Agricultural and Food Chemistry. Horseradish is one of nature's best sources of glucosinolates – it has up to 10 times more than broccoli, the next-best source. It also acts as a digestive stimulant.

Lemongrass: Can be helpful for discomfort with menstruation, vomiting, diarrhea, muscle spasms, and fever. For fevers, combine with ginger, sugar, and cinnamon. Good for children's digestive system. Externally, great for lumbago, chronic rheumatism, ringworm, lice, athletes foot, scabies, and sprains. Mix with pure coconut oil to apply as a liniment.

Mustard: A stimulant known to be helpful in cases of respiratory complaints. Yellow mustard and mustard seed contain health-protective isothiocyanates.

Nutmeg: A small amount, about the size of a pea, can be taken once daily over a long period to relieve chronic nervous disorders and heart problems. Internally helps with digestion, diarrhea, and vomiting, bloating, indigestion, colic. Externally, it's good for eczema, rheumatic and abdominal pain.

Oregano: Oregano is the most antioxidant dense herb out of 27 fresh culinary herbs. It offers many antibacterial benefits and can help strengthen the immune system. It can help repel mosquitoes. Oregano may be effective against multi-drug resistant bacteria.

Paprika: Good source of Vitamin C. Acts as antioxidant, paprika is a mild form of cayenne pepper, which serves as a carrier for other nutrients and may help reduce blood-platelet stickiness and lower the risk of cancer.

Parsley: Expels worms, relieves gas, prevents tumors, and enhances digestion. It's used to stop bedwetting, used as a diuretic, to relax spasms, and clear toxins in the body, menstrual complaints, urinary tract problems, arthritis, anemia, anorexia, colic, lactation. Externally relieves itching.

Rosemary: Stops gene mutations that can lead to cancer and may help lower heart attack risk by stopping damage to the blood vessels. Commonly used as an aspirin substitute for headaches. Good as a mouthwash for gums and sore throat. Externally used in baldness shampoos, increases circulation, and scalp stimulation. Rosemary is warming, both a circulatory and liver tonic.

Sage: Contains monoterpenes that prevent the spread and progression of tumors. Internally it is helpful for indigestion, gas, night sweats (especially menopausal), excessive salivation, profuse perspiration, anxiety, and depression. Used externally, helps with insect bites, throat, mouth and gum infections, combats greasy oily hair and scalp and is also helpful with acne.

Tarragon: Anti-fungal, anesthetic, stimulates appetite, and relieves flatulence.

Thyme: A tea made with thyme is commonly used for acute

bronchitis, whooping cough and laryngitis. It is also beneficial for the treatment of diarrhea and lack of appetite. Other uses include headache, mucus, stomach worms, hangover and respiratory problems. Externally, its antiseptic properties make it a useful mouthwash and cleansing wash for the skin. It will also destroy fungal infections such as athlete's foot and skin parasites such as scabies, crabs and lice. Not used during pregnancy.

Turmeric: A warming analgesic, antioxidant, anti-inflammatory, antiseptic and astringent that helps control free radicals and therefore protects against cancer. It promotes bile, relieves a congested liver and gallstones and aids digestion. Turmeric can also help to reduce tumors and uterine fibroids.

At the Health Food Store

Alfalfa leaf: An excellent source of chlorophyll, vitamin C, and minerals. The herb has a neutral flavor and helps improve anemia and digestion.

Aloe Vera: Studies support the use of Aloe Vera for the healing of first to second degree burns. Also used externally to improve skin's appearance. Used internally for gastro intestinal problems. Not given during pregnancy.

Anamu: A pain reliever, used for arthritis, osteoarthritis and diabetes.

Anise seed: Has a pleasant, licorice-like flavor. Improves digestion, freshens breath, reduces gas, nausea and coughs due to its expectorant properties.

Astragalus: Used to boost the immune system by minimizing toxins caused by chemicals or radiation.

Barley Greens: Used for energy, nutrition, and fights aging and rheumatism.

Bayberry: Fights colds, coughs, excess mucus, fevers, and bleeding gums.

Bee Pollen: Used for allergies, quick energy, and nutrition.

Billberry: An antioxidant and astringent used to treat bruising, varicose veins, retinal blindness, poor night vision, cataracts, poor circulation, Raynaud's disease, rheumatoid arthritis, gout and periodontal disease, and circulation complications due to diabetes.

Black Cohosh: Used for natural estrogen, in treating hot flashes and women's reproductive problems, as well as whooping cough, asthma, and sometimes depression. Not safe for pregnant women.

Black Cumin (Nigella sativa): Traditionally used in Islamic medicine as a cure for a variety of ailments including bronchitis, asthma, rheumatism and related inflammatory conditions. It is also known to increase milk production in nursing mothers, digestive and eliminative problems, and parasite infections. The oil is used to treat skin conditions such as eczema and boils.

Black Horehound: Used for motion sickness, female problems and respiratory ailments.

Black Walnut: Fights parasites/worms, skin rashes, lupus, and eliminates toxins.

Blackberry Leaf: has astringent properties, is a source of blood-building iron, and has been used to treat diarrhea.

Burdock: Used to reduce swelling and deposits in joints, as a blood purifier, and for gout and eczema.

Butcher's Broom: helps with circulation, leg cramps, and varicose veins.

Calendula: Used traditionally (and verified by science) for abdominal cramps and constipation.

Catnip: A sedative used for cold and flu symptoms because it is good for breaking a fever and easing trembling. It can also be used to calm cigarette cravings, upset stomach and even hiccups. Catnip tea can help you sleep, but it can also make you sweat, so it is used as a rub for arthritis pain.

Chamomile: Used to calm upset stomach, reduce headaches, improve appetite and even ease the symptoms of drug withdrawal. Used externally for wounds and burns. Essential oil of chamomile was shown to be a promising antiviral agent against herpes simplex virus type 2 (HSV-2).

Chicory root: is mildly cleansing to the liver and colon. When roasted, it tastes like coffee – without the caffeine.

Coltsfoot: Used for coughs, asthma, whooping cough. Externally for skin disorders, insect bites. Not used during pregnancy.

Creeping Thyme: Used for upper respiratory ailments. Gaseous indigestion, colic and hangovers. Not used during pregnancy.

Dandelion: Good for liver detoxification, hepatitis, anemia, and a number of other uses.

Dill: used to treat colic and other digestive disorders. Dill stimulates the movement of the digestive system and relaxes the stomach.

Echinacea (Purple Coneflower): Immune system booster. Studies demonstrate that it can limit the length and severity of rhinovirus colds. Second, it neutralizes invading microorganisms. Researchers have shown that Echinacea stops staph, strep, fungal infection and a variety of viruses.

Elder Flowers: Increase perspiration by gently dilating the pores. Elder flowers are also excellent for the prevention and treatment of colds and flu.

Eyebright: Used to improve vision, eye strain, cataracts, allergies, and sties.

False Unicorn: Used as an ovarian/uterine tonic and to treat menstrual problems and prevent miscarriage.

Gingko Biloba: Used to improve memory and attention span, and to treat Alzheimer's and stroke sufferers. Studies have shown it to be effective in increasing peripheral blood flow, making it useful in treating age-related brain disorders, cerebral and vascular insufficiency, Raynaud's disease, chronic bronchitis, emphysema and to prevent strokes.

Ginseng: Used to increase energy and endurance, decrease stress and depression, and as a male stimulant.

Goldenseal: Treats infection, cleanses urinary system, and is a natural insulin.

Gotu Kola: Considered "brain food," used to improve memory and treat mental fatigue, depression, and nervous breakdown.

Green tea: Components may inhibit growth of breast cancer cells and may heal scars faster. Tea's antioxidant catechins are linked to reduced heart-disease risk. Tea may also help inhibit other cancers. Just make sure you buy an organic brand, because 1 out of 6 store-bought varieties of green tea contain DDT, a pesticide that actually CAUSES cancer.

Hibiscus: Purified extracts of the seeds may have some antihypertensive, antifungal and antibacterial effect. Hibiscus flowers have a tart flavor and are rich in vitamin C. Hibiscus has a cooling effect, which makes it an excellent choice in herbal iced teas. It provides a beautiful rose color to a tea blend.

Hops: Reduces cramps, spasms, digestive disorders, and desire for alcohol.

Horsetail: Used to reduce hair loss, stop split ends, and to fight tumors.

Juniper Berries: A diuretic used to strengthen kidneys.

Kava Kava: A sleep aid, fights anxiety, chronic fatigue and panic attacks.

Lady's Mantle: Used for female ailments. Externally used for sores and minor injuries.

Lemon Balm: Studies show it helps protect the brain from excessive external stimuli, so it has a calming, anti-anxiety effect. Not only tastes nice but also has antiviral properties, making it good for colds and flu. Used externally for cold sores, insect bites, and as insect repellant..

Lemon Verbena: Has antiseptic properties and has been used throughout history for digestive disorders, colds, and flu.

Licorice: Available in many stores as "chew-sticks," licorice root has been used to adjust blood sugar, increase energy, reduce cough and sore throat, and to reduce plaque (by chewing).

Meadowsweet (or Queen of the Meadow): Used for a variety of anti-inflammatory and antimicrobial purposes due to presence of salicylic acid (the basis for aspirin). Effective for fevers and inflammations, pain relief, ulcers and as a bacteriostatic (limits the growth of bacteria).

Milk thistle: Research suggests that milk thistle extracts both prevent and repair damage to the liver from toxic chemicals and medications, as well as helping to reverse the effects of hepatitis and cirrhosis.

Motherwort: Used for heart palpations, female problems. Not given to pregnant women.

Mullein: Added to tea blends to relieve congestion, coughs, hay fever and sinusitis. Mullein has a bittersweet taste, reduces inflammation and soothes irritated mucus membranes.

Nettle Leaf: Extremely rich in nutrients, including iron and beta-carotene, Improves kidney, adrenal function, benefit allergies and has a salty flavor.

Oat Straw: The young stem of the oat plant has a pleasant, sweet flavor. Oat straw is highly nutritive (especially high in calcium) and supports the nervous system, helping to relieve depression, insomnia and stress.

Passion Flower: Used for insomnia due to overwork or exhaustion. Combined with valerian and hops it brings on a very restful and sound sleep. It eases nerve pain brought about by neuralgia or shingles, and eases withdrawal symptoms from antidepressants.

Pau D'arco: Also known as lapacho, is effective at preventing colds, flu and bacterial infections. Can also soothe painful joints, boost energy levels and stimulate activity of enzymes in the liver, enhancing the ability to remove toxins from the blood. In Brazil, it is used to treat leukemia, cervical cancer, and skin cancer. Studies suggest that the herb may also be effective against breast cancer.

Pennyroyal: Used to ease indigestion, feverish colds, and skin irritations. Not for pregnant women.

Peppermint: Used as a decongestant for upper respiratory ailments, indigestion, and ringworm. Peppermint oil can have benefits for individuals with irritable bowel syndrome and it helps relieve nausea and flatulence. Peppermint has antiseptic and diaphoretic properties, making it a great choice for colds, flu and fevers.

Psyllium: A strong source of fiber, taken internally to "scrub the colon" and clean out the digestive tract, therefore reducing the risks of certain cancers. Psyllium husks (or "Psyllium hull") are effective for constipation and also slow diarrhea by absorbing excess water.

Raspberry Leaf: Rich in nutrients, especially calcium, magnesium and iron. It has long been regarded as an excellent tonic for women during menstruation and pregnancy. However, raspberry is also nourishing for men and has a pleasant, black tea-like flavor.

Red Clover: Considered helpful for aiding all of the organs of elimination, benefiting the kidneys, cleaning the blood, expelling phlegm from the lungs and improving health in general. It is flavor is mildly sweet and salty.

Rooibos: Rooibos tea, a traditional South African beverage, is a rich, reddish brew that tastes like black tea but contains no caffeine, is low in tannins, and high in vitamin C, minerals, antioxidants, and a number of important phenolic compounds. Rooibos has traditionally been used for skin ailments, allergies, asthma and colic in infants. Studies suggest that aspalathin, a Rooibos constituent, can help diabetes by stimulating insulin secretion and glucose uptake in muscle tissue.

Rose Hips: May provide benefits in the treatment of osteoarthritis. Rose hips show anti-COX activity. Rose hips have a pleasant, tart flavor, contain vitamin C, and have mild antiseptic properties to help ward off colds and flu.

Rose: Rose tincture has been used to treat infertility, impotence, and low sperm count. It encourages regular menstrual cycles, and eases painful periods. Rose calms and nurtures, soothes anger and irritability. But if you're a man who frequently aggravates your woman, you already knew that.

Sasparilla: Used for testosterone production, muscle development, hair growth, and fighting impotency.

Saw Palmetto: Can be used to treat prostate problems in men, promote breast development in women, and eliminate colds and mucus.

Senna: Used for constipation. It's the main ingredient in Ex-Lax.

Skullcap: It can be used as a remedy for anxiety, stress, tension headaches, neuralgia, and nervous breakdowns or exhaustion.

Slippery Elm: Treats acid reflux, indigestion, ulcers, excess mucus, and even diaper rash.

Southernwood: Used for female problems, de-worming, digestive problems, and hair loss.

Spearmint: The type normally found in the fresh herb section of your grocery, is antioxidants and anti-carcinogens, aids digestion and headaches and has mild antiseptic properties. Like any mint, it makes a great iced tea.

Spirulina: An excellent source of nutrition, protein, vitamins, and minerals.

St. John's Wort: Used internally for mental ailments such as depression. Some studies say it works; some say it doesn't. Incompatible with some prescribed medications.

Tea Tree Oil: Can be used to treat acne and skin conditions in general. (See a full article on its many uses at www.HoodHealthHandbook.com)

Uva Ursi: Used for spleen, bladder, and kidney infections, diabetes, and gonorrhea.

Valerian: Used for insomnia, anxiety, tension headaches, and migraines. It can also relax abdominal and other tight or knotted muscles, and be applied externally for skin disorders.

Wild Yam: Used to reduce PMS and menstrual irregularities.

Willow bark: Can be used for a variety of anti-inflammatory and antimicrobial purposes due to presence of salicylic acid and tannins.

Witch Hazel: Used to treat gastro intestinal ailments and women's problems. (See "Cheap Stuff to Make Your Life Easier")

Yarrow: Used for colds and fevers to clear the pores and allow you to sweat, and in treatment of nosebleeds and chickenpox.

Yerba Mate: Traditionally used in South America, as a tea, to boost energy and stamina without causing the jitters that caffeine can cause. Anecdotal reports suggest that yerba mate is also effective against asthma and allergies.

Don't Get Carried Away (Literally)

If you have a serious health condition and are considering an herbal remedy, don't discontinue any ongoing medical treatment (See "Traditional Medicine vs. They Medicine"). Many physicians today are just now learning about herbs as medicine. If your doctor isn't, you can help educate him/her by being prepared with all the information about the herb you are considering. Or find a doctor that's both competent AND on the same page with you. Herbal professionals, naturopathic doctors, Traditional Chinese Medicine practitioners, Ayurvedic Medicine practitioners, and other professionals are trained in the proper uses of healing herbs.

When used properly, most herbs are safe, effective, and without side effects. To promote safer and more effective herbal therapy, before you start the herbal regimen, make sure you understand the potential risks involved in self-treatment these can include:

- ❏ Misdiagnosing your ailment
- ❏ Taking the wrong herb
- ❏ Worsening your condition by not going to the doctor
- ❏ Taking an herb that counteracts or interacts with prescribed medical treatment
- ❏ Taking an herb when you shouldn't (e.g., when pregnant)

It is very important to familiarize yourself with the herb's actions and side effects before you start taking it. Any sign of an adverse side effect, like a stomachache, rash or other allergic reaction, should be a warning sign, not a challenge to keep truckin on.

Herb Journal

ITEM TAKEN	
DATE	
❏ INTERNAL ❏ EXTERNAL ❏ TEA ❏ POULTICE	
AMOUNT	
REASON	
NOTED RESULTS	

Finally, keep a journal of what you are trying, the amounts and the effects it is having, and share it with your medical practitioner (Physician, Naturopath, Herbalist) so that they can take that into account when prescribing a course of action. An example of an Herbal Journal is below.

Season your meals according to your health goals or medical condition. Develop a specific recipe for an ailment.

THE HEALING POWER OF FRUITS
BY SUPREME UNDERSTANDING

The following list is a sampling of the health benefits of fruits. Some of them might really surprise you.

Apples: Contain essential nutrients and vitamins that may help protect the body from certain illnesses, including the common cold. Apple juice may also improve brain function, protect the heart, and inhibit various types of cancer.

Apricots: Helps your heart, fights fatigue, prevents infection, improves your skin, hair, and nails, regulates your blood pressure, and keeps your digestion moving smoothly, all in only about 16 calories. Rich in beta carotene they can also cleanse your system of nicotine leftovers. Dried apricots have three times the amount of fiber and vitamins.

Avocadoes*: Known to prevent birth defects, lower cholesterol, dilate blood vessels, and lower blood pressure. They are one of the richest sources of glutathione, a powerful antioxidant, shown to block thirty different carcinogens and to block proliferation of the aids virus in test tube experiments, A good source of vitamin E. well worth the high fat content.

Bananas: Help fight cancer, heart disease and a long list of other ailments. Banana peels make excellent fertilizer, but also contain a compound that may shift the immune balance of your skin to help relieve warts. People have claimed to heal warts by pressing the inside of a peel against their skin. **Blackberries:** Interferes with the metalloproteinases that contribute to skin wrinkling. Also acts as an antibiotic by blocking the attaching of bacteria that cause urinary tract infections. Contains chemicals that curb diarrhea. Also has antiviral activity and high in natural aspirin.

Blueberries: Blueberries help prevent and treat bladder infections by making it hard for bacteria to stick to urinary tract walls.

Cantaloupes: One cup of cantaloupe provides about 103.2% of the daily value for beta carotene. Because of its high vitamin C, it also fights infection, and stimulates white blood cells. Its folate content is very important in the production of new cells, especially during pregnancy. Green and yellow (cantaloupe and honeydew) have anticoagulant blood-thinning activity.

Cherries: A good source of perillyl alcohol, which helps prevent cancer. Heart-protective anthocyanins give cherries their color.

Cranberries: May treat urinary tract infections and bladder infections.

Eggplants*: Contains a host of vitamins, minerals, and phytonutrients. An anthocyanin phytonutrient found in eggplant skin called nasunin is a potent antioxidant and free radical scavenger that has been shown to protect cell membranes from damage.

Elderberries: May speed the recovery from type A and B influenza.

Figs: Help to prevent cancer. Both fig extract and fig compound, benzaidehyde, have helped shrink tumors in humans. Figs also have laxative, anti-ulcer, antibacterial and anti-parasitic powers.

Grapes: Contains many antioxidant and anticancer compounds. Red grapes are high in antioxidant quercetin, and are antibacterial and antiviral. Grapeseed oil also raises good type HDL cholesterol. Purple grapes (especially the skins) and juice offer three heart-guarding compounds: flavonoids, anthocyanins and resveratrol. (Green grapes are not rich in them)

Kiwis: Kiwi consumption has been linked to a decrease in respiratory-related health problems among children, including asthma. Enjoying just two kiwifruit daily may significantly lower your risk for blood clots and reduce the amount of fats (triglycerides) in your blood, therefore helping to protect cardiovascular health. Kiwi fruit also contains more vitamin C than oranges.

Mangoes: A single mango has your entire recommended daily amount for beta-carotene, 57 mg of vitamin C, and plenty of cancer-fighting antioxidants and heart-healthy carotenoids.

Noni: Used in the Pacific and Caribbean islands for the treatment of inflammation and pain. Human studies indicate it may help prevent cancer.

Oranges: One orange provides an impressive 50 g to 70 g of vitamin C, 40 mcg of folic acid, 52 mg of calcium, as well as beta carotene and Vitamins B1, B2, B3, and fiber. Tangerines provide similar benefits.

Papayas: The nutrients in papaya promote heart health, boost immune systems, increase male fertility, aid digestion, prevent emphysema, and protect against colon cancer. Papaya contains the digestive enzyme, papain, which is used like bromelain, a similar enzyme found in pineapple, to treat sports injuries, wounds, other trauma, skin disorders, and allergies.

Peaches: The heavy dose of fiber in peaches acts as a gentle laxative, aids digestion, and may also help combat cancer. A study in China found that men and women who ate peaches more than two times per week had less risk of developing cancers of the mouth than those who did not eat peaches.

Pears: Pears are high in fiber, particularly lignin, an insoluble fiber that helps to move cholesterol out of the body, and pectin, a soluble fiber which binds to cholesterol, also causing it to be removed from the body. The insoluble fiber also helps reduce the risk of colon cancer. Pears also contain minerals called boron that plays an important role in keeping bones strong.

Pomegranates: Contains tons of phytochemicals like potassium, which is great for lowering your blood pressure. Studies also suggest that pomegranates can inhibit cancer cell growth, slow the progression of prostate cancer and reduce the risk of atherosclerosis (See "Heart Disease").

Prunes (Dried Plums): Famous for their laxative effect, prunes are known for normalizing blood sugar levels, protecting against many ailments (heart disease, breast cancer, colon cancer, etc.), and helping with weight loss.

Raspberries: High in fiber, as well as vitamin C, natural aspirin, ellagic acid and anthocyanins. They appear to have anti-viral and anti-cancer properties, with studies suggesting they may have a role in preventing oral cancer.

Squash*: Very high in vitamin A, contains fiber, vitamins C, B6, B1, potassium, folate, and other phytonutrients which may help prevent cancer, heart attack, stroke, and high blood pressure. The copper found in summer squash is helpful for reducing the painful symptoms of rheumatoid arthritis.

Strawberries: Contain lots of ellagic acid and anthocyanins, and are rich in vitamin C and fiber. They also display anti-viral and anti-cancer activity, particularly against liver cancer. In one study, strawberries topped a list of eight foods most linked to lower rates of cancer deaths among elderly people. They also protect against macular degeneration and rheumatoid arthritis.

Tomatoes*: A major source of lycopene, an antioxidant and anti-cancer agent that intervenes in devastating chain reactions of oxygen free radical molecules. Tomatoes are linked to lower rates of pancreatic cancer and cervical cancer. Lycopene – even as found in ketchup – may also lower the risk of cardiovascular disease. Organic ketchup (which is darker) contains up to 60% more lycopene per gram than regular brands. Researchers have also found that organic ketchup has the highest levels of vitamins A, C, and E.

Watermelons: Contains high amounts of lycopene and glutathione, antioxidant and anti-cancer compounds, and also displays mild anti-bacterial, anti-coagulant activity. Watermelon boosts energy production, while preventing erectile dysfunction, macular degeneration, and prostate cancer.

*Fruits that are often thought of as vegetables

Eat fruits raw, dried, or frozen in a homemade smoothie. Try to eat a new fruit a week and make a list of fruits you will eat daily.

THE HEALING POWER OF VEGETABLES
BY SUPREME UNDERSTANDING

The following list is a sampling of the health benefits of vegetables.

Alfalfa: One of the most popular sprouts, Alfalfa is a good source of vitamins A, B, C, D, E, F, and K and is rich in many minerals, as well as many enzymes needed for digestion. Alfalfa sprouts are high in phytoestrogens – known to have preventive elements for cancer, heart diseases, menopausal symptoms, and osteoporosis.

Artichokes: High in fiber, as well as a flavonoid that has been shown to reduce skin cancer. May also reduce cholesterol levels.

Arugula: This green contains cancer-preventative compounds known as isothiocyanates.

Asparagus: High in the antioxidant glutathione, which appears to lower cancer risk.

Beets: Beta-cyanin, which gives them their reddish-purple color, is a disease-fighting antioxidant. Beets are richer than spinach in iron and other minerals. Helpful in cases of anemia, tuberculosis, constipation, poor appetite, obesity, tumors, gout, and pimples. Also helpful in the elimination of irritating drug poisons.

Beans: (Including legumes, navy, black, kidney, pinto, soybeans, black-eyed peas and lentils) One-half cup of cooked beans daily reduces cholesterol an average 10% and regulates blood sugar levels. An excellent food for diabetics. Linked to lower rates of certain cancers. Very high in fiber.

Broccoli: Abundant in antioxidants, including quercetin, glutathione, beta-carotene, vitamin C, lutein, glucarate, sulforaphane. Extremely high in cancer fighting activity, particularly against lung, colon and breast cancers. Like other cruciferous vegetables, it speeds up removal of estrogen from the body, helping suppress breast cancer. Rich in cholesterol reducing fiber. Has anti-viral, anti-ulcer activity. High in chromium, which helps regulate insulin and blood sugar. Most protective when eaten raw or lightly cooked.

Brussels Sprouts: Possesses some of the same powers as its relatives, broccoli and cabbage. Anti-cancer, estrogenic and packed with various antioxidants (including plenty of Vitamin C) and cancer-fighting indoles.

Cabbage: (including Bok Choy) Contains numerous anti-cancer and antioxidant compounds. Speeds up estrogen metabolism, is thought to help block breast cancer and suppress growth of polyps, a prelude to colon cancer. Eating cabbage more than once a week cut men's colon cancer odds by 66%. As little as two daily tbs. of cooked cabbage protected against stomach cancer. It has anti-bacterial and anti-viral powers. Some of these important compounds are destroyed by cooking. Raw cabbage, as in cole slaw, appears to have stronger overall health value. Raw cabbage juice helps heal ulcers in humans.

Carrots: High in beta carotene, with powerful anticancer, artery-protecting, immune-boosting, infection-fighting, antioxidant qualities. A carrot a day slashed stroke rates in women by 68%. The beta carotene in one medium carrot cuts lung cancer risk in half, even among formerly heavy smokers. Also reduces odds of degenerative eye diseases (cataracts and macular degeneration as well as chest pain (angina). The high soluble fiber depresses blood cholesterol and promotes regularity. Cooking can make it easier for the body to absorb carrot's beta carotene.

Cauliflower: Another great source of anti-cancer indoles, fiber, and vitamin C. Cauliflower provides special nutrient support for three body systems that are closely connected with cancer development as well as cancer prevention: (1) the body's detox system, (2) its antioxidant system, and (3) its inflammatory/anti-inflammatory system. To preserve these anti-cancer nutrients, raw is best, steamed is second best.

Celery: A remedy for high blood pressure. Also has a mild diuretic effect. Contains eight different families of anti-cancer compounds, such as phthalides and polyacetylenes, that detoxify carcinogens, especially cigarette smoke.

Cucumbers: Good for fevers, constipation, skin eruptions, high blood pressure, rheumatism, obesity, acidosis and is a mild diuretic.

Green beans: Contains a variety of antioxidant carotenoids, including beta-carotene, lutein and zeaxanthin.

Greens: (Including collard, kale, mustard, turnip) These greens are packed with anti-cancer, antioxidant compounds (lutein, zeaxanthin, and isothiocyanates), beta carotene, vitamin C, and 93 to 226 mg of calcium per cup. Like other green leafy vegetables, these are all associated with low rates of all cancers.

Kale: A rich source of various anti-cancer chemicals. Has more beta carotene than spinach and twice as much lutein, the most of any vegetable tested. Kale is also a member of the cruciferous family, endowing it with indoles that help regulate estrogen and fight off colon cancer.

> **Did You Know?**
> Hot sauce curbs appetite. Eating just one meal that contains capsaicin not only reduces levels of hunger-causing ghrelin but also raises GLP-1, an appetite-suppressing hormone, says new research in the European Journal of Nutrition. Putting hot sauce on food also speeds up metabolism, burning off calories. Contrary to popular belief, hot peppers do not harm the stomach lining or promote ulcers.

Leek: Effective on diarrhea and back pain.

Onions: An exceptionally strong antioxidant. Thins the blood, lowers cholesterol, raises good-type HDL cholesterol, wards off blood clots, fights asthma, chronic bronchitis, hay fever, diabetes, atherosclerosis and infections. Anti-inflammatory, antibiotic, antiviral, thought to have diverse anti-cancer powers. Specifically linked to preventing human stomach cancer.

Okra: Originating in Africa, okra is a low-calorie source for many nutrients, effective for the prevention of neural tube defects in developing fetuses, mainly due to its high content of vitamin B6, calcium, fiber, and folic acid. Unlike fiber from grains, okra's fiber is easy on the stomach. It can ease digestion and constipation, help irritable bowel syndrome, sooth the gastrointestinal track, and can help to heal ulcers. Okra can also help prevent heart disease, cancer, and diabetes, and help treat asthma and sun stroke.

Peas: A good source of the carotenoids lutein and zeaxanthin – both of which help protect against age-related eye disease.

Peppers (chili, hot): Capsaicin (which makes peppers "hot") helps dissolve blood clots, opens up sinuses and air passages, breaks up mucus in the lungs, acts as an expectorant or decongestant, and helps prevent bronchitis, emphysema and stomach ulcers. Also a potent painkiller, alleviating headaches when inhaled, and joint pain when injected. Antibacterial, antioxidant (anti-cancer) activity.

Pepper (green): Bell peppers have been shown to be protective against cataracts, blood clot formation, and the risk of heart attacks and strokes, probably due to their vitamin C, capsaicin, carotenoids and flavonoids.

Peppers (red, sweet): An improved version of the green pepper, with twice the vitamin C content and more vitamin A.

Potato (white): When eaten with the peel, provides 5g of fiber, 43% of the day's vitamin C requirement, anticancer protease inhibitors, and a major dose of potassium, which may help prevent high blood-pressure and strokes.

Pumpkin: Extremely high in beta carotene, the antioxidant reputed to help ward off numerous health problems, including heart attacks, cancer, cataracts.

Radishes: Chewing activates the heat-producing but healthy indoles and isothiocyanates.

Lettuce: (Including Romaine and other dark lettuce) The darker the green, the more carotenoids. There's also 40% of the RDA for folic acid in 2 cups of Romaine. Iceberg lettuce contains much less nutrients.

Seaweed: Seaweed contains the broadest range of minerals of any food – the same minerals found in the ocean and in human blood, such as potassium, calcium, magnesium, iron, and iodine. Seaweed also contains vitamin C, fiber, beta-carotene, and pantothenic acid and riboflavin – two B-vitamins needed for your body to produce energy. Sea vegetables have been shown to cleanse the body of toxic pollutants, improve hair growth, enrich the bloodstream, and enhance metabolism.

Spinach: Contains many antioxidants and cancer fighters, containing about four times more beta carotene, more than half the RDA for folic acid, and three times more lutein than broccoli. Rich in fiber that helps lower blood cholesterol. Some of its antioxidants are destroyed by cooking. Eat raw or lightly cooked.

Squash (Winter, Butternut, Summer): Due to their carotene properties, winter squash exert a protective effect against many cancers, particularly lung cancer. Summer squash is less nutritious, but studies have shown that juice made from them is equal to juice made from pumpkins, leeks, and radishes in their ability to prevent cell mutations. Summer squash are most helpful during the summer due to their higher water content. They protect against dehydration and the carotenes help protect against UV damage from the sun.

Turnips: Turnips are root vegetables known to lower the risk of obesity, high blood pressure, diabetes, and cancers of the stomach, pancreas, bladder, and lung diseases, as well as cataracts. Turnip greens are more nutrition dense than the root. The greens provide an excellent source of vitamins A, B6, C, E, folic acid, calcium, copper, fiber, and manganese.

Watercress: One of its compounds detoxifies a major carcinogen in tobacco and as such may help prevent lung cancer. Also contains carotenoids.

Yams (Sweet Potatoes): Yams, also native to Africa, supply elements that are important for optimal glandular function and benefit the respiratory, urinary and nervous systems. Their sugar content is absorbed slowly, so they actually help maintain blood sugar levels as well as blood pressure. In addition, due to their high fiber content, yams help control the body weight, by the uniform distribution of weight without transferring extra weight to the hip area or the waistline.

Are You Eating Enough Fruits and Vegetables?

It's been recommended that you eat at least 5 servings a day of fruits and vegetables. And if you have a healthy, plant-based diet, you'll probably be eating more than that (about 9 to 11, or more). But are you?

Applesauce	Dates	Dried Fruit	Asparagus
Baked Potato	Peppers	Carrots	Papaya
Steamed Vegetables	Pears	Cantaloupe	Berries
Kale/Collards	Grapes	Cauliflower	Apples
Green Salad	Pineapple	Mushrooms	Garlic
Squash/Zucchini	Grapefruit	Onions	Avocado
Strawberries	Salsa	Eggplant	Tomatoes
Tropical Fruit	Bananas	Spinach	Spinach
100% Fruit Juice	Oranges	Sprouts	Beans
Bean or Pea Soup	Cabbage	Cucumbers	Broccoli

Above, circle the fruits and vegetables you have eaten in the last week. Give yourself a point for every serving. (A serving is defined as 1 cup of raw leafy vegetables; ¾ cup of 100% fruit or vegetable juice; ½ cup cut–up-fruit or cooked vegetables; 1 medium whole fruit; ½ cup cooked beans or other legumes or ¼ cup dried fruit.) Count the total and read below for your score.

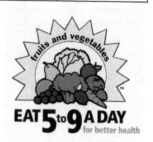

EAT **5** to **9** A DAY
for better health

Scoring

35 or more:	You're eating at least 5 servings a day of fruits and vegetables. Unless you're also eating 30 servings of ribs a

Healthy	day, you probably have a pretty healthy diet.
20-34: Not Bad.	You're almost there, so you should try to increase the variety and servings of fruits and vegetables you eat, starting today. Consider fruits and vegetables you liked as a child, but haven't incorporated in your meals in a while.
10-19: Um, no.	It's time you visit the produce department right away. That's the place on the side of the supermarket with all the colorful round things. Pick up some fruits and vegetables and cook something better, starting tonight.
9 or less: Your diet sucks.	I know, it's harsh. Maybe the table just didn't list those "special" fruits and vegetables you DO eat, but I'm more willing to bet that you really don't eat any fruits or vegetables beyond the toppings at Pizza Hut. It's time for a change. I guarantee your health is suffering, perhaps silently, but it's suffering.

For more details on the health benefits of these foods (and others), visit www.whfoods.com (which provides the George Mateljan Foundation's "World's 130 Healthiest Foods") or www.everynutrient.com

You can also find detailed nutritional data on just about ANY food product (including processed and packaged foods) at www.nutritiondata.com

Focus on variety. Some vegetables will taste better sautéed and others may be enjoyed raw. Experiment.

THE HEALING POWER OF HOT SAUCE
BY SUPREME UNDERSTANDING

Why do Black people love hot sauce? And why do white people prefer mayonnaise? Yeah, those are stereotypes, but there's some truth to em. Historically, Europeans have dined on bland food. (See "Get Off the Cow Titty") **Throughout most of Europe, the cuisine remains relatively bland to this day** (especially in the UK…I almost died of starvation out there!). **It was only after prolonged exposure to the Moors, the Chinese, Indians, Egyptians, and other Original people that Europeans got excited about spice.** If you remember, that's what Christopher Columbus set out looking for in 1492. Foreign spices were both a status symbol for "culturally seasoned" Europeans (much like today), but were also used by the poor whites to preserve meat through cold winters, and to cover up the taste of spoiled (or heavily salted) meat and fish.

The only place where white people are really big on hot sauce is in the South. Why? Because of Mexican influence in the Southwest and Black influence in the Southeast. **If you see the big picture, you'll see that Original people throughout the world have a love for spicy food.** You'll be hard-pressed to find some indigenous culture that doesn't have a hot pepper of choice.

But why? **There's actually some serious science to hot sauce.** That heat really keeps us healthy. You've probably heard that eating too much spicy food will give you an ulcer. It turns out that not only is that a myth, but the opposite is true. Capsaicin actually stimulates blood flow to the stomach and increases its mucus lining, which appears to help heal ulcers. Hot sauce also may kill off some forms of cancers (especially prostate cancer), lower triglycerides (an unhealthy fat), reduce high blood pressure, and spice up a diabetic diet (which forces you to give up a lot of things…but not spice).

The Health Benefits of Hot Sauce (and Hot Peppers)

Treat a cold. Hot sauce, hot peppers, and other spices can be used to clear the sinuses (See "Cure for the Common Cold, Pt. 2"). (You can make super mucus-unclogger with a handful of jalapeño peppers, onion, ginger root, horseradish root, garlic bulb, and organic apple cider vinegar thrown in a blender. You'll only need one teaspoon at a time…trust me)

Helps with weight loss. A study published in the *British Journal of Nutrition* has discovered that hot sauce (or hot peppers in any form), when added to breakfast foods or appetizers at lunch, causes people to eat less during meals and for hours afterwards. **Aside from acting as an appetite suppressant, red pepper also seems to increase the number of calories burned, particularly after high-fat meals.** Capsaicin also improves digestion by stimulating stomach secretions and has a laxative effect.

Combat food poisoning. Studies have found that many hot spices – from mustard seed to green chilies – are anti-microbial, meaning they can kill off bacteria like E. coli, L. monocytogenes, and Salmonella, common food-borne pathogens which can cause severe illness and even death in some cases.

Battle depression. Every time you eat something hot, you release endorphins, the natural "happy drug" that your body produces. **Endorphins relieve pain and promote a sense of wellbeing.** They're often called "natural pain killers" or "the runner's natural high."

How Hot Can it Get?

Peppers are rated based on Scoville Units, which measures the amount of capsaicinoids (capsaicin) in parts per million. Capsaicin is the compound that gives chilies their heat. The chart below rates chili peppers, with 0 being mildest and 10 highest heat. Pepper spray is typically 2,000,000 Scoville Units, and Police grade pepper spray clocks in at 5,300,000, but both are off the chart for obvious reasons. Pure capsaicin is 16,000,000 Scoville.

Scoville Chile Heat Chart (Rtg. = Rating)

Type of Pepper	Rtg.	Heat Level
Sweet Bells; Sweet Banana; Pimento	0	Less than 100 Scoville Units
Cherry; New Mexico; Anaheim	1	100-1,000 Scoville Units
Ancho; Pasilla; Espanola; Anaheim	2	1,000 - 1,500 Scoville Units
Sandia; Cascabel	3	1,500 - 2,500 Scoville Units
Jalapeno; Mirasol; Chipotle; Poblano	4	2,500 - 5,000 Scoville Units
Yellow Wax; Serrano	5	5,000 - 15,000 Scoville Units
Chile De Arbol	6	15,000 - 30,000 Scoville
Aji; Cayenne; Tabasco; Piquin	7	30,000 - 50,000 Scoville
Santaka; Chiltecpin; Thai	8	50,000 - 100,000 Scoville
Habanero; Scotch Bonnet; Fatalii	9	100,000 - 350,000 Scoville
Red Savina Habanero; Indian Tezpur	10	350,000 - 850,000 Scoville
Naga Jolokia	10 +	1,000,000+ Scoville Units

What Do I Do When it's Too Hot to Handle?

It's mostly psychological. But the most effective way to relieve that burning sensation is with dairy products, such as milk and yogurt. A milk-based protein called casein binds to capsaicin, making it less available to "burn" the mouth. Chewing something, especially rice, also helps lessen the burn, which is why rice typically accompanies spicy food throughout the world.

Hot sauce clears out the mucus, bacteria, fat, and weak emotions from the body. Think of it as a cleanse for optimal functioning.

MAGIC MUSHROOMS

BY SUPREME UNDERSTANDING

When you start talking about the health benefits of fruits and vegetables, it's easy to forget about these guys. **Their meaty texture makes them a great substitute for meat** (and for processed GMO soy substitutes). In fact, you can make a portabella mushroom sandwich that will put most burgers to shame. Not only that, but they're good for your health. **Mushrooms are widely recognized as both a heart medicine and cancer remedy in Asia.** Studies have shown mushrooms can help prevent and/or treat cancer, viral diseases such as influenza and polio, high blood cholesterol, sticky blood platelets and high blood pressure.

Button Mushrooms (Crimini, Portabella, White): Button mushrooms actually contain more antioxidants (and protein) than some of the most colorful vegetables. **They are the richest source** (of any food) **of the powerful antioxidant L-ergothioneine.** Button mushrooms are also rich in vitamins and minerals that are essential for proper functioning of the antioxidant system, including selenium, copper and niacin. Moreover, these phytonutrients are well maintained even after mushrooms are cooked. Several studies have shown button mushrooms' potential for protecting against certain cancers. The high potassium can aid in preventing and controlling high blood pressure, and the high copper levels may help osteoporosis, osteoarthritis and rheumatoid arthritis, breast and colon cancer, cardiovascular disease and bone and connective tissue conditions.

Shiitake Mushroom: These mushrooms, which you can usually find in any supermarket, taste great in any dish – almost like meat. Except shiitake mushrooms do the opposite of meat and, instead of giving you cancer and bacteria, studies have shown that they stop the growth of tumor cells and the spread of pathogenic bacteria and fungi. Shitake mushrooms may also help lower cholesterol and blood pressure.

Reishi Mushroom: Reishi is used in Chinese medicine for its immunogenic, antibacterial and anti-inflammatory properties. It is said to promote a healthy heart and prostate and to be a powerful anti-cancer agent. **Reishi has also been shown to help treat allergic reactions, chronic bronchitis, coronary heart disease, hypertension, arthritis and muscular dystrophy.**

304

Maitake Mushroom: Maitake has also been shown to be beneficial for AIDS patients and has helped lower blood sugar levels in diabetics. It has also been shown to stimulate immunity, reduce high blood pressure, shrink brain tumors and fight prostate cancer. Maitake is considered an adaptogen, which means it aids the body in adapting to physical and emotional stress.

Mushrooms are a great meat substitute. They're great sautéed, marinated, and even raw. Get them dried and toss them into a soup.

A SIMPLE GUIDE TO LEGUMES
BY SINCERE JUSTICE ALLAH

Legumes are peas, lentils and beans. Because they're such a healthy source of many nutrients, you should strive to eat 2 or more servings/a day. (Each serving is about a cup of cooked beans, cup of soy milk or 4 ounces of tofu or tempeh.) **All the following beans will help stabilize blood sugar, lower bad cholesterol, and give you a boost of energy.**

Eat a variety of legumes every day

Black beans are definitely popular in many Mexican dishes. Black beans contain folate, fiber, manganese, protein, magnesium, thiamin, phosphorus and iron, as well as provide multiple antioxidants.

Garbanzo beans, also known as Chickpeas, are found in popular dishes such as hummus (Mediterranean) and chana masala (India). Chickpeas contain folate, fiber, protein, manganese, copper, phosophorus and iron.

Kidney beans are usually found in chilis, soups, stews and salads. They contain a good source of folate, fiber, manganese, protein, iron, phosphorus, copper, potassium, magnesium and thiamin, and can improve memory. **Be sure to cook them as they contain toxins when eaten uncooked.**

Lentils are easy to make and go well with soups and stews. Lentils contain folate, fiber, manganese, iron, protein, phosphorus, copper, thiamin, and potassium **(Note: Lentils don't need to be soaked prior to cooking).**

Lima beans are found in soups, stews, and salads. Also, found in a dish known as succotash – lima beans combined with corn and bell peppers. Lima beans contain folate, fiber, manganese, protein, potassium, iron, copper, phosphorus, magnesium, and thiamin. Lima beans keep you youthful with antioxidants.

Navy beans are also known as white beans. They're often found in soups, salads and chili. Also, they once were staples of the U.S. Navy, hence the name. Navy beans contain folate, fiber, protein, phosphorus, copper, magnesium, iron, and thiamin, and can help improve memory.

Peas are found in common dishes like split-pea soup and rice and peas. Peas contain folate, fiber, manganese, protein, thiamin, potassium and phosphorus.

Pinto beans are often used in Mexican dishes as refried beans. Pinto beans contain fiber, folate, manganese, protein, phosphorus, iron, magnesium, potassium, copper and thiamin..

Soybeans are found in many products such as soy sauce, soy cheese, soy milk, mock meats, tofu and more. Soybeans contain plenty of protein, isoflavones, fiber, high levels of essential fatty acids, vitamins and minerals.

Choosing dried, canned or frozen?

In terms of the type of legumes you want to get, there are dried, canned and frozen varieties. Canned isn't the best choice (because of aluminum), but besides that, there isn't a strong difference in the nutritional value of canned versus dried beans, except in the amount of salt. However, rinsing the canned beans through some water can lessen the amount of salt.

Preparing Dried Legumes

1 cup of dried beans will make about 2-3 cups cooked.

Basic: Rinse dry beans in water to get out any debris. Soak beans overnight to cut down cooking time and make them softer. Over soaking beans more than 12 hours can cause beans to ferment. Remember to drain beans before cooking.

Place beans in pan, where they'll be cooked. Cover pan with 3 inches of water. Bring to a boil and boil again for 2 more minutes. Remove from the heat, place cover on top of pan and let beans stand for 1-2 hours. Then proceed with your recipe.

Remember; add any salt, sugar, or acidic foods like tomatoes after beans have been cooked because they will harden the uncooked beans.

Cooking the Beans

Place beans in pan and add water. Adding oil can reduce amount of foam the beans will create. (Note: **Do not use soaking water as they contain toxins**)

Bring beans to a boil.

Reduce heat and let simmer until beans are tender.

Beans/peas are ready to eat when you can poke them easily with a fork. Anticipate 1.5 to 2 hours to cook beans fully.

Storing Legumes

Dry legumes can last up to 2 years in a cool, dry place. Nutritional value and flavor degrade and cooking times increase as legumes sit on the shelf longer.

Cooked legumes can be covered and refrigerated for 4-5 days. Most legumes can be made frozen (except lentils) making beans last for 6 months in freezer.

If you are turning vegetarian and have questions about a source of protein...This is it. They make a cheap and healthy dip or spread.

AN ESSENTIAL GUIDE TO GRAINS
BY DIERDRA BAPTISTE

What is a Whole Grain?

Most of us are familiar with grains because of the breads we eat. Often these breads are made from a stripped down, processed version of the original grain that lacks most of its original nutrients. **A grain is considered "whole," on the other hand, when all three parts – bran, germ and endosperm – are present.** Most people do not know that whole grains are often an even better source of the nutrients usually thought of associated with some fruits and vegetables. Vitamin E, magnesium, B vitamins, fiber, iron and fiber and other antioxidants can be found in the whole grain.

What are the Benefits?

Daily regular consumption of whole grains has shown to reduce the risk of heart disease by lowering blood pressure and cholesterol levels. They also reduce the risks of some types of cancer and for people living with diabetes, it helps somewhat to regulate blood glucose. **It is also shown that those who eat whole grains regularly tend to weigh less than those who don't.** Additional benefits include prevention of childhood asthma as well as breast cancer and helping the body repair itself. **An 8 year clinical trial showed that Black**

women who ate whole grains consistently had a 31% lower rate of diabetes than their counterparts who ate less. It is recommended that five servings of whole grain be consumed daily for maximum benefit.

Brown Rice: It is packed with vitamins B1, B2, B3, B6 and iron and just one cup will serve a significant portion of your RDA of manganese, magnesium, selenium and tryptophan. Converting brown rice to white rice (stripping the outer layer to leave only the endosperm) removes 67% of the vitamin B3, 80% of the vitamin B1, 90% of the B6, and more than half the iron, manganese and phosphorus as well as all of the dietary fiber and fatty acids. All of this is added back to white rice, chemically, as "enriched" as required by the FDA.

Oats: A species of cereal grain with high fiber content, noted to remove cholesterol from the digestive system that would otherwise end up in the bloodstream. This promotes heart health. It is the only cereal that contains protein, one found similar to soy protein.

Wheat: A grass species and the husk of the grain, separated when milling white flour, is called bran. Wheat germ is the embryo portion of the wheat kernel and is a concentrated source of vitamins, minerals, and protein, including phosphorus, potassium, folate and zinc.

Wild Rice: It's high in protein, lysene (an amino acid) and fiber, while low in fat. It is also a good source of the minerals and vitamins potassium, phosphorus, thiamine, niacin and riboflavin. It's not actually rice but related to grass and is grown in the water.

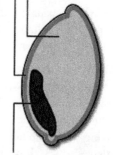

Whole grain kernel

Bran
"Outer shell" protects seed
Fiber, B vitamins, trace minerals

Endosperm
Provides energy
Carbohydrates, protein

Corn: A staple food for most Native American peoples. Elsewhere in the world it's known as Maize. It is a grass species and was domesticated by the Aztec and Mayan cultures. It is high in fiber, promoting heart health and also improves memory, lung health and energy production.

Bulgur: A cereal food made from several wheat variations, but most often from durum wheat. It's common in Middle Eastern and Greek cuisine.

Rye: This is a grass grown as a grain. It's a member of the wheat species and is closely related to barley and wheat. It can be eaten whole, either as boiled rye berries, or by being

Germ
Nourishment for the seed
Antioxidants, vitamin E, B vitamins

rolled, similar to rolled oats. Rye is an excellent source of manganese, phosphorus, magnesium and proteins and is also a good source of dietary fiber. It also contains lignin phytonutrients, important in aiding the body fight disease.

Spelt: A form of wheat is an excellent source of B12 as well as manganese, copper, thiamin and niacin. With these combinations of vitamins and minerals, those who suffer from diabetes, atherosclerosis and migraine headaches may find an increase intake of Spelt helpful.

Amaranth: A leaf vegetable (not a grass) and cereal from a traditional food plant in Africa. **The amaranth seed is gluten free so it's edible for gluten intolerant individuals.** It's high in vitamins A, K, B6, C, Riboflavin and folate as well as minerals calcium, iron, magnesium phosphorus, zinc and copper.

Sorghum: A grass species rich in vitamin B complex as well as Beta carotene. Africa grows more than half the world's sorghum and it's a staple for more than a half a billion poor people worldwide.

Barley: A cereal grain and is an excellent source of fiber, selenium, phosphorus, copper and manganese. It's known for its robust flavor.

Quinoa: High in protein and the amino acid lysene, which promotes tissue repair and growth, it is a grain like crop grown for its edible seeds. When prepared it has a nutty flavor and is fluffy in texture.

How to Find Whole Grains

Any natural food store or farmer's market should carry these grains and others. Additionally, most "regular" supermarkets now stock a wide variety of whole grains. However, in supermarkets, you have to be careful with package labeling. **Any foods labeled with words such as "multi-grain," "100% wheat," "cracked wheat," "bran" "seven grain" or "stone ground" are usually not whole grain.** Also, just because it's brown does not necessarily mean that it's whole wheat or whole grain, **because some companies are simply adding brown food coloring to get that "healthy look."** To determine if a packaged food product contains whole grain or not, look for the word "whole" in the ingredient list. The Whole Grain Stamp is also a good indicator. One with a "good source" on the stamp contains at least ½ a serving of whole grains, while one with an "excellent source" on the stamp contains at least 1 serving of whole grains.

Like everything that's processed for you, the most nutritious part is removed. Whole foods let the body keep the best parts to itself.

CAN CERTAIN FOODS FIGHT CANCER?
BY EARTH EM'MAYA JEWEL

At **EatDrinkBetter.com**, the authors provide a list of **"10 anti-cancer foods."** The list includes popular celebrities in the health food world, including garlic, dark leafy greens, grapes, green tea, tomatoes, blueberries, flaxseeds, mushrooms, cruciferous vegetables (such as broccoli, cauliflower, cabbage, Brussels sprouts), and whole grains.

But don't believe the hype! There is no such thing as an "anti-cancer" food. Recent studies reveal that it's *overall* eating habits and not a single element in a particular food that fights cancer by itself. Many researchers and cancer specialists believe that up to 60% of the 500,000 YEARLY cancer deaths in America can be prevented if Americans adopt healthier overall diets and lifestyles. According to Rachael Stolzenberg-Solomon, a researcher at the National Cancer Institute, "The easiest and least expensive way to reduce your risk for cancer is just by eating a healthy diet."

Eating a variety of healthy foods on a regular basis can not only fight and prevent cancer, it can even reverse cancer. Cook with herbs and spices and drink plenty of fresh, pure water. If you have to have alcohol, drink organic red wine in moderation. Eat more foods that have omega-3 fatty acids. Cold water fish like salmon, flaxseed oil, and walnuts all are rich in this essential vitamin. Foods that are high in antioxidants are known to lower the risk of cancer. See our information on legumes, grains, fruits, vegetables, and herbs.

Compounds known as inhibitors can keep the abnormal cells from growing. Some vitamins and phytochemicals in plant foods are known to be inhibitors. Therefore adding them to the diet on a daily basis increases your odds of beating or not getting cancer.

A healthy lifestyle is a holistic one. Just as our food needs to be whole, our way of living needs to cover the full spectrum of health.

TAKE YOUR VITAMINS?

THE SCIENCE TO SUPPLEMENTS AND MULTIVITAMINS
BY C'BS ALIFE ALLAH

You don't necessarily "need" to take vitamins. A healthy plant-based diet can give you everything you need. Fresh fruits, vegetables, and legumes contain not only all the vitamins and minerals found in those supplements, but also fiber and other naturally occurring substances that may help protect you from chronic diseases. Additionally, those foods are more easily digestible than supplements, and they can give you energy. So whenever possible, your nutrients should come from natural sources (like fresh food) instead of supplements. Despite this, sometimes it's helpful to supplement our diet.

Why? Many of us don't get enough vitamins and nutrients, due to nutritional ignorance. If you ask the average person, they don't know what the nutritional needs of their body are, so no matter your eating style, you may have a gap in your nutrition.

If you think you need dietary supplements, a general vegan multivitamin may be a good way to go but make sure you do research. Some supplements are nothing more than colored chalk. Others mix everything under the sun, yet end up being ineffective, and some mix known destructive chemicals with vitamins, which does double damage. On one hand they don't offer you any type of supplemental assistance, and on the other hand they cause more problems in your body. Be sure to talk with your physician or dietician before starting or stopping any supplements.

Now, too much of anything thing is not a good thing. Supplements are typically the only way you can get TOO MUCH of a vitamin. Popping vitamins in abundance (or supplements with an "overdose" in them) is not healthy. According to Dr. Joe Fuhrman:

> The judicious use of supplements can be utilized to offer nutritional insurance and protection as well as better assure ideal levels of some difficult to obtain nutrients, but many nutritional supplements cause more harm than good. Remember more is not always better. Almost daily, I see people placing themselves at increased health risk from supplement excess; too much Vitamin A, too much B6, too much beta carotene, too much iron, too much selenium, too much fish oil, too many herbal concoctions and laxatives (called bowel cleansers). People can easily hurt themselves with too much supplementation. We want to supplement intelligently and not incur the risks of excessive nutrients.

Resources

For general resources on satisfying your body's nutritional needs, look up the following online: "Essential Nutrients in the World's Healthiest Foods" by the George Mateljan Foundation; "Filling Your Plate with

Fabulous Phytochemicals" by NutritionMD.org; "Staying a Healthy Vegan" by Vegan Outreach; "The New Four Food Groups" by Physicians Committee for Responsible Medicine; "The Vegan Food Pyramid" by ChooseVeg.org; "World's Healthiest Foods List" by the George Mateljan Foundation; and "Your Health" by Physician's Committee for Responsible Medicine

Recommended Reading

The China Study: The Most Comprehensive Study of Nutrition Ever Conducted and the Startling Implications for Diet, Weight Loss, and Long-term Health by T. Colin Campbell and Thomas M. Campbell II; Eat More, Weigh Less by Dean Ornish, M.D.; Food for Life: How the New Four Food Groups Can Save Your Life by Neal Barnard, M.D.; and The Vegan Diet as Chronic Disease Prevention: Evidence Supporting the New Four Food Groups by Kerrie K. Saunders

Get familiar with the nutrients in your food. This way you know if you need to supplement or look for food with those missing nutrients.

CHEAP STUFF TO MAKE YOUR LIFE EASIER

BY MECCA WISE

Today we are encouraged to spend large amounts of money on overpriced products and prescription medication that contain harmful chemicals and have adverse side effects. Instead we can use something safe, practical and inexpensive. Products such as hydrogen peroxide, baking soda, rubbing alcohol, apple cider vinegar, castor oil, coconut oil, witch hazel and Epsom salt are age old and were used by our grandparents and their parents and can prevent, eliminate, and treat illnesses before we need that trip to the doctor. Below you will find a list of these products and ways to use them to treat some of our common ailments.

Hydrogen Peroxide ($0.79 for 16 oz)

Hydrogen Peroxide is a disinfectant and is one of those products that can be used for just about anything. Whenever I feel my throat getting scratchy due to the onset of a cold, I immediately gargle with some. I use it at times when I feel that my teeth can be a bit whiter, and Yes, I have gotten compliments. Every time I get a cut on my hand, I use it. Whenever, I feel irritated down below, peroxide is there to save the day. Wanting to keep, my clothes clean and white, but eliminate the use of Clorox in my home, I reach for the peroxide. I've used it on my carpet for stains, on my sink counter for germs and in my bathroom for mold. I've even recommend it to a friend who had athletes foot, not only did it stop the itch but it brighten his toe nails.

- Fight colds: Gargle ¼ cup at onset of a cold
- Brighten teeth: Swish a capful in your mouth for a few minutes a day (this will also kills germs in your mouth)
- Treat cuts: Use a q-tip to clean cut
- Fight Yeast infections: Pour a couple of cups in your bath water and soak, use equal parts in a douche bag, or use a needleless syringe to insert directly
- Fight athletes foot: Soak your feet in a 50/50 solution
- Clean laundry: Pour a half to a whole cup into your laundry water, not directly on clothes
- Clean carpet: Dilute with water and apply to stain
- Remove blood stains: Pour a capful directly onto the stain
- Clean fruits and veggies: Use ¼ cup into a sink of cold water and scrub fruits and veggies to remove viruses and bacteria and neutralize chemicals (rinse well)
- Fight mold and kill germs on kitchen counter tops, bathroom surfaces: Mix half water, half peroxide in a spray bottle
- Treat Acne: Use a q-tip to apply directly to acne

Castor Oil ($1.49 for 4 oz.)

This oil is not only a used as a laxative but also has anti-inflammatory, antibacterial, antiviral, and anti-fungal properties. It is known to treat many skin diseases, encourages hair growth and stimulates the lymphatic system.

- Treat constipation: Take 1-4 tablespoons
- Treat skin conditions such as ringworm, athlete's foot, eczema, dry skin, sunburn, and warts: Rub on affected area (repeat as necessary)
- Alleviate Arthritis pain: Rub directly onto painful joints
- Promote Hair growth: Rub onto thinning areas
- Condition hair: Saturate hair and leave on for an hour
- Stimulate lymphatic system/treat cysts and ulcers: Create a castor oil pack (You can Google how to make one)

Coconut Oil

Have you heard the saying that breast milk is the best milk? Well **the fatty acids in coconut oil are identical to a group of fats found in breast milk**, have antiviral, antibacterial, and antifungal properties, as well as strengthen the immune system and assist with the absorption of nutrients.

- ☐ Boost Energy: Mix a tablespoon of this vitamin and mineral packed oil in your food
- ☐ Moisturize skin: Rub directly onto dry/wrinkled skin
- ☐ Treat skin conditions: Massage onto areas affected by eczema or fungus
- ☐ Promote overall health: Cook with it, put it in your smoothies, and put it on your salad to protect against heart disease, cancer, diabetes, liver disease...it also aids in digestion and weight loss.

Epsom Salt ($2.79 for 4 lbs.)

The use of Epsom salt has been around for years and extends beyond soaking.

- ☐ Constipation relief: Dissolve 2-4 tablespoons in 8 oz. of water
- ☐ Exfoliant: Rub salt on wet skin
- ☐ Muscle Relief: Pour 2 cups in bath water to relieve sore muscle and eliminate harmful toxins from the body

Apple Cider Vinegar ($3.19 for a quart)

Apple cider vinegar is packed with nutrients, vitamins, minerals, fiber, essential acids and enzymes. It's an excellent source of potassium and great for the immune system with its anti-bacterial and anti-fungal properties. All vinegar is not made equal though, so use organic raw unfiltered. Externally, it can be used full strength, but when you drink it, be sure to dilute it.

- ☐ Digestion/upset stomach/acid reflux/mild food poisoning: Drink 2 tablespoons in water with 1 teaspoon of honey
- ☐ Arthritis: 2 teaspoons with 2 teaspoons of honey to break down calcium deposits in joints
- ☐ Asthma: Sip on 1 tablespoon of apple cider vinegar in water
- ☐ Eczema: 2 teaspoons with 2 teaspoons of honey three times a day
- ☐ Heartburn: 2 teaspoons of acv in water before meals
- ☐ High blood pressure: 2 teaspoons with honey in water
- ☐ Insomnia: 2 teaspoons in water before sleep
- ☐ Kidney and Bladder: 2 teaspoons in water six times a day
- ☐ Obesity: 2 teaspoons with water in morning and before each meal; sip with meals

Basically just use about 2 teaspoons in a glass of water a couple times a day if possible, add two teaspoons of honey if you are not a vegan and just watch your overall health change for the better, Not to mention it can be used for fatigue, headache, hair loss, and just about anything else you suffer from.

Rubbing Alcohol ($1.00 for 16 oz.)

Alcohol is a sterilizer and cleaning agent.

- [ ] To clean cuts and scrapes: Apply to cut
- [ ] To clean windows: Mix with baking soda and vinegar
- [ ] To remove marker, coffee or lipstick stains: Apply to stain (don't use on leather)
- [ ] To dry out and relieve mosquito bite itch: Use a q-tip to apply to bite
- [ ] To remove adhesives: Pour some on a cotton ball and apply

Witch Hazel ($1.99 for 16oz)

Witch Hazel is a natural astringent that reduces inflammations and constricts capillaries.

- [ ] Treat sunburn/prevent peeling: Apply to affected areas
- [ ] Heal Bruises: Apply a compress to bruise
- [ ] Treat a bug bite: Apply a small amount to q-tip to relieve itching
- [ ] Heal diaper rash: Apply to baby's bottom with a cotton ball
- [ ] Relieve pain and swelling of Varicose Veins: Soak wash rags in witch hazel and put on legs
- [ ] Refresh tired/red eyes: Place compress over CLOSED eyes for 10 minutes
- [ ] Treat dry skin: Apply immediately after a shower
- [ ] Treat Wrinkles: Apply to fine lines of the face
- [ ] Relieve Hemorrhoids: Apply to affected area to relieve itch. It also tightens and heals the skin
- [ ] Heal cuts: Apply to clean and heal a cut
- [ ] Treat bags under eye: Carefully apply under eye to tighten skin
- [ ] Sooth/prevent razor burn: Apply before or after shaving
- [ ] Sooth poison Ivy and Poison Oak: Apply to affected areas
- [ ] Treat Acne: Use a q-tip to apply to pimples

Cornstarch ($1.19 for 1 lb.)

Cornstarch is a safer alternative to baby powder/talcum powder. Talcum powder is made from the mineral Talc, which is crushed into fine particles, which can cause allergies and lung cancer if inhaled. **If applied to the genital area, talcum powder has been known to cause a variety of feminine cancers, the most prevalent being ovarian cancer.** Particles of talc have been found in these cancer tumors. So it goes without saying that – despite the name "baby powder," talcum powder isn't safe for your baby's bottom. Cornstarch might cake up a bit more, but it does everything baby powder should, and safely.

- [ ] Removes grease spatters from walls: Pour on cloths and rub grease spots

- Removes grease spills from clothing: Let sit for 20 minutes
- Underarm deodorant: Use alcohol to remove bacteria, then apply cornstarch.
- Rid bloodstains: Saturate the spot with cornstarch/let dry and rub off
- Rid roaches: Mix equal parts of cornstarch and plaster of Paris and place in crevices.
- Freshens Carpet: Sprinkle on rug and freshen wait 20 minutes and vacuum

Replace what you can with these products. The amount of toxic chemicals you will be free from will greatly improve your health.

WHAT IS ACUPRESSURE?
BY DIVINEGOD B ALLAH

Acupressure is a safe form of self-care, done using finger pressure, massages, and strokes rather than needles, using the same principles and meridian points as acupuncture in traditional Chinese medicine. Acupressure is a two-step process. Step One is finding and locating the right pressure point. Step Two is properly massaging the pressure point.

How Is It Done?

Pressure points are about the size of a pin head, and are tenderer than the surrounding area. After you've identified the point, stimulate it using the tip of your index finger, your middle finger, or both side by side. In some spots it may be easier to use your thumb. The points should be stimulated as deeply as can be endured in a digging kind of massage. A few seconds of pressure, repeated several times, will often be enough. You should push until you feel some discomfort

Within about 30 seconds of activating an effective pressure point you should feel a sense of calmness, warmth, and or a slight flush of perspiration on the eye brows or shoulder area, along with a light headed feeling. This reaction is a good indication that you found the right point. If you do not get fast, satisfactory relief, you most likely:

- Did not find the point for your symptom. Look for another point.
- Did not find the point at all. Make sure you feel the twinge when you search and press.
- The point may not have been stimulated properly. Use the different finger techniques mentioned above (tip of index, middle finger, etc.)

For even better results stimulate two pressure points at once, one with each hand, while the part of the body stimulated is stretched to effect maximum energy flow between the points. Or you can duplicate the pressure on both sides. Immediately after locating and massaging a point on one side, repeat in the other side. In most cases the points only need 15 seconds of attention apiece to get fast relief.

Acupressure for Common Ailments

- [ ] Sore Back? Press on either side of the lower spine, just around the corner from the bottom rib. Press both sides at the same time. A little pressure to the tip of the tail bone can also ease and lift an aching back.
- [ ] Headache? A finger press right between the eyes can relieve a headache.
- [ ] Menstrual pain? Press about an inch below your belly button.
- [ ] Irritating hiccups? Press a point just above the breast bone to halt hiccups.
- [ ] Leg cramps? Just apply strong pressure to the points behind the knee, Center of the calf, and where the Achilles tendon joins the calf muscle.
- [ ] Insomnia? Press point below the little finger at the first crease of the wrist. Also press two fingers right at the natural hairline on either side of the spine.
- [ ] Loud cough? Press the points just below the collarbone. The same pressure points also help ease an asthmatic cough.
- [ ] Sore throat? Press the center of your forehead about midway between the eyebrows and the natural hairline.
- [ ] Need temporary relief of a toothache? Press right above the corner of the jaw of the affected side.
- [ ] Need more athletic energy? Press the nape of the neck, hard and quickly, just before the event.
- [ ] Lower abdomen problems (bowel disorders, indigestion, etc.)? Run your thumb up the inner rear edge of the shinbone toward the knee. At about 3" up, you will feel that unmistakable tingling that announces the point.
- [ ] Neck tension? With your palm down, bend your hand back slightly to locate (and remember) where your hand and wrist meet. Measure two thumb widths towards your elbow which (should be about two inches.) Using your middle finger, press very deeply in the small hollow between your two arm bones. Repeat on the other arm.
- [ ] Neck and shoulder tension? Locate your elbow, go down about two inches toward your hand, on your upper forearm. Search deeply in the muscle until you feel a very tender spot. It will be quite tender with even moderate pressure.
- [ ] Need more headache relief? Place your right hand palm facing the floor. Squeeze your right thumb and right index together, a fleshy mound should pop up on the back of the right hand between them. Place the bent knuckle of the left index finger on top of the mound. Keeping the knuckle in place, relax the right hand and press deeply in the area until you feel the tender point. The more it hurts, the better it is likely to be for your headache.

- Need to suppress hunger? Locate the cleft between the bottom of the nose and the top of the upper lip. Pinch it when you are hungry, within moments your hunger will be gone.
- Bad menstrual cramps? Pinch either side of your foot in the groove under and slightly behind the anklebone. Then take your other hand and firmly press the center of the big toe on the same foot.

The body can heal itself. All it needs is a push in the right direction.

THINK YOURSELF WELL?

BY SUPREME UNDERSTANDING

Does Prayer Heal?

According to the *Washington Post*, "Prayer is the most common complement to mainstream medicine, far outpacing acupuncture, herbs, vitamins and other alternative remedies." But scientific studies have failed to confirm that prayer does anything miraculous for people. Don't get me wrong. Many scientists and medical professionals accept that prayer can help recovery, not due to divine influence but due to psychological and physical benefits. Namely, praying, meditating, and knowing you are being prayed for "may help reduce stress and anxiety, promote a more positive outlook, and strengthen the will to live," according to a study by CentraState Hospital. But it doesn't appear to make a difference what you're praying to or focusing on. A 2008 study concluded that the regular practice of "Surya Namaskar" (a Hindu "Salute to the Sun") had a positive impact on cardio-respiratory health. (See "Sun Salute")

A 2001 study in the *British Medical Journal* reported that by praying the rosary or reciting yoga mantras at specific rates, baroreflex sensitivity improved significantly in cardiovascular patients. That makes sense, if you reconsider where the source of all divine power really is. The point is, if grandma wants to pray while she's sick, let her. It won't make the cancer go into remission, but it may give her the will to live a little longer so she can fight a little more. The problem isn't what people do in addition to getting treatment. The problem is what people do INSTEAD of getting treatment. **When people focus all of their hope for healing on forces outside of themselves, they disregard their own body's ability to heal itself.** Instead, the next time you're sick, after you begin pursuing a real course of treatment, meditate and focus on your body doing its job. The power's all in you.

Faith Healing

Even with the pleasant explanation above, I know some of us still believe you can be miraculously cured through faith. That's understandable, because it happens in nearly every church and on every TV church program there is. Plus, I'm sure you have friends who believe their personal "experience" is enough to counter hundreds of scientific studies that haven't found anything miraculous. **Is faith healing real? In one word – No.** And the people who are saying "no" aren't in on some conspiracy against God. The real conspiracy is people making money by having you believe they're the only ones who can fix you. Western medicine does it, and so do most religions. The truth is not at either extreme. In fact, the truth is right in the center, where you are. **Everything you need to heal is IN you, and in nature. But there's a process to it. There is no "quick fix."** Those preachers on TV "laying hands" on people, curing them of blindness, diabetes, cancer, and pigeon-toes…it's not for real. In fact, there are dozens of books exposing these frauds and their tricks, like **James Randi's *The Faith Healers*.** The most common method is simply putting actors (called "plants") in the audience. That crippled old man learns how to walk in a new church EVERY Sunday. But it's more than just a scam, because people are dying. In churches that don't allow their members to get outside treatment, sick people die of problems that could have been easily fixed. In other cases, families spend so much time trying to "faith heal" a sick relative that they ignore conventional methods that could have worked. Just Google "faith healing deaths." I guarantee there were dozens in the news just this month alone.

It's All in Your Head

"The oneness of mind and body holds the secret of illness and health." – Arnold Hutschnecker

At the same time, we can't discount the power of the mind. In *How to Hustle and Win, Part Two*, I explained:

Are you hot? Cold? Hungry? Tired? Angry? Depressed? Worried? Why? It's all in your mind! None of it is actually real. It may feel real, but it's only as real as you allow it to be. Did you just lose your job? Well, that's real. But how you deal with it is up to you. You can choose to be upset about it, or you can choose to be excited about what the future now holds. Most people, unfortunately, choose negative feelings over positive feelings. But you have to understand that there is a choice.

When it's chilly outside, you probably complain that it's cold. That complaint only makes you feel colder. You gave it power over your mind, and now you're convinced to feel cold. But there are people who live in the Arctic circle and the Himalayan mountains. They don't whine about the cold. You can say that they're used to it, but there's more to it. Many of these people are disciplined. There are monks who can set themselves on fire without screaming, so what's your problem? You're stressed because you're not getting along with someone the way you want to? You mad cause your finances ain't perfect? Get over it. Think differently. And that will make all the difference in the world.

When my stomach starts growling for food, I remind myself that many people go days without food. And I tell my body not to complain. If it's cold outside, I breathe differently and think myself warmer. If that seems out of your reach, then you've been brainwashed into believing that there is something out there more powerful than your mind. And there isn't.

Pain, heat, cold, hunger, and a number of other "conditions" are based significantly on YOUR perception. Meaning, you can think yourself into pain, and think yourself out of it. In double-blind trials involving over a thousand people suffering from chronic pain, relief was felt not just by those given painkilling drugs but also by half of given such drugs but in fact received dummy pills (placebos). **Studies on depression have found people did as well on placebos as on the actual anti-depressants.** Tons of other conditions are psychosomatic, that is, they result from interactions occurring between the mind and body. And that's why placebos and perception make such a difference. Placebos have been shown to be effective in a wide variety of conditions, including anorexia, depression, skin diseases, diarrhea, palpitations and many more. **In about a third of all people, most pains are relieved by placebos.** Placebos work best against headache-type pain (over 50% effectiveness), and are actually far more effective against severe pain than mild pain.

A lot of it is in your head. You can "think yourself well" from many ailments or "believe yourself to death" on things you can't!

MODERN-DAY SNAKE OIL

DO HEALTH FADS AND MIRACLE CURES ACTUALLY WORK?
BY SUPREME UNDERSTANDING

Back in the late 1800s, clever salesmen would travel from town to town, promising healing and pain relief through their miraculous snake oil. **No matter what your affliction, whether back pain or gout, these old school hustlers would tell you that the snake oil could fix it.** They would even employ a fellow hustler to emerge from the audience, supporting these extraordinary claims. Because of the human tendency to believe things like this, snake oil merchants would make tons of money in every town they visited, never to return. **Eventually, this kind of marketing fraud became known as "selling snake oil," meaning selling a product that promises fantastic results but doesn't deliver.** What's ironic though, is that snake oil, real snake oil at least, is one of the few products from its era that actually worked. If you had constant pain and you got a real bottle of snake oil, that bottle contained oil from the Chinese water snake, which is actually highly effective in numbing pain because of its high EFA content. Chinese laborers often brought little bottles of this stuff when they came to the American West to work on the Transcontinental Railroad. The white settlers saw the Chinese treat their pains using this oil, and then saw Pueblo Indians using their own snake oil, made from rattlesnakes...and you know how the story goes. Whites took this old indigenous knowledge and used it to get rich. But most of the snake oil sold then didn't even contain real snake oil. In 1917, tests of a federally seized shipment of Snake Oil Liniment revealed it to be mostly mineral oil containing about 1% fatty oil (thought to have been beef fat), along with some red pepper (probably to impart a soothing warmth to the skin) and possible traces of turpentine and camphor (perhaps to provide a suitably medicinal smell). It didn't do anything close to what real snake oil would do. But for many people, the belief that it was working was enough. How else would the thousands of snake oil salesmen stay in business? How else would a new snake oil hustler (then called a "grafter") be able to come to town right behind the last one, and still make sales?

Now, what does this have to do with us right now? Well, do you think the hustle ever stopped? **The game didn't change; it's just new players** (and products). I can think of a few products that typically promise amazing results and don't deliver, but I don't want to upset some of us who have gotten attached to our "miracle cures," even when I tell people that scientific studies have shown that certain products do almost nothing to promote health in humans, they don't want to hear it. They cry conspiracy, even though there are many natural products that have fantastic results in scientific studies, so why would there be a conspiracy against one specific "natural" product? In most cases, it's more likely that all those studies are not funded by some secret "anti-miracle" organization...and the product simply doesn't do all that it promises. It should be a clue that most of those extraordinary claims without extraordinary evidence (besides "testimonials" wink wink) are being made by people who are selling a product or a book.

"Many "miracle" products appear to have no scientific basis for use in humans, though they may be supported (or not) in rat studies! So many products are sold with – at best – an intent to help, and – at worst – an intent to simply generate income for the manufacturer or vendor." – Shanda Hodge

There are also many services that can be considered snake oil. Many of them also derived from ancient traditions we once used and understood. But now they've been "rediscovered" "reinvented" and "repackaged" by white folks, who sell these "ancient" products and services back to us (we typically don't catch on until the trendy white hippy crowd is doing it though). But the version we get is usually nothing like what our ancestors used, and the explanations we use are typically nothing like the way our ancestors understood them. Ain't that deep? Take our sh*t and sell it back to us, yet we buy your watered down version because we don't know our history.

So many of these products, services, and traditions don't do anything to promote health, and some are actually dangerous. Typically the dangerous ones didn't have ANY place in our culture, (like consuming "monoatomic gold," which actually has no proven health benefits, but comes with some serious health risks[28]) or attempting breatharianism (living without eating or drinking, only breathing), which makes no damn sense, period. If the human body could survive without food or drink, we wouldn't have a damn digestive system. I don't want to crusade against too much more, because people get real sensitive about their 'snake oil' when they believe it works for them. So let me say this, and hope everyone understands where I'm coming from. **There's nothing wrong with snake oil, especially if you can get the real thing. And this isn't 1880, so now you can actually research any product or service's claims by scouring the internet. Just make sure you're consulting independent sites and checking out critical perspectives.** You can even start at Wikipedia if you don't know where to start.

Maybe that stuff doesn't really work but you're belief in it is helping you feel better. So long as it's not expensive or dangerous, continue.

PH BALANCE: A MATTER OF MINERALS
BY NASIM ALLAH

If you remember those little strips of litmus paper from High School chemistry class, pH is a measure of how acidic or alkaline something is. The pH scale typically ranges from 0 to 14. 7.0 is neutral; anything below is acidic and anything above is alkaline. **The pH of our blood is slightly alkaline, ranging around approximately 7.4...no matter what you eat.**

The pH level of blood is maintained through the use of minerals stored in our bones and tissues, and the minerals we obtain through our diet. After food is digested and nutrients are assimilated, an ash-like residue of minerals is left over. **Minerals such as calcium, iron, magnesium, and potassium are stored in bones and muscles, and if necessary, can be extracted to maintain the alkalinity of**

---

[28] The "benefits" of monoatomic gold appear to go mainly to the seller, not the user. The fact that these "gold sellers" are now talking about even greater benefits in "monoatomic platinum" should be a clue that it's all about money!

the blood.

This occurs in diets too high in protein. Excessive amounts of amino acids (what proteins are broken down to) are converted by the body into organic acids that can potentially acidify the blood. However, the blood does not become acidic because minerals are used to neutralize the organic acids.

Our body automatically compensates but in the process can off-set and obstruct the development or maintenance of bones, muscles, and organs. **By extracting minerals to buffer acidic levels rather than to build and maintain bodily structures and functions, we begin to experience mineral deficiencies.** In fact, many scientist are beginning to link osteoporosis (a disease in which bones become extremely weak and fragile) with high protein diets due to the potential loss of calcium.

Since our blood's pH level is automatically balanced, it doesn't matter if our food is acidic or alkaline. **All food is subject to acidic and alkaline-based conditions during digestion.** When food enters the stomach, it has entered an acidic environment and when entering the intestines, it's entered an alkaline-based environment. No amount of vegetables can affect the acidity of the stomach, and no amount of meat can affect the alkalinity of the intestines. In fact, food only has an effect on the pH level of urine, which is confined to the bladder, but what you eat still matters.

A meal made up of processed foods and empty calories will not have the nutrients necessary to compensate for a potential acidic rise in pH and can create deficiencies.

Grains, bread, milk, and meats are often promoted as acid foods, while fruits and vegetables are promoted as alkaline foods. It is interesting to point out that so-called "alkaline-forming" foods are very high in minerals and vitamins while so-called "acid foods" mostly consist of empty calories or high amounts of protein. It is the mineral content and nutritional profile that matters, the body itself handles the rest.[29]

There are no dietary measures you need to take to "balance your pH." Eat more fruits and vegetables to prevent mineral deficiencies.

---

[29] Note from Supreme: If you notice, there are a lot of "revolutionary" approaches to health, coming from people selling books, courses, and supplements, yet no matter what kind of terminology they use (or what categories they've created), they all seem to promote the same thing we're talking about in this book (without the fancy words and techniques): Eat less junk food, fast food, fried food, and meat. Eat more vegetables (and a plant-based diet in general).

10 REASONS TO GET A MASSAGE

BY C. WISE "TAWA" HAAKIM ALLAH

I've been practicing Massage Therapy for over 30 years. After attending massage academy, I've been doing so professionally for the past 11 years. Just like most other people in the hood, before learning massage professionally, I once thought of massage as merely something you do before sex. But the longer I practiced massage and the more I learned about its healing effects, **I came to truly realize that massage is one of the most amazing tools of preventative medicine, as well as general healing.** Most of us know that massage can reduce pain and stiffness and put our bodies at ease. But there's more to it than muscle relaxation. Here are ten reasons why massage – in terms of healing – is "the truth."

> **Did You Know?**
> Massage increases circulation, and thus can be a very powerful detoxifying vehicle, helping cleanse the body of many pathogenic germs by way of the lymphatic system. Massage is also great for mental wellness and emotional balance, as it releases hormones from the brain that attribute a sense of goodness and wellbeing.

Increases attentiveness and learning which has positive implications for those with ADD, ADHD, or learning disabilities.

Reduces stereotypical and off-task behavior in people with autism and increases their normal behavior.

Assists in overcoming addictions, like cigarettes, and drug/alcohol use.

Reduces stress, migraine headaches, and alleviates pain.

Promotes healing for all psychiatric diagnosis.

Assists in the improvement of skin conditions.

Lowers blood pressure, anxiety, and hostility levels in individuals with hypertension.

Promotes overall peace for the giver and receiver. Therefore when used with couples it can reduce domestic disputes.

Depending on where you go, a professional massage (Shiatsu, Swedish, etc.) can be costly. Yet if you ask around, there are always places with reasonable rates. However, giving and receiving massages with friends, family, or significant other, can be FREE. Some of the best massages will come from children! They love giving them and walking on their parents' backs!

Instead of paying your youth, you can barter with them. Give them a massage as well, and they will love and appreciate you a whole bunch more. **Learning how to give and receive massage with your mate is also very powerful. It helps to keep families' together, and**

show your mate you care. It's also a great way to reduce your stress and hostility. I'm sure that if there were more healing massages in the hood, there would be far less violence.

Simple Steps to do a Healing Holistic Back Massage

Here are few suggestions to give a good back massage.

Preparation. Before starting your massage session you want to create an atmosphere of peace. Clean and clear your working space of any clutter. Light some candles, play some soothing music, burn some incense or aromatherapy oils, and place a nice comfy blanket or mat on the floor (or prepare your bed or couch for the workspace). Finally, have natural hypoallergenic oil such as apricot or olive oil nearby. **Before you begin, put in your mind that you are the Giver and they are the Receiver.** Ask the receiver where their area of most need is. This is where you'll begin. Tell them that you'll do your best to bring lasting relief to them.

Grounding/Centering. The first thing you want to do is make sure your mind is right to give a massage. Otherwise, whatever is on your thoughts will be transferred to the person receiving the massage. A simple grounding exercise is to sit or stand with your hands right beneath your bellybutton (not touching). With your eyes closed, visualize a ball of light and energy building up in your belly. Take a series of deep breaths until you feel energized, peaceful, and relaxed.

Briskly Rub Hands Together. This serves, but is not limited to heating your hands and it draws the energy that you were centering to your hands.

Connecting. A smooth start for a massage has greater results than a brisk beginning. Simply take a deep breath, and then gently and slowly rest your hands on the receiver's back. Keep them still in a resting position until you feel a connection with the receiver.

Rocking. This step is very important because just as a mother relaxes her child by rocking them, so will you relax your receiver for the massage session. Gently rock the receiver for about three minutes. This releases chemicals that stimulate relaxation and prepares the receiver to be at ease.

Oil Application. Pour a small amount of oil in one hand and rub your hands together until the oil feels warm. Don't rub too much because the oil will penetrate your skin. And never pour the oil directly on the receiver as cold oil can startle your receiver and interfere with her/his relaxation. Slowly glide the oil upon your receiver's back using light pressure until you've equally applied oil on the entire back. Gradually increase the pressure of your gliding motion, monitoring the receiver's comfort and avoiding pressure on the spinal vertebrae or any bony area. **(Never apply pressure on bony areas during a massage)** Always start with light touch and increase the pressure based upon receiver's comfort.

If you are working the shoulders, use a kneading motion. Place the shoulder muscle in your hands and sort of knead it like kneading dough to make bread. Repeat the same process on the next shoulder and the back of the neck. **(Avoid pressure on the spine or front of the neck).**

Using a friction motion, place your hands on the muscles of the shoulder blade and gently rub the muscle in a circular motion, applying enough pressure to work that muscle against the bone without applying pressure to the bone.

Beginning at the top of the back with your knuckles and fingers on the erector spinae (thick muscle on the sides of the spine), use gradual pressure as you slowly glide your hands down the spinal muscle all the way to the lower back. **(Avoid any pressure on the spine and the bones of the lower back)** Do this about three times, increasing pressure to the receiver's comfort level.

Place both hands face down on either side of the receiver's lower back. Use slow pumps of alternating pressure (or lean in), to press with one hand deep, one hand light, to the receiver's comfort level.

Use your kneading motion again to work the oblique sides of the back, from the lower back on up to the armpits. Do this on both sides, using firm pressure, to your receiver's comfort level.

Use a tapping motion across the entire back area, gently patting receiver's back using the edge of an open hand or a closed fist, avoiding too much pressure on any boney area.

Peaceful Finale. Finally, rock your receiver as you did in the beginning for about three minutes. Then tell them thank you, as you want to show your gratitude for them allowing you to practice this Holistic Massage on them.

There are many books and videos available online, at the bookstore, or your local library that can teach you more about the art of massage, including topics like sensual massage, acupressure, and self-massage.

Two websites that offer free tutorials are www.MassageFree.com and www.SelfMassageForAthletes.com

---

Use massage to improve the quality of relationships. It's always great to learn a new skill set, massage is a great one.

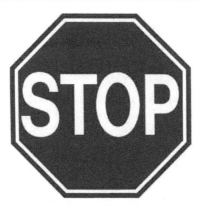

Take a break.
Put this book down for a minute.

Do NOT go back to reading this book until you do one (or more) of the following things:

- ❑ Call somebody who is going through some rough sh*t and make sure they are okay.
- ❑ Eat something that your body is telling you it needs, or drink some water.
- ❑ Wrestle, spar, or slapbox someone to make sure you "still got it."
- ❑ Take a walk through your neighborhood and see if somebody needs help with something.
- ❑ Clean up a part of your house, or organize some f*cked up part of your life.
- ❑ Tell somebody about this book and what you're learning. Invite them to come read it.
- ❑ Give this book away to somebody who needs it and get another copy for yourself.
- ❑ Cook something good, and make enough to share. Invite people.
- ❑ Check yourself out in the mirror and pick something to improve.
- ❑ Identify ten positive things about your life and stop forgetting them when you're stressed.
- ❑ Tell somebody you love them, cause it might be your last chance.

This has been a PSA from 360 and SDP.
Once you're done, carry on.

19 WAYS TO GET HEALTHIER FOR FREE

BY DENIZ LOPEZ

Getting healthy doesn't have to blow your budget. Here's 19 ways you can improve your health for free.

Join your local library for the workout DVDs. Most libraries have a big selection, the perfect antidote to a pricey gym routine. And because the key to sticking with exercise is to keep it interesting, you can switch it up cheaply as often as you want. The library is also a quiet place to distress.

Order a free health calendar. Get one from the National Women's Health Information Center (www.womenshealth.gov). The 2010 calendar lists recommended health tests, surprising symptoms of serious health conditions, and advice on how to read drug labels and get a second opinion.

Surf for deals. Sites like www.Thunderfap.com, www.FreakyFreddies.com, and www.Freemania.net have free-by-mail samples and coupons for all kinds of basic need items.

Get a free radon test. Radon, an odorless natural gas present in many homes, is the leading cause of lung cancer deaths among nonsmokers. Visit the EPA's Web site to check for free or low-cost test kits in your state.

Click off the weight. Studies show that interactive online-weight-loss programs help people drop pounds and maintain weight loss, too. To get diet counseling, try www.SparkPeople.com. You can access calorie-counting tools at CalorieCount.about.com.

Strike a pose. Try your Downward Dog for free – or pretty cheap – thanks to the Internet. Every week, Yoga Today streams a free, one-hour class. (Downloads cost $3.99) Why yoga? It hikes flexibility and strength, provides help for relieving stress and controlling weight, and lowers risks of heart disease and sleep problems.

Bargain hard. Many health clubs and gyms are willing to cut you deals or give you free passes to try their facilities. Bally, Gold's Gym, and 24 Hour Fitness all offer free 7-day trials. Remember: Everything is negotiable. And once you're a member, train with a buddy to cut trainer costs in half, or sign up for 30-minute training sessions instead of hour-long ones. Besides being cheaper, the shorter workout may move faster and be more intense.[30]

---

[30] NOTE: Also, check out your local neighborhood park and park recreation centers. Often they have aerobics, weigh rooms, ball courts, and programs going on there for free that you can take advantage of.

Do a smoke checkup. Some local fire departments offer smoke alarms (a potential lifesaver, considering up to 20% of the alarms installed in people's homes don't even work) for free or at discounted prices. Speaking of smoke; if you're trying to stop smoking, call 1-800-784-8669 to find a coach who'll help you kick the nasty habit for free. Quitting will not only save you money but also lower your risks for heart disease and cancer.

Create a medical family tree. Start planning a healthier future today by asking relatives about their health conditions and creating a free Family Health Portrait. (See "Knowing Your Family's Health History")

Save $170 in the shower. That's how much you can cut from your water bill each year by taking shorter, cooler showers, according to the EPA. Your budget and your skin will thank you. Hot water causes blood vessels to expand, causing you to lose more moisture. To keep your skin soft and supple, limit showers to around five minutes and think warm, not hot.

Snag free health apps. There are about 3,000 iPhone applications designed to boost your health and fitness – and many are free. MyNetDiary has 91,000 foods in its database to help you plan healthy meals, and its community forum is reviewed by a registered dietitian. Free Menstrual Calendar helps you predict your periods and fertile days. FitnessKeeper uses GPS tracking for runners who want to keep tabs on their distance, speed and calories burned. Vibrating Massager literally turns your iPhone into a feel-good massager. I could go on. Even rapper David Banner has an iPhone app that will allow fans to benefit from what he learned during his personal weight-loss and fitness journey. "David Banner's Work Out or Die" offers subscribers videos of the various workout strategies that Banner has found effective and a host of tools to support their decision to attain and maintain a healthy lifestyle.

Moisturize for free. Stop by cosmetic or lotion stores and try their free samples. Keep it natural/organic to avoid any chemicals that might do you harm.

Eat healthier, no cookbook required. There are tons of free cookbooks and recipes online with the health conscious person in mind.

Tweet for discounts. Follow your favorite stores on Twitter and get hot sales alerts and great advice.

Try a new sport. If you've romanced the idea of skiing, hiking, rock climbing – get out there and try it out. Many places will offer free or discounted trials if you tell them you've never tried these things before.

Give and get for free. Loads of useful items are available for free on the grassroots network Freecycle.org, a smart online location for secondhand giveaways. The site's goal is to keep good stuff in use instead of letting it get thrown away and end up harming the environment. Keep in mind: Available items change daily!

Sign up for a free pedometer. www.JustKeepMoving.com, a healthy-lifestyle site, will send you a pedometer (while supplies last) if you register. Studies show that using the simple gadget is an effective weight-loss tool.

Talk it out. There is a free self-help group out there for whatever is bothering you, whether it's physical or mental. Find a searchable database of about 1,000 support groups for people dealing with acne, addictions, allergies, breast cancer, headaches, infertility, eating disorders, OCD, parenting, and many more issues at www.mentalhelp.net

Go outside. At least 20 minutes per day of direct sunlight gives your body much needed Vitamin D, which boosts your immune system, keeps your skin looking good, and even helps ward off depression by increasing mood and creating higher levels of energy.

Next time you're on your computer or smartphone check out some of these free resources.

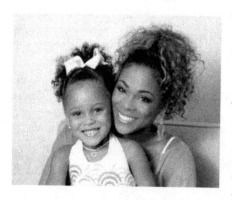

GET A SECOND OPINION

BY SUPREME UNDERSTANDING

Just because someone is a licensed doctor doesn't mean they have all the answers, or the only answer. Often, doctors are trained and conditioned to see things a certain way, so it's difficult for them to consider a possibility outside of that scope. **This is why it's essential that you get a second opinion when you're concerned about what a doctor has told you.** A good doctor won't be offended if you tell them so, either. In fact, many will recommend another doctor, but I suggest you look outside of that circle and **ask a doctor with no connection to your current doctor.**

A perfect example can be found in the story of T-Boz of TLC. T-Boz

(Tione Watkins) has had sickle cell anemia all her life. Doctors told her that she wouldn't live past 30 or have children. They were wrong about both. So when she learned she had a brain tumor (which took away her ability to speak for months) she battled in secret for nearly three years before finding doctors who could actually help.

She told *People Magazine*, "Because of my sickle-cell disease, I have a high tolerance for pain. By 2006, I'd have headaches for six years. I thought it was stress. But when my vision went blurry, I got an MRI." Turned out, she had a large acoustic neuroma (a noncancerous tumor) on her brain's vestibular nerve, which affected her balance, hearing, sight and facial movement. "I thought, "God, why now?" I told the doctor my goal was not to die – I had to be there for [my daughter] Chase."

She went to doctor after doctor. They all refused to remove the tumor, citing sickle-cell-related complications, like lung or heart failure. They said it was impossible to fix. But she never lost hope. She kept looking for a solution. Finally, Dr. Keith L. Black (a Black neurosurgeon who has been called "a god" for his life-saving work) told her that he thought surgery was possible if they worked with a blood specialist. Watkins explained:

> Dr. Black asked me in what order did I want to save these three things: my hearing, balance and facial movement. I said save my facial control first and hearing second, because you wouldn't be able to tell if I can't hear well just from looking at me. At least I'd have hearing on one side. Then save my balance last. But I worried about it. What if I couldn't sing or dance? Music is my heart…The surgery took about seven hours. (I had written my will – I might not have made it.) When I awoke, I could hear and looked normal. But then I had a sickle-cell crisis. With the pain meds and steroids, they said I kept flopping and hitting my head. They gave me IV fluids in order to stop it.

> After I was released, more than a week later, the ride to my L.A. apartment was like vertigo to the 10th power. I had to sit up in bed for two months. They propped me up, but I kept sliding down, which made my head swell. It was so painful. At one point, fluid poured out my nose. I was readmitted. I couldn't walk or really see. I heard screeching noises. They said "We may have to cut you open again" I was like, "No!" I prayed, and the fluid stopped, so I got out. When I was eating pancakes four days later, they fell out my mouth. I couldn't feel my cheek. I couldn't blink, walk or form words. When I saw my face was distorted – I cried.

> Two weeks later Chase, who stayed with my aunt in Atlanta, and I were on iChat and she was like, "Mom, you look pretty." I don't know what she saw, but it made me feel better. In rehab, I had to relearn how to walk and how to say my ABCs. I can relate to deaf people: You think you're saying "where" but your mouth goes "whaa." When Chase visited me, she'd hold my cheeks and kiss me. She didn't treat me like I looked funny.

Thanks to speech and dance therapy, Watkins even started performing again.

If you say "sick kids," you always get me...To this day, the headaches are unbelievable. My facial nerves jump, and I want my smile back. But if that's all? No problem. I fight to be here daily because I want to see Chase get married and have kids. I want to party and laugh. I'm doing a solo album, and I want to tour. I have to see if I can do it. I'm still here. It will take way more to stop me.

Don't lose all hope because of one doctor. Some doctors have different solutions. The right doctor is the one with the solution.

I'M NOT A DOCTOR, I JUST PLAY ONE WITH YOUR LIFE

BY DIERDRA BAPTISTE

ARE YOU OVERWEIGHT? DO YOU SOMETIMES LOSE IT AT THAT SPECIAL MOMENT? DOES YOUR LEG DO THIS? DO YOUR EYES BLINK? CAN YOU SMELL MORE THAN OTHERS? THEN YOU MAY BE SUFFERING FROM BEING HUMAN. ASK YOUR DOCTOR IF PACLAMETHAHYDRENE IS RIGHT FOR YOU!

We're all familiar with the ads and commercials claiming cures for this, relief from that and enhancements for everything else. It's to the point where if you breathe, eat, sh*t and sleep, then you may need to ask your doctor if (insert brand name) is right for you. Usually backing these products is some person in a lab coat stating to be a doctor of some sort with letters after their name. Hell, sometimes there isn't even the claim of a medical profession. Just a random Joe-Schmuck actor in a white jacket. But it works because **we're conditioned to believe that anyone wearing one knows what they're talking about and is full of knowledge and integrity.** Truth is, a lot of doctors are full of something, but it ain't knowledge...or integrity.

The U.S. is one of only TWO countries in the world that allows pharmaceutical companies to market directly to consumers. And out of those two countries, the people of the U.S. are the only ones dumb enough to believe everything they see on TV. As a result, the money spent on direct-to-consumer advertising has more than quintupled in the 7 years between 1997 and 2005 since the FDA changed the guidelines, from $700 million in 1997 to more than $4.2 billion in 2005. It's been money well spent, because the pharmaceutical companies saw an 80% increase in their sales. The FDA, regulates (and I use that term loosely) these drugs, but prescription drug fraud is just as common as the over-the-counter pseudo-med scams. And we know they have more side-effects, risks, and costs than the thing we're trying to cure. **So don't think every doctor has your best interest in mind. Some are just acting on behalf of their pharmaceutical philanthropists.** (See "I'll Be Your Pusher")

Selling Drugs for a Living

"Doctors give drugs of which they know little, into bodies, of which they know less, for diseases of which they know nothing at all." – Voltaire

How can you tell if your doctor is just a drug-dealer in a lab coat?

- ☐ If your doctor doesn't take the time to listen to what's bothering you, nods his/her head at everything you say while filling out a prescription before you even finish.
- ☐ If your doctor doesn't encourage you to take any other proactive measures to improve your health.
- ☐ If your doctor can't explain what foods or herbs could improve your condition, but can somehow tell you all about what herbs NOT to take.
- ☐ If your doctor doesn't even ask if you're interested in addressing your health through natural methods.
- ☐ If you can get a refill from him/her before you should have run out.
- ☐ If you can get a refill from his/her partner without any discussion, chart review, etc.
- ☐ If your doctor is pushing the new drug that you just saw on the TV in the waiting room (the same drug name printed on the pen you used to sign in...before you sat down and read a pamphlet from the pharmaceutical company who made it).
- ☐ If you arrived early or on time for your appointment at 10 am, but aren't seen until 10:20, yet you're still out of there, 5 prescriptions deep by 10:35.

"The art of medicine consists of amusing the patient while nature cures the disease." –Voltaire

These people aren't doctoring you, they're doctoring their wallet. **Along with checking the time of your visit, make sure you check your health insurance EOB** (explanation of benefits) **when it arrives in the mail.** You were seen for 15 minutes, but I guarantee you were billed for the entire hour. And for each prescription that's filled, the consult is billed at a higher rate due to complexity of the exam, intake of information, etc. Oh yeah, scammers.

Be Proactive

"Never go to a doctor whose office plants have died." – Erma Bombeck

Most doctors who are as described above have a track record of either being sanctioned or not being in a particular location very long. This is because it's only so long before there's a problem with one of those 500 drugs they prescribe, or with the overall lack of attention they apply to their patients. So you definitely want to check your doctor out before you see them. **The best way to find a reputable doctor for yourself and your family is, of course, to ask around, but there are other resources available to us.**

There is the **NPI Registry**. NPI stands for National Provider

Identification. All medical providers are required by law to have this number for identification and reimbursement purposes. The website for this system is (https://nppes.cms.hhs.gov) and is run by the Health and Human Services Dept. of the U.S. Government. This is a tool you can use to FIRST determine if the person you just met (or were recommended) even HAS a current license to practice medicine.

Additionally, you may also look up any provider in your home state by going to your state's government website. For instance, in Massachusetts, its Mass.gov and from there, any information would be listed under the Division of Professional Licensure. It's probably different for each state, but with a quick search using terms like "physician," "licensing" "medical board," etc., you'll be able to find what you need. The state sites often give plenty information, including malpractice suits, settlements, revoked licenses, etc.

There are plenty of doctor review sites online, but after checking out a few of them, it seems the best site (though not the prettiest) is **www.RateMDs.com**, which **provided not only ratings, but personal testimonials about the doctors we looked up.** And some stories were simply tragic. One of the doctors we searched for was an OB/GYN who nearly killed Mecca Wise, Supreme Understanding's wife, during her pregnancy. The reviews told the story Supreme wished he'd known beforehand. In fact, one of those reviews led us to this last resource...

Google. Yup. Simple as that. **Google the doctor's full name** (try using quotation marks around their name if it seems common). You might find records of malpractice lawsuits (we found one case where the OB/GYN above botched a circumcision with horrific results, and at least five other cases), sanctions, and even license revocation proceedings. Just as you would with any NATURAL health approach, do your research. Don't trust somebody with your life just because they're wearing a white lab coat.

Don't trust someone in a lab coat any more than you would a stranger. You need to know everyone you do business with.

STUFF YOU'LL DIE WITHOUT

WATER, SUNLIGHT, OXYGEN, AND REST

Historically, we've always valued Sunlight, Water, Rest and Air. We even developed complex mythologies around them, even personifying them as divinities named after the Sun, the Moon (rest), the Sea, and the Sky. **We didn't worship the Sun; we just valued its role in keeping us alive!** Now we hide from it, and we're sick as a result, with the majority of people of color in the U.S. deficient in Vitamin D. **Since ancient times, we used to base our civilizations around our water sources, but you know we don't even drink water anymore...at least not unless it's got sugar in it.** But at least we get enough sleep, right? Wrong. Research says most of us are either getting too much or too little! And neither is healthy. So the following articles all deal with one of the four "other" essentials (Sunlight, Water, Rest, and Oxygen) besides diet and exercise, and how we can improve the quality (and quantity) of their presence in our lives.

Don't neglect these four essential elements. Plan to get them as you would plan for a diet or exercise program.

THE FUEL OF LIFE

BY YVETTE GZ

"Water is life's mater and matrix, mother and medium. There is no life without water." – Albert Szent-Gyorgyi, Biochemist, 1937 Nobel Prize for Medicine

Water is not only important to quench your thirst; every system in the human body depends on it, from your brain and digestive system, to your blood and body temperature. **Your body is MOSTLY composed of water, about 50-70% of it to be more exact** (this can change, depending on your age, health, and level of water intake). Water makes up your blood, brain, lungs, glands, muscle and organ tissue. You need water to sweat, flush toxins out of your body, carry oxygen and nutrients in your bloodstream throughout your body, regulate your temperature, and digest food properly. Unfortunately your body doesn't produce water, so you have to provide it with the right amount daily.

The circulatory and respiratory system: This consists of your heart, blood vessels, and lungs. Your blood is 90% water; it acts as the solvent to dilute salts, minerals, oxygen and nutrients so that your cells can absorb them. If those contents are not diluted, your body will have a serious problem trying to absorb what it needs and this can end up causing heart problems and high blood pressure. The thing is, whenever you're depriving your body of something or changing a routine, it adapts to it. Therefore, drinking less water will make your blood vessels slightly shrink so that you won't lose water too fast, but that also causes high blood pressure and possibly, heart problems. (See "Heart Health")

The respiratory system: Even your lungs get affected if you don't drink enough. You lose 20 ounces of water a day by breathing alone, and your lungs need moisture to absorb oxygen and transfer other gases like carbon dioxide and nitrogen. **So avoid lung and breathing problems by keeping your system watered.**

The excretory and urinary system: Your kidneys, bladder, large intestine and sweat glands. You can poison yourself to death if you're not drinking enough water to get rid of the toxins and wastes in your body. Those toxins can come from food, alcoholic beverages, smoke, or even your environment. And of course, water is the best agent to flush them out. You also need it in your digestive track to carry out proper digestion and transport foods easily, or else you could end up with constipation, kidney stones, and other difficulties. Just as nutrients need to be dissolved in water to be absorbed, acids and wastes need to be dissolved to be transferred out of your body.

Last but not least, your brain needs water because it's composed of it. That's why you get headaches when you go for long periods of time without drinking. When you get heated from exercising or hot weather, you need to cool your body down by sweating, or else you could damage your organs or even die of sunstroke and other forms of hypothermia, which is another word for over-heated. **Sweating is your body's way of regulating your temperature by excreting heat out while giving your skin that cooling-off feeling.** And yep you guessed it, you need water to make sweat.

Oh and here's a little beauty tip. **Water acts as a rejuvenating agent by keeping your skin and body hydrated.** You're about ¾ water when you're born but go through an age-related dehydration and end up ¼ water by the time you're 90, which is why most old people look wrinkly and dried up…like going from a fresh grape to a raisin. The best way to slow down the aging process and keep looking young and fresh is by drinking lots of water.

The amount of water needed per day varies from person to person. A common technique is to take your weight in pounds, divide it by 2, and drink that amount in ounces. So if you weigh 140 lbs., drink at least 70 ounces daily. If you live in a hotter climate, exercise a lot, or are pregnant/ breastfeeding, you'd have to drink a little more. Just make sure to not overdo it, because even too much of a good thing is bad. **Drinking TOO much water can lead to hyponatraemia, which is what happens when all your minerals and salts get completely diluted and almost nonexistent.** Even though water is important, you still need those nutrients for your body to function properly. You can find out if you need more water by observing yourself. **If you experience fatigue, lack of energy, headaches, pain in joints, or your urine is not clear to pale yellow, you need to drink more.** Also, it's best to start drinking BEFORE you get thirsty. Thirst is more of a warning than a suggestion; try to not let your body get to that point because it is a sign of dehydration.

Water is the vital building block of life. Drink it consecutively throughout the day. A cup an hour is a great way to stay hydrated.

THE IMPORTANCE OF WATER
BY EARTHIASIA

You are What you Drink

The earth's surface is covered approximately 3/4ths by water and our body shares a similar composition, being composed of about 70% water. Knowing this relationship, it isn't hard to see why water is one of the most important compounds on this planet.

With the current state of our planet, clean water is becoming increasingly difficult to obtain. This is because **our drinking water is far from pure, containing some two hundred deadly commercial chemicals.** Within this list is chlorine which is supposed to clean our water, but causes hardening of your arteries, and – when mixed with other chemicals – can become a carcinogen. Aluminum Sulphate is added to clarify water and has long been associated with memory loss and possibly Alzheimer's. Among these chemicals you have bacteria and parasites that the chlorine in the water leaves behind. Giardia and cryptosporidium are parasitic to the intestines of animals and humans. Once in the body, these parasites then multiply and cause infections. To the above mixture you can add inorganic minerals which make your water hard and leaves a film that stains your shower.

All of this information is given to you so you can have some reference point if you care to look into the water that's being supplied to your home, not to send you screaming and heading for the hills. If you go to the **EPA** and look up water contaminates, you can get a list some of the toxins in the water and their **Maximum Contaminant Level Goal** (MCGL) – Which is the amount of a contaminant that can be in drinking water without having what the EPA deems an adverse effect on health. Then they give you the Maximum Contaminant Level (MCL) which is the amount allowed in the water.

What they don't give you is how much is really in the water. With all of that said it is imperative that we look into alternative waters sources to tap water. Don't fret, I'm not going to leave you with problems without any solutions. So let's explore the different types of water sources and different purification techniques available to us.

A spring is a place on the earth's surface where groundwater emerges naturally. The water source of most springs is rainfall that seeps into the ground uphill from the spring outlet. **While springs may seem like an ideal water supply, they need to be selected with care, developed properly, and tested periodically for contaminations.** Spring water moves downhill through soil or cracks in rock until it is forced out of the ground by natural pressure. The amount of available water from springs may vary with the time of year and rainfall. Groundwater obtained from springs is similar to water pumped from shallow wells. Like shallow wells, springs may be contaminated by surface water or other sources on or below the ground surface. **Spring water is readily available in supermarkets and corner stores.** You must be aware of the brand that you buy some products labeled as spring water are nothing more than filtered water with no greater filtration than that of a home filter system such as Brita.

An alternative to spring water is distilled water. This method is one of the most effective methods when it comes to water purification. This is because it mimics the water cycle which is the natural process of evaporation of water by the sun followed by condensation produced by the rain. This is how the distillation process works. Contaminated water is vaporized into a sterilized steam and then it condenses back in a pure state. All of the waterborne contaminants are left behind.

What you should be cautious with regarding distilled water is that this process takes everything out of the water leaving it void of any minerals, which some schools of thought see as a problem while others see this as a benefit. An easy solution to this problem is charging your water or leaving it exposed to oxygen and or sunlight. (See "Pure water tip").

Home Water Purification Systems

Another option for having safe water is using a proper filter. There are good, mediocre and poor filters on the market so you have to do your homework. What you should be sure of is that it removes chemical compounds, like THMs and heavy metals (like lead). **Boiling water is not a sufficient purification technique.** This is because it does not remove the chemicals in the water and can actually concentrate the metals like lead in the water.

When it comes to home water purifiers there are a lot of options. When it comes to price, the water pitchers are probably the most affordable. They however are among the least effective because they leave behind a wide range of contaminants. Multimedia filters are going to be more valuable when it comes to removing certain elements from your drinking water. This is because in addition to carbon filtration they use second filtration sources that will further the purification process.

Then you have reverse **osmosis filters** which are quite pricey. This technology is based on cell biology. Just like everything else it has its advantages and disadvantages. One of the main advantages, besides its removal of most contaminants, is that it doesn't use any electricity. So you don't have to worry about it raising your bill. One of the major disadvantages is the amount of water that it wastes (2-4 gallons of tap water is wasted for every one gallon that gets filtered). You also have **Water Ionizers** that will filter your water and make it alkaline. It turns the pH. of the water from neutral or 7ph to around 9.5ph.

No matter what your choice of filter is, you have to make sure that you consume enough water to fit your lifestyle. **It only takes your body to lose around 2-3 liters** (10 cups) **to become dehydrated.** Severe dehydration can cause fainting, seizures, comas, and even lead to death!

Just ask Solange Knowles! According to her Twitter updates, Solange (younger sister of Beyonce), passed out from dehydration after taking a dose of Nyquil. When she woke up, she was in the hospital, where she was hooked up to an IV, being treated for dehydration and low blood pressure. Yes, you can have LOW blood pressure too, and that's not

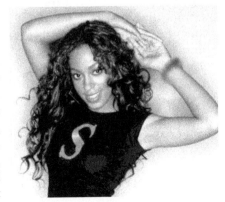

good either. She tweeted:

> Woke up to 8 random people over me, laid out on the floor in baggage claim!
> …Guess I passed out! Scary. Hooked up to IV now. Apparently I'm super
> dehydrated…My mom is the best. LOL…She's like, ain't nothing wrong with
> this girl, she need some water and rest… Pull up the car! LOL.

Upon leaving, doctors ordered her to rest and drink lots of water.

A few ways to increase your water intake is cut back on the amount of
soda that you drink so if you drink three a day have one and replace
the other two with water. If you are a juice drinker you can dilute your
juice with water to up your intake. This doesn't replace the water you
need to drink but it can help. Get creative, challenge yourself and stay
hydrated.

Although it's important more that you drink water, you should be mindful of its quality. Come up with a plan to get clean water.

FINALLY, SOME SUNSHINE!
BY YVETTE GZ

A large majority of people of color are
dangerously vitamin D deficient
(about 98% of Blacks and 90% of
Mexicans and Latinos in America).
This is due to the following reasons:

- ❏ Most of us are lactose intolerant and can't get vitamin D from dairy products.
- ❏ Some voluntarily cut vitamin D sources like dairy products, fish, and eggs out of our diets.
- ❏ Most importantly, we're not getting enough sunlight.

> **Did You Know?**
> Sunlight is a prescribed treatment for jaundice. Sunlight can also help with a cold. Proper exposure to the sun is vital for a healthy immune system because exposure to sunlight increases your white blood cell count. This is your body's primary defense against foreign agents. Sunlight can increase your circulation by increasing the blood flow to the skin. So if you have sore and aching muscles, a little sunlight can help with that too.

The reason why we suffer from this deficiency the most is because of
our melanated skin. **The more melanin you have, the more
sunlight you need to absorb to function properly.** It's no wonder
most people of color are naturally located in the tropics and warm
climates. You can easily live your entire life without milk, fish, or eggs
if you get sufficient sunlight because your body produces vitamin D on
its own. **Sunlight is actually the best source of vitamin D.** If you're
relying on your diet alone, only 50% of what you eat gets absorbed.
You'll have to eat a whole lot of dairy products and fish to get even
half of what the sun gives you, plus you could be poisoning yourself
even more by increasing your cholesterol intake. By getting more
sunlight, on the other hand, you're lowering your cholesterol, because

sunlight converts it to vitamin D, all through your skin alone!

White people are known to have the least amount of melanin (after albinos) which is why they don't need and can't take too much sunlight. In fact even a minor amount of it can cause skin damage in very pale people. That's why you always hear white people saying "too much sunlight can damage your skin and cause skin cancer" and "if you want to look younger stay away from the sun, use more sun-block, etc..." Mind you, "too much sun" to them is over 10 minutes of sunlight per week. Don't pay much attention to those sources because your skin is different, and most of the times they exaggerate in order to sell more sun-block products or even promote light/fair skin. But just like water, too much of a good thing can be harmful. **If you're sweating too hard or feel like your skin is baking, then it might be time to get yourself some shade. In fact you don't even need to reach that level.**

Our children are affected just as badly as we are, especially since they don't go outside to play anymore. It appears that letting our children stay indoors playing video games has 92% of all Black children deficient in vitamin D, according to a new analysis published in the journal *Pediatrics*. By comparison, 80% of Hispanic children and about 67% of white children have insufficient levels of the vitamin.

What's the Big Deal about Vitamin D?

The most important role vitamin D plays is in the absorption of calcium, phosphorus, magnesium, iron, and zinc. Your organs need those to maintain a healthy status and carry out their tasks, especially your bones, intestines, kidneys, liver, and brain. **Without vitamin D, your calcium intake is almost useless because your body can't absorb it. Research has also shown that vitamin D plays a role in killing cancer cells and preventing heart diseases.** (See "A Guide To Vitamins")

For some time, scientists have noticed a connection between multiple sclerosis (MS) and the equator. MS is a slowly-progressing autoimmune disease that

> **Did You Know?**
> A Vitamin D deficiency can cause high blood pressure, artery disease, tuberculosis, obesity, fatigue, memory loss or poor brain function and lead to calcium deposits in the arteries (atherosclerosis). Research has noted that northern countries (due to harsher winters) have higher levels of cardiovascular disease, and that more heart attacks occur in winter months. Regions with more cloud cover in the northern latitudes tend to have two to three times higher cancer rates (prostate, breast, and colon) than in sunnier areas. (Vitamin D deficiency can also allow cancerous cells to grow and induce something called seasonal affective disorder, a form of depression or mood change that occurs during the winter when there's less sunshine. See "Why are you so S.A.D.?")

affects the nervous system. **The further one lives from the equator, the higher the risk of developing MS.** Researchers at the Harvard School of Public Health found that vitamin D may protect against MS. They examined the data collected from the Nurses' Health Studies from over 187,000 women. Those who received good doses of vitamin D a day had a 41% lower chance of developing MS. It is believed that MS occurs when the body's immune system turns against itself, and vitamin D may work by calming overactive immune cells.

As a person of color (especially if you have darker skin), you need about 6 times more sunlight than the average white person. It's hard to say exactly how much since it depends on your complexion, but no less than 40 minutes per week is needed (about 2-5 minutes per day is appropriate). Remember, having some melanin in your skin decreases the risk of skin cancer, so it's not something you have to worry about unless you're going overboard.

All you need to do is go outside! Take a walk with your spouse, play a basketball game, or eat a meal, but leave the long sleeves behind.

THE PINEAL GLAND
BY ROBERT BAILEY

People have called it the "third eye," "the Black Dot," and even the "seat of the soul." But what IS the Pineal Gland? You're about to find out.

The endocrine system is one of your body's 11 systems. It's a system of glands responsible for secreting hormones that serve to regulate and maintain bodily functions. Of these glands, the pineal gland is the true master gland. It's through the pineal gland and the melatonin hormone that we get our melanin.

Located near the center of the brain, the pineal gland gets its name from the pinecone, which it resembles. It is reddish-gray and about the size of a pea or grain of rice, yet, together with the pituitary gland, it has a profuse blood flow, second only to the kidneys. In fact, unlike much of the rest of our brain, the pineal gland is not isolated from the body by the blood-brain barrier system, allowing it to secrete melatonin directly into our bloodstream. **What's even more unique about the pineal gland is that the "third eye" label may be a literal reality.** Schwab and O'Connor, in their 2005 article in the *British Journal of Opthalmology*, write:

> If the development of the third eye seems mysterious, the function is even
> more obscure. Most observers believe the organ to be a solar dosimeter [a way

to measure exposure] useful for photoperiod recognition for circadian and seasonal rhythms, but there may be more to this murky organ than first meets the eye...In animals that have lost the parietal [third] eye, including mammals, the pineal sac is retained and condensed into the form of the pineal gland...This central dorsal third eye is much older than reptiles and probably belongs to our watery beginnings as chordates...The structure is probably older than the Devonian period leading perhaps as far back as the protochordates. But, since the pineal complex seems to be in decline even among the reptiles and in subsequent radiations, it may be going the way of the appendix and, hence, is a very lonely eye indeed.

Translation: It appears the pineal gland was once literally a "third eye." In fact, a study by Lucas and colleagues, published in volume 284 of the journal *Science*, suggests that our pineal gland, even encased inside the brain, can still somehow "see" and respond to light and darkness, even in the absence of the other two eyes. Another study published in 2008 in *The Journal of Experimental Biology* discovered that some eyeless fish actually navigate using only their pineal gland.

What Does It Do?

Our pineal gland is the first gland developed in our bodies. It grows until about 1–2 years of age and doesn't grow any more, though, its weight increases gradually from puberty onwards. The pineal gland plays a number of roles. Some of which include your inner eye (sensing light and darkness), compass, pacemaker (sets the pace for anything in the body that depends on time or speed) and biological clock (keeping track of time). (See "Get Some Damn Rest")

The pineal gland is stimulated by several things, allowing it to function properly. Some of which includes light (specifically natural sunlight), temperature, and food (raw green vegetables rich in chlorophyll, which is food for your pineal gland. Chlorophyll is melanin in plant form), and sleep (important for the production of melatonin, which reaches its max at midnight).Your pineal gland secretes the hormone melatonin into your body in response to darkness and serotonin in response to light.

Melatonin

Melatonin affects your circadian rhythms (your internal clock), boosts memory, organizes your biological system (mentally and spiritually), and is responsible for dream sleep or REM (Rapid Eye Movement). According to Dr. Uzzi Reiss, in his book *Natural Hormone Balance*, a healthy pineal gland produces 2.5 milligrams of melatonin every twenty-four hours. **Melatonin is produced in abundance in people of color because our pineal gland is not as calcified as that of Caucasians.** It should be noted however, that you won't get an optimum amount if you don't sleep at night during its peak hours of production. When you do sleep, strive to make sure it is completely dark with no light. As soon as the pineal gland senses light, the production of melatonin shuts down, even if you sleep in a pitch black room during the day.

Some of melatonin's other known properties include its ability to polymerize into melanin and improve the symptoms of Parkinsonism. According to Carol Barnes, at high dosages, it stimulates contraction of the smooth uterine muscles and the secretion of breast milk. It induces sleep, imagery and the feelings of well-being.

Scientist have found If you produce too little melatonin at night or too much during the day, you will start suffering from depression. SAD (Seasonal Affective Disorder) is a disorder in which too much melatonin is produced, causing profound depression, oversleeping, tiredness, weight gain and sadness.

Serotonin

Serotonin is secreted during the day as soon as the pineal eye senses the dawn. Serotonin gives us an abundance of energy and acts as a neurotransmitter, relaying signals from one area of the brain to another. **It helps us to repress or forget things that are very painful.** In the gut, serotonin regulates intestinal movements, while in the central nervous system it regulates mood, appetite, sleep, muscle contraction, and some cognitive functions including memory and learning.

Some of serotonin's characteristics include the ability to polymerize into melanin, cause muscles to contract and regulating blood pressure.

Tryptophan is an essential amino acid for serotonin and must be supplied through our diet. Serotonin levels drop when fasting and in situations when food is not available. Foods such as chicken soup, dark chocolate, asparagus, avocado, pecans, pineapple, eggplant, spinach, walnuts, oats, and coffee (if you use it sensibly),flaxseeds/flax oil, buckwheat, whey protein, bananas, sour cherries and high quality eggs are just a few of a number of foods that can help to raise your serotonin levels. The main thing is to eat foods rich in tryptophan content. **An increase in the ratio of tryptophan to phenylalanine and leucine will increase serotonin levels.** Fruits with a good ratio include dates, papaya and banana. Foods with a lower ratio inhibit the production of serotonin. These include whole wheat and rye bread.

Calcification

Calcification is a process in which calcium salts build up in soft tissue, causing it to harden. Limestone, calcium, and especially, fluoride deposits contribute to the calcification of the pineal gland, affecting the brains ability to function. Exposing your head to sunshine will help stimulate a calcified pineal gland.

Even a calcified pineal gland is stimulated by light; use this information to enlighten even the most hard-headed individual to live a healthier life.

GREENERY

HOW TO FIND NATURE IN THE HOOD
BY C'BS ALIFE ALLAH

<table>
<tr><td>

Did You Know?
Racial differences in calcification have been noted, with Original people having little to no calcification and white people having 60-80% calcification or greater. Adeloye and Felson's 1974 study found that calcified pineal was twice as common in white Americans as in Blacks in the same city, but that Black Americans had more calcification than Blacks in Africa.[31]

</td></tr>
</table>

The metropolitan cities of ancient Africa, India, South America, East Asia and Moorish-influenced Europe were built in harmony with the environment. The food sources of the city surrounded each city or – in some cases – were integrated with the structure of the city itself. In Zimbabwe the structures were built with inspiration from termite hills that caused them to work as miniature air conditioners. The Aztecs had floating gardens that surrounded the periphery of their cities. All of these civilizations had high technology yet none had experienced the Industrial Revolution.

The European perspective of time being linear (rather than indigenous conceptions cyclical time) translated to white people being focused on consuming without any regards for conservation. (See "We Started This Captain Planet Thing")

Coming to America

"The consideration of man's body has not changed to meet the new conditions of this artificial environment that has replaced his natural one. The result is that of perceptual discord between man and his environment. The effect of this discord is a general deterioration of man's body, the symptoms of which are termed disease." – Professor Hilton Hotema

Europeans were notoriously afraid of the dark. European culture has many traditions centered on this fear, from being 'shut in' (locking up everything in the house – doors, gates, shutters, etc.) to werewolves and other evil creatures roaming in the dark of night. Thus, when they came to the New World, they saw the wilderness as their enemy and as something to conquer. **So they became focused on "clearing the wilderness."** Though some wrote ballads about how the 'noble savage' (aka the Indians) lived in harmony with the environment, they

---

[31] For specifics, see Chapter Three of *Geographical Neurosergery*, available online at book.neurosurgeon.org

kept a-chopping away.

Uh oh, what do we do now?

The population explosion on the East was in full effect during the growth of New York and other older East Coast cities. The frontier was still the frontier and approached only by a relative few. The cities on the East Coast started to become very crowded with no place to go to 'be alone' (another element of European philosophy – individualism and isolation). It got so bad that people started gathering in cemeteries to 'get away.' **It was these conditions that led to the creation of the first public parks like Central Park.** This seemed ideal – little islands of nature in the midst of the city. And it was, until they realized that parks need upkeep. Many parks went through periods of disuse because the politicians of the time didn't think they were important, or because of lack of funds or mismanagement. By the 1950s, Blacks began slowly moving into these communities, and sharing these public resources. Then came the great white flight. Whites left the cities – en masse – for suburbs.

And new parks, swimming facilities, hiking and wilderness programs soon became available in the suburbs. Meanwhile, the racial politics that relocated these resources to the suburbs also kept those from the inner city from having access to them (and it could be argued that the people in the inner city needed them the most). Before long, parks in inner cities fell into total disrepair. Naturally, the residents themselves were blamed for the conditions.

How can someone from the ghetto catch some rays and greenery?

"Fresh air impoverishes the doctor." – Danish Proverb

Here are some little things that you can do to offset the lack of nature.

Take a long trip on the bus. Set aside a day to just ride the bus in its entire circuit. Many buses go far out into places that are a little more rural. This is usually the rule no matter what bus you are riding. You start to see how 'small' the urban bubble really is.

Go to the beach. Yes, some beaches are notoriously filthy and you can't swim in them yet sea air is good air. It clears out a lot of the pollutants that many are exposed to in the inner city. You get to breathe a little deeper and waves are just kind of hypnotic.

Find the greenhouses in the city. There are always some official greenhouses that you can visit in your city. You're going to have to do a little digging, yet they do exist. Some of these places are privately owned while others are owned by public groups. Both types usually want to show off all of their hard work.

Go to the park. Most of us only go to the parks on July 4th. Get a gang of people together and just go to the park on a day during the week or on the weekend. Many parks have been taken over by criminal elements yet this is only due to the fact that a large segment of the public hasn't found a use for the park. Find the use for your park and put it into effect.

Get some plants. House plants can improve the quality of air. They actually can remove pollutants from the air. The best houseplants for this are:

- ☐ Philodendron scandens `oxycardium', heartleaf philodendron
- ☐ Philodendron domesticum, elephant ear philodendron
- ☐ Dracaena fragrans `Massangeana', cornstalk dracaena
- ☐ Hedera helix, English ivy
- ☐ Chlorophytum comosum, spider plant
- ☐ Dracaena deremensis `Janet Craig', Janet Craig dracaena
- ☐ Dracaena deremensis `Warneckii', Warneck dracaena
- ☐ Ficus benjamina, weeping fig
- ☐ Epipiremnum aureum, golden pothos
- ☐ Spathiphyllum `Mauna Loa', peace lily
- ☐ Philodendron selloum, selloum philodendron
- ☐ Aglaonema modestum, Chinese evergreen
- ☐ Chamaedorea sefritzii, bamboo or reed palm
- ☐ Sansevieria trifasciata, snake plant
- ☐ Dracaena marginata , red-edged dracaena

Hit up a Home Depot, Lowes, or a local nursery and cop a couple (or more) of these plants and add some greenery to your living space. It's really not that expensive and it may help you in the long run.

Look for a hiking trail, beach, or park near your community. After a few trips you'll see what is natural and unnatural in life.

SUN SALUTE

BY C'BS ALIFE ALLAH

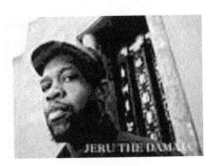

Jeru the Damaja once did an interview where he said that missing the sunrise was tantamount to heresy, as you are missing the actual creation of a new day. I can roll with that. When you rise in tune with the sun, you set your internal clock right. The day's digestion and mental elevation go smoothly. You crap right, you sleep good, and headaches are nothing but a myth to you because you don't experience them.

I ain't no Muslim, Christian or any other kind of religious person, so I can't get with prostration. The only time I like to get down on the ground like that is if I am B-boying, playing Capoeira, or using some esoteric position out of the Kama Sutra. However, there is one more reason by which I get down on the ground. That is in the morning when I do my Sun Salute.

Sun Salutation is a series of short yoga movements that one does in the morning. At first, one might be under the illusion that it's a pagan form of Hindu sun worship. I am not denying that some may have approached it that way in the past. Shoot, a lot of the forms of praying may actually have root in the *asanas* (that's yoga positions) that only later became identified with petitioning an astral being in a religious context. The science of it though, is that the sun is also a means of monitoring time; internally and externally. When dawn comes that lets me know that it is time for me to do that series of movements for the maintenance of upkeep of my physical and mental landscape.

I do have to let you know that doing yoga is something that we men do (See "Yoga's Not Just for Hot Chicks"). **Sitting around with your boys, crushing your internal organs slouching, while playing PlayStation 24/7 isn't masculine bruh.** Making your rounds at the club or bar the highlight of every week ain't a measurement of your testosterone level either.

There are a billion and one benefits of a daily yoga routine like this. I can just tell you what it does for me. It massages my inner organs and makes sure that my blood flow is on point while activating several glands. I've never had high blood pressure (the doctors are still surprised because – at 36 years old – a Black man in America is 'supposed' to have some hypertension going on). I never had internal problems – no heart, liver, kidney, stomach or intestinal pain. My energy level is consistently good. I sleep and dream well. And my gonads are golden right now, with style and stamina. Again, let me reiterate. **Most impotence problems are caused by lack of blood flow so if you can get that right, your woman won't be complaining** (or going somewhere else). A "Sol (meaning sun) Controller" makes sure that he is in "sole control" of his body and is the sole provider of his body's needs. **Many of us are masters of breaking down our body, yet for some reason we don't seek to become masters of healing our body.**

Instead of me writing a whole separate section on instructions, let me point you to some websites that are up to par.

This site (www.yogapose.org/sun_salutation_yoga_poses.html) will outline the positions and also instruct you on the proper breathing that needs to go along with each posture (breathing is KEY). This site (www.proliberty.com/pranayoga/SuryaNamaskar.applet.html) is a flash animation that will give you that visual perspective that you need.

Along with exercise, have a daily "healing" routine. The body like all things needs maintenance.

THE SCIENCE OF BREATHING

BY SWAMI SUPREME UNDERSTANDING

"To insure good health: eat lightly, breathe deeply, live moderately, cultivate cheerfulness, and maintain an interest in life." – William Londen

Of the things you can't live without, oxygen is number one. But we take oxygen (and the air it's packaged in) for granted, mostly because it's one of the few things white people have not figured out how to charge us for (yet).

But just as all food ain't good food, and all water ain't good water, all air ain't good air. **Depending on where you are, there's differences in the quality of the air you're breathing.** If you're Black or brown then it's likely that either: (A) you live in an overpopulated urban area that's more "grey" than green, and lacks natural means of recycling your air supply, or (B) you live in a Southern city that's less grey, but still polluted by factories and toxic dump sites poisoning the air. (We'll explore all that, and why it's like that, in an upcoming book, *Chemical Genocide*) Combine those factors with the amount of time you spend indoors or in your car, and you're probably not getting enough clean air in your system. So what do you do? Go somewhere green. Get into nature. Take a flight if you have to! (See "Greenery")

Regarding getting the most out of the oxygen around us, Dr. Craig Sommers writes in *The Raw Foods Bible* (www.rawfoodsbible.com):

> Everyone knows that we can live without food for quite a while but without oxygen we lose consciousness and die very quickly. What most people don't know is that we can control the amount of oxygen that we bring to our tissues, and that the amount has a potent effect on our health. Most people breathe much more shallowly than is optimal. For example, our brain is between 1 and 3 percent of our body weight but requires about 20 percent of our oxygen intake. The brain needs oxygen to perform all its tasks, and if there is an insufficient supply, our thinking process will be impaired. However, slow, deep breathing that fills our lungs with this life-giving substance allows our bloodstream to absorb more air and to transport it to our brain for optimal brain function.

Experts in the field say that our bodies require oxygen to produce as much as 95% of the energy that we need. If adequate amounts of oxygen are not available, it may result in a lactic acid buildup. Scientists have found that injecting calm people with lactic acid can cause them to experience panic attacks. So it seems that lactic acid buildup from inadequate oxygen (due to shallow breathing and/or poor circulation and from spending time in low oxygen environments such as sealed rooms) can be a primary cause of anxiety.

For vibrant health, the bloodstream must be able to carry optimum amounts of oxygen. Research has shown that a diet containing saturated fats from animal products (including cow's milk and fish) and hydrogenated or cooked vegetable fats lessens the oxygen-carrying capacity of the blood, resulting in less oxygen to the brain, muscles, organs and so forth. Research has also shown that a diet high in dark green, leafy vegetables increases the oxygen-carrying capacity of the blood, resulting in more oxygen delivered to vital organs.

Deep breathing increases the amount of oxygen delivered to the lungs for absorption into the bloodstream and ultimately into the tissues of the body. Most people take very shallow breaths and do not use the full capacity of their lungs. I recommend full inhales and exhales whenever possible. Breathing through the mouth is like drinking from a dirty puddle without filtering the water first. The reason for this is that your lungs need warm moist air.

When we breathe through the nostrils the air is warmed, moistened and filtered through the sinuses. The sinuses produce mucus to catch airborne debris. If we breathe through the mouth we bypass this wondrous filter. That is why it is important to breathe through your nostrils.

It has been said that our lymphatic system is the body's sewer system. It cleans up most of the waste products of cellular metabolism. The body contains about four times as much lymphatic fluid as blood. If our lymphatic system were to shut down for only 24 hours, we would die. The lymphatic system does not have a pump like the bloodstream has. The only way that the lymph fluid gets pumped through the tissues of the body is by muscular movement such as exercise and/or deep breathing, which both move the lymphatic fluid extremely well.

So breathe deeply and remember that air is free!

How to Breathe Properly

To breathe RIGHT, you gotta divide your breath into three parts; lower abdomen (belly), middle abdomen (midsection), and chest.

When you inhale, breathe in through your nose, not your mouth. Take in the air slowly and deeply and let it fill you in parts. First fill up your lower abdomen (belly) with air, then your middle abdomen (midsection), and last the chest. Think of it like you are filling a large pouch with water. You'll actually let your belly stick out when you inhale.

When you exhale, you're emptying the pouch. Breathe out the air from top to bottom. That is breathe out the air in your chest first, then the air in your middle abdomen, and lastly the air in your lower abdomen. Exhaling should take double the time it took to do the inhale. You had to physically push your belly out when inhaling. However, when done correctly, there is no need to pull your belly in because it happens naturally.

Don't feel rushed to take your next breath. You don't need to. Most people feel a natural (or conditioned?) urge to inhale immediately after exhalation. But when you grow out of this, you will be able to reach that higher level of consciousness all the yoga experts talk about.

You can even take an online test to see how "well" you're breathing at www.breathing.com/tests.htm

Yawning and Sighing

People try to avoid yawning and sighing because they're considered impolite. But it's actually very important NOT to suppress these functions. Here are Janet Goodrich's views on the benefits of yawning from her book *Natural Vision Improvement*:

> Yawning brings fresh oxygen into body cells including the eyes and brain. Yawning contracts then releases the muscles related to the eyes. A really good yawn will contract and expand muscles from the top of your head to the tips of your toes – including the shoulder or trapezius muscles, the eyes (orbicularis oculi), the neck (neck flexors), the belly (the abdominals and solar plexus area). Yawning is capable of changing emotional states from negative to positive…Yawning stimulates the production of refreshing tears that bathe naturally tired eyes and moisten chronically dry eyes. Yawning helps to cleanse the liver and to balance the energy in the liver meridian.

So whenever you have to yawn, go ahead. And make it a BIG yawn, opening your mouth wide and even making that annoying noise while you exhale. The same with sighing. DO it big and noisy. It's all part of healthy breathing, and your body does those things because it needs something you just ain't providing otherwise.

Recommended Reading

The Science of Breath by Yogi Ramacharaka (recently republished by Supreme Design Publishing's sister company Two Horizons Press)

Make it a habit to breathe deeply and you'll soon be able to see deeper into everything.

SLEEP – THE COUSIN OF DEATH?

BY SUPREME UNDERSTANDING

"I never sleep, cause sleep is the cousin of death" – Nas, "It Ain't Hard to Tell"

About 700 BC, Greek poets Homer and Hesiod both referred to sleep as the brother of Death, as did Virgil hundreds of years later. The Hebrew Talmud says sleep is 1/60th of death, and Shakespeare made the same connection much later. But Nas didn't need any of them for his insight. "Sleep is the cousin of death" is actually a traditional African proverb from the Congo. You knew all that wisdom started somewhere. But is it "true" wisdom? Is it really bad to get plenty of

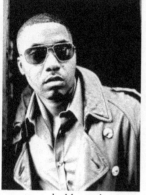

sleep? Sure, Nas was talking about remaining vigilant, not necessarily how many hours of rest he got, but let's look at things literally for a minute.

We all should know it's ridiculous to sleep 12-13 hours a day, but in case not, I'll let Ghostface Killah tell it. This is what he had to say in his audiobook, *The World According to Pretty Tony*:

Y'all motherf*ckers sleepin too much man, especially sleepin all night, sleepin all day... like y'all ain't got nuttin to do! Y'nahmean, yo, sh*t is too valuable out here, man, time is money man! Y'all niggas spend a lot of y'all time in bed, man! Sleepin, man, not doin nuttin, man!...Nahmean, it's time to get up with some new ideas, man! Y'nahmean, y'all niggas don't even know how to invent sh*t, man! Think of an invention! Make a new toilet bowl or somethin, man! You know what I'm sayin? Do somethin, man! Y'all motherf*ckers, man, y'all niggas kill me, man, it's time to get up, man! Snap out that bullsh*t! Walkin' around here dead, man, word up! One!

The average "successful" person in my community only gets 6 to 7 hours of rest/sleep a night. This ranges from people who run their own businesses to dopeboys who are making enough money to get out the game. I average about 6 hours. I'm not impressed, because I heard Minister Farrakhan only gets 5, and he's old enough to be my grandfather. The people I know who get a lot more...let's just say they're not developing any new inventions, to say the least.

Now, if you're in the first group, you might be concerned that you're not sleeping long enough, not realizing that 6 to 7 hours is currently the population average. **Many of us believe that 8 hours of sleep is required for health, but there is little medical basis to recommend sleeping 8 hours or more.** For example, a classic study found that long sleepers (8 hours or more) reported less energy and had more psychopathology than short sleepers.

"Early to bed, early to rise, makes a man healthy, wealthy and wise." – Benjamin Franklin

But we know that sleeping too little can cause stress and poor mental performance. In fact, **studies have shown that people who sleep for less than 6 hours each night are 12% more likely to die prematurely** – before the age of 65 – than those who get the recommended 6 to 8 hours a night.

But is sleep literally the "cousin of death"? I'll let you decide for yourself. The following is a list of 6 "problems" associated with sleeping 9 or more hours each night.

1. Higher risk of death. Although it's a common belief that 8 hours of sleep is required for optimal health, a six-year study of more than one million adults ages 30 to 102 has shown that people who get only 6 to 7 hours a night have a lower death rate. Individuals who sleep 8 hours or more, or less than 4 hours a night, were shown to have a significantly increased death rate.

2. Long Sleep and Depression. Depression is linked to both long and short sleep. Most depressed people are at risk of insomnia and sleeping too little, but about 15% sleep too much. This is probably due to lethargy and lack of excitement for life.

3. Seasonal Effectiveness Disorder. Light and temperature are big factors in controlling our internal body clocks. Winter days are shorter, causing our bodies to "hibernate." From a physical standpoint, there is no need for the extra sleep during winter. In fact, sleeping more during the winter months further aggravates the symptoms of S.A.D. (See "Why are you so S.A.D.?")

> **Did You Know?**
> The start of daylight savings time can be bad for your health. That one hour loss of sleep is serious! The number of serious heart attacks jumps 6% to 10% on the first three workdays after the start of daylight saving time. Men are more likely to commit suicide during the first few weeks of daylight saving time than they are during the rest of the year. And the number of traffic accidents spikes on the Monday after the clocks move forward.

4. Less Energy. That's right. **Studies have shown that long sleep is associated with decreased energy.** Have you ever noticed that a 10 hour sleep can leave you feeling MORE tired than a 7 hour sleep? Truly restorative sleep comes from sleep QUALITY not quantity. Your body tries to compensate poor quality sleep by sleeping longer. Good sleep quality comes from good sleep habits and lifestyle habits. Excellent sleep quality will leave you feeling refreshed/energetic after only 6 or 7 hours of sleep.

5. Lack of Exercise. Daily exercise increases your core body temperature, allowing for a larger drop in body temperature at night, which improves sleep quality. Sedentary activity can cause a slight increase in sleep duration.

6. Poor Diet. Eating habits and sleep habits go hand in hand. A poor diet is usually full of fatty, artificial foods, which sap your energy and make you feel tired. Poor diet means poor energy. Poor energy means more sleep. If eaten before bedtime, these foods will greatly decrease the quality of sleep.

Unfortunately, none of these associations really answer the question "Is too much sleep harmful?" Although long sleep is associated with a higher risk of death, is it the sleep ITSELF that's harmful? Or do certain health issues cause long sleep? Though most scientists agree that there's nothing harmful about sleep ITSELF, those who sleep more than nine hours have something wrong with them that causes the heavy sleep, and will eventually lead to early death. So **sleep itself is not harmful, according to sleep researchers, but the problem may be found in what's making you sleep so much.**

Attaining Deep Relaxation

It is also important to understand the bedroom is a place where you can rest and relax. Research has led me to believe that the most beneficial position for deep relaxation is lying on your back with your arms by your sides, palms facing up, legs straight out, and toes pointing to the sides. Your breathing is deep but relaxed and the **mind is relaxed** as well as the physical body. **Studies have shown that for most people, only three months of 20 minutes per day spent in deep relaxation causes blood pressure to normalize, overall energy to increase, moods to improve, sleep to improve and both hands and feet to become warmer.** This result suggests that relaxation improves circulation. Deep relaxation can be done in bed for ten minutes upon waking in the morning and for ten minutes before going to sleep. If something happens to stress you out at any time during the day, relaxing deeply can really help.

Learn How to Create Restful, Sound Sleep

Wear a mask/sleep in complete darkness or as close as possible. (See "The Pineal Gland") No TV right before bed, even better, get the TV out the bedroom. It is too stimulating to the brain, taking you longer to fall asleep. Eat a high-protein snack several hours before bed. This can provide the L-tryptophan, needed to produce melatonin and serotonin. Also eat a small piece of fruit. This can help the tryptophan cross the blood-brain barrier.

Avoid caffeine. A recent study showed that in some people, caffeine is not metabolized efficiently and therefore they can feel the effects long after consuming it.

Avoid alcohol. Although alcohol will make people drowsy, the effect is short lived and people will often wake up several hours later, unable to fall back asleep. Alcohol will also keep you from falling into the deeper stages of sleep, where the body does most of its healing.

Lose weight. Being overweight can increase the risk of sleep apnea, which will prevent a restful night's sleep. Don't drink any fluids within 2 hours of going to bed. This will reduce the likelihood of needing to get up and go to the bathroom or at least minimize the frequency. Make sure to exercise daily.

Take a hot bath/shower or sauna before bed. When body temperature is raised in the late evening, it will fall at bedtime, facilitating sleep.

Keep your bed for sleeping. If you're used to watching TV or doing work in bed, you may find it harder to relax and to think of it as a place to sleep.

Have your adrenals checked by a good natural medicine clinician. Scientists have found that insomnia may be caused by adrenal stress. If you are menopausal or perimenopausal, get checked out by a good natural medicine physician.

Put work away at least one hour (but preferably two or more) before bed. This will give your mind a chance to unwind so you can go to sleep feeling calm, not hyped up or anxious about tomorrow's deadlines.

Sleep Disorders

Improper rest as a result of sleep disorders[32] can cause much stress in your life (which feeds upon itself to make it harder to sleep). Lack of sleep will have you to become irritable, aggravated, and confused; the nervous system and the whole body are eventually affected. Over time, it contributes to many health problems such as diabetes, hypertension, and weight problems and can reduce your life span. It has also been estimated that improper sleep has been a factor in 60% of driving accidents, because fatigued drivers were not as alert and their reactions were slowed down.

Insomnia (sleeplessness). Insomnia is defined as having difficulty falling asleep and/or staying asleep that leads to a negative impact on the next day. It is a medical condition that touches the lives of approximately 20 million adults in the U.S. Symptoms of insomnia include difficulty falling asleep, waking up frequently during the night, difficulty returning to sleep, waking up too early in the morning, daytime sleepiness, difficulty concentrating and irritability. Sleeplessness can cause memory problems and mood problems.

---

[32] There are 33 major sleep disorders (classified under three groups)—the most common include: Intrinsic (hypersomnia, narcolepsy, sleep apnea); Extrinsic (alcohol-dependent sleep disorder, food allergy insomnia, inadequate sleep routine); and Circadian rhythm (advanced sleep phase syndrome, delayed sleep phase syndrome, jetlag, shift work sleep disorder).

Worker fatigue has been linked to major international disasters such as the Chernobyl nuclear meltdown, the Challenger explosion, and the Exxon Valdez Alaskan oil spill. **Insomnia should not be allowed to continue; medical advice should be obtained.**

Sleep apnea is a serious disorder that causes people to stop breathing while they sleep. Each time this temporary pause in breathing occurs, the body responds by waking up for a very short period of time. People who suffer from sleep apnea may stop breathing hundreds of times every night. According to statistics, more than 1 in 2 people with Type II Diabetes have sleep apnea. Eight out of every 10 people who have sleep apnea have not been diagnosed for it. Get treated.

Sleepwalking (somambulism) occurs when only part of the brain is asleep, needs special care. Children who walk in their sleep are probably highly sensitive, and of excitable temperament. Never make fun of a child who walks in their sleep. If possible, lead them gently back to bed without waking them; if they must be wakened, the process should be quiet and gradual.

Bedwetting, without a doubt, is a symptom of a very deep, inherited sleep disorder. It is oxygen deprived sleep, and it is definitely not healthy. Bed wetter's spend most of their night in the very deepest stage of sleep, known as stage 4. The body receives less oxygen during stage 4 than it does during any other stages of sleep. Therefore, if the body is receiving less oxygen all night, that includes the brain. When the brain experiences lower levels of oxygen at night, symptoms like lack of focus, reading comprehension, being easily distracted, class clown syndrome, fatigue, irritability and daydreaming may ensue. The symptoms can mirror those of ADD/ADHD. You've got to ask yourself how you would function after a poor night's sleep. **Once we change the sleep disorder the bedwetting goes away, and most often so will the ADD/ADHD symptoms,** or at the very least, they will improve.

Frequent Urination (Nocturia or Adult Nocturnal Enuresis). Nocturia is defined as being awakened at night one or more times in order to pass urine, referred to as (sleepless nights). This can occur at any age, although it's less frequent in the age range below 60 years, and becomes more common as the person becomes older. Some causes are gender specific. For example, nocturia in men is often linked to an enlarged prostate that blocks the flow of urine from the bladder. The onset of nocturia in women is generally linked to the consequences from childbirth, menopause, and even pelvic organ prolapse. Sometimes nocturia is a symptom of a greater medical problem that alters the way in which the body functions during sleep. Targets include diabetes, high blood pressure, heart disease/congestive heart failure, vascular disease, varicose veins or swelling due to fluid accumulation in lower extremities.

Sleep Paralysis, also known as night terrors, or nightmares (the dark side of dreams), are caused by dreams of fear, pain and irrational bad feelings which occur mostly because some problem disturbs you unconsciously but seriously. These nightmares can become a serious problem when you wake up terrified–so you don't sleep out of fear. Sometimes nightmares can indicate really serious problems like depression. While the body is resting, the muscles that move the body are "turned off" during REM sleep, which prevents you from acting out dreamed actions in reality, resulting in a Non-REM sleep paralysis after waking. This is caused by a failure to re-activate the muscles immediately (lasting a few seconds, but sometimes it can go for a minute), which causes the "scary feeling" when you know you're awake but you can't move. The hallucinatory element to sleep paralysis makes it even more likely that someone will interpret the experience as a dream, since completely dream-like objects may appear in the room alongside one's normal vision.

It's estimated that sleep paralysis (which is often coupled with panic disorder (PD) and post-traumatic stress disorder (PTSD)), has been experienced at least once by 51.6% of Afrikan Americans. **Western scientists have proposed this condition as an explanation for stories of alien abductions, ghostly encounters, witch hexes, and/or demon-possession during sleep.** There may be some historical fact to this theory. Until very recently, Afrikan American elders would often say that nightmares and the incapacity to move were caused by "the devil riding your back." It is believed that the origin behind these superstitions can be found in the period of the Afrikan American experience when we were simultaneously "put to sleep" during the "waking nightmare" of chattel slavery. As a result, sleep paralysis (called a "culture-bound syndrome" common among Afrikan Americans) is a lasting vestige of the trauma, anxiety, and life stress experienced disproportionately by Afrikan Americans.

If you're sleeping too long, your job is to know why. It can be an underlying health condition. Try to get 6-7 hours.

HOW TO STAY AWAKE NATURALLY
BY RODNEY JONES

With more and more of us getting less and less sleep, it's tempting to reach for a Red Bull or an espresso when we feel sleepy at work. But consuming caffeine to combat sleepiness can lead to a vicious cycle. **Caffeine can reduce your sleep time, alter the normal stages of sleep, and decrease the quality of your sleep.** I think we can safely call caffeine legalized cocaine (notice the similarity in spelling? Things that make you go hmmmm). Caffeine is a helluva drug. (See "Addicted to Caffeine" in Volume 2)

"The higher your energy level, the more efficient your body. The more efficient your body, the better you feel and the more you will use your talent to produce outstanding results." – Success coach Anthony Robbins

How can you stay awake naturally? Try some of these 12 jitter-free tips to take the edge off sleepiness.

1. Get Up and Move Around to Feel Awake. In one well-known study, Robert Thayer, PhD, a professor at California State University, Long Beach, studied whether people were more energized by eating a candy bar or taking a brisk 10-minute walk. Though the candy bar provided a quick energy boost, participants were actually more tired and had less energy an hour later. The 10-minute walk increased energy for two hours. That's because walking pumps oxygen through your veins, brain, and muscles.

2. Take a Nap to Take the Edge Off Sleepiness. There are two things to remember about naps: Don't take more than one and don't take it too close to your bedtime. "Nap between five and 25 minutes," says Barry Krakow, MD, author of "Sound Sleep, Sound Mind: Seven Keys to Sleeping Through the Night." It's best to nap about six or seven hours before you would go to bed. If you must take a late nap close to bedtime, make it a short one.

Napping on the job can be touchy. If you need to nap at work, do it during your break and use a vibrating alarm clock, if necessary, to make sure it doesn't spill over into your work time. Sleeping at your desk is usually not a good idea, but many companies now provide nap rooms for employees. If you can't sleep try resting your eyes for 10 minutes. That helps too.

3. Give Your Eyes a Break to Avoid Fatigue. Continuous fixation on a computer screen can cause eyestrain and worsen sleepiness and fatigue. Look away from the screen for a few minutes periodically to relax your eyes

4. Eat a Healthy Snack to Boost Energy. Healthy snacks such as fruit will provide better overall energy in the long run. Changing your diet overall can also change how easily you get fatigued and exhausted. Mike Tyson, after switching to a vegan diet, boasted "I get these explosions of energy. I don't know how long they last, but they're like explosions. So powerful." Coming from Iron Mike, that means something.

5. Start a Conversation to Wake Up Your Mind. If you're fading fast, engaging in conversation can get your mind moving again. "Talk to a colleague about a business idea, politics, or religion," says Barry Krakow. "It's a very strong behavioral stimulator – especially when it's a conversation about politics." And if you fall asleep on somebody right in their face, they're probably boring. Find someone else. You may not like talking to liars, but they ARE fun to listen to.

6. Turn Up the Lights to Ease Fatigue. Dim lighting aggravates fatigue. Studies have shown that exposure to bright light can reduce sleepiness and increase alertness. Try increasing the intensity of your light source at work. But keep in mind that studies have also found that warm yellow lights and sunlight are much better for you than UV/fluorescent lights.

7. Take a Breather to Feel Alert. Deep breathing raises blood oxygen levels in the body. (See "The Science Of Breath") The idea of deep-breathing exercises is to inhale to the abdomen, not the chest. You can do them at your desk, sitting up straight, try this exercise up.

This technique, called stimulating breath, is used in yoga for a quick energy boost and increased alertness: Inhale and exhale rapidly through your nose, keeping your mouth closed but relaxed. Make your in-and-out breaths short – do about three of each cycle in a second. Then breathe normally. You can do this for up to 15 seconds the first time and then add on five seconds each time after until you reach a minute.

8. Switch Tasks to Stimulate Your Mind. In 2004 Finnish researchers who studied people working 12-hour night shifts found that monotonous work is as harmful as sleep loss for alertness. At work or home, try to reserve more stimulating tasks for your sleepy times. Or switch to more engaging work responsibilities when you feel yourself nodding off. Speaking of which, get off that computer and that Blackberry more! The radiation is bad enough, but staring at those screens can really fatigue you.

9. Drink Water to Prevent Tiredness. Dehydration can cause fatigue. Drink plenty of fluids and eat foods such as fruits high in water.

10. Get Some Daylight to Regulate Your Sleep Cycles. (See "The Pineal Gland")

11. Exercise to Increase Energy and Reduce Fatigue. In a 2006 analysis of 70 studies involving more than 6,800 people, University of Georgia researchers found that exercise was more effective in increasing energy and reducing daytime fatigue than some medications used to treat sleep problems. Regular exercise also improves quality of sleep.

When to See a Doctor About Your Sleepiness

If you find that you can't stop nodding off when you need to be alert, consult a doctor or sleep specialist. You may have an underlying sleep disorder such as excessive sleepiness or narcolepsy, which can be treated. Your doctor may prescribe medications to help you with a sleep disorder. If you have trouble falling asleep because of stress or other reasons, cognitive behavioral therapy can help you develop good sleep habits and relieve sleep anxieties.

Feeling energized does not need to come with side effects. Follow these easy (and mostly free) suggestions to remain awake naturally.

BAD POSTURE DOES MORE THAN MAKE YOU LOOK LAME

BY SUPREME UNDERSTANDING

"They see a woman standing up on her own two/
Sloppy slouching is something I won't do" – Queen Latifah, "Ladies First"

Posture refers to the body's alignment and positioning with respect to gravity. Whether we are standing, sitting or lying, gravity exerts a force on our joints, ligaments and muscles. When standing, proper posture involves having your body in alignment so that the pull of gravity is evenly distributed and no one structure is overstressed. This includes:

❏ A straight line from your ears, shoulders, hips, knees and ankles

❏ Head is centered

❏ Shoulders, hips and knees are level

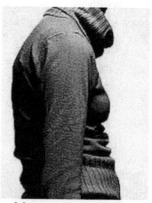

When you have poor posture, the body's proper vertical position is out of alignment and the back's natural curves become distorted. **Poor posture forces your muscles to work hard just to hold you up. You waste energy just moving, leaving you without the extra energy you need to feel good.** This can also cause wear and tear to your muscles and bones. Your problems can range from fatigue, tightness and joint stiffness to degenerative osteoarthritis and major spine-related problems when you're older. **Plus your abdominal organs sag, crowding and making more**

work for your heart and lungs. And because your abdominal organs are shifted out of place, it makes your gut look bigger than it actually is.

"A good stance and posture reflect a proper state of mind." – Morihei Ueshiba, founder of Aikido

Sometimes, screwed-up posture develops because of an accident or fall. But more often, it develops from environmental factors or bad habits. In urban communities, we often develop poor posture on purpose. **The way we stand, sit, even lay down at night, gradually affects our normal posture.** You weren't born crooked, but you've probably made yourself that way.

Common Posture Problems

Forward head posture: known as anterior head carriage, here your

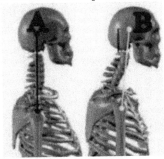

neck cranes forward and ears don't line up with your shoulders. This condition is worsened by bending our heads constantly to use computers and cellphones.

Rounded shoulders: Common among stick-up kids, goons, and others putting on menacing demeanors. As NORE once rapped "You monkey-walk, I'm hunchback, creep quiet." But also common among people with low-self-esteem, as it's basically the opposite of having your chest out. As a result, it's also common among women who – as young girls – changed their posture to minimize how noticeable their breasts were.

Arched lower back: Your back should have a natural "S" arch, but there's a limit. This condition is common among women who arch their backs unnaturally to "fake" a booty.

Excessive anterior pelvic tilt: Also known as 'protruding backside,' which is also common among women. As Guru once rapped, "Your girl don't really got no ass, she just pokes it out."

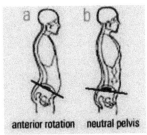

anterior rotation   neutral pelvis

Excessive posterior pelvic tilt: Or protruding pelvis, common among brothers trying too hard NOT to stick out their ass, and instead pushing their hips forward, showing off their fancy belt buckles. Also common because of the posture required to walk with sagging pants, also known as the 'duck walk.' Because of the variety of ways we stand to "look cool" our hipbone (pelvis) can actually tilt to the left or right as well, and get stuck that way.

Test Your Posture

To figure out if you have good posture, take the following posture tests.

The Wall Test – Stand with the back of your head touching the wall and your heels six inches from the baseboard. With your butt touching the wall, stick your hand between your lower back and the wall, and then between your neck and the wall. If you can get within an inch or two at the low back and two inches at the neck, you are close to having excellent posture.

The Mirror Test – Stand facing a full length mirror and check yourself out.

The Unbiased Review – Have someone else check you out from the side and look for the following:

> **Did You Know?**
> In a recent study reported by NPR, researchers used an MRI to study three sitting positions. Their findings: The best one is "leaning way back like you would on a La-Z-boy at a 135 degree angle." Yup, that's right. Hunching over was worse for your back, but the worst position for your back was sitting upright at a 90-degree angle. This position puts pressure on your lower back and has long-term consequences.

☐ Your head is straight rather than slumped forwards or backwards

☐ Chin is parallel to the floor

☐ Shoulders are in line with ears and leveled.

☐ Knees, ankles, and feet are facing forward.

☐ Slight forward curve to your lower back, hips leveled.

> *"We leaning with a slouch, on a European made couch/*
> *I'm a walking night club, cause there's a disco ball in my mouth"*
> *– Paul Wall, "North to tha South"*

Slouching is Better?

With all this talk about posture, it's only natural that we talk about "sitting up straight." Young people of color seem to have a real hard time with this. Whether driving, on our couch, or at a desk, we lay back in our seats, in a position our elders call "slouching" (even though "slouching" really means you're drooping forward). I've heard people speculate that Black people "slouch" like this because this is how Blacks were seated in the slave ships, with no headroom to sit upright. Well, that turns out to be an urban legend. In fact, if you've ever looked at those wooden seats from West Africa, they're built so that you lean back. And I can show you historical pictures of brothers and sisters throughout Africa, leaning back looking gangsta.

> *"I stand tall, like buildings on Van Dyke" – RZA, "Tragedy"*

Here are eight more reasons to have a 'correct' healthy posture:

1. It portrays a better, more confident image. The first thing you notice about people ain't their eyes, their hair, or even their clothes. It's the way they stand. And it screams messages about who they are. Someone who stands tall gives off an aura of pride and self-confidence, while someone who slumps and stoops looks like he's ashamed to be taking up space. Which one of them "looks like money" to you?

2. Breathing becomes easier and deeper. Try this: Sit down and bend over and try to breathe in. Notice how it is harder to breathe. This is an extreme example of how our muscles and tendons get over restricted and make our breathing more shallow and strenuous.

3. It improves circulation and digestion. Good posture increases lung capacity, aiding oxygen transport and nutrition around the body. Upright open posture also allows more room in the abdominal cavity; this improves your health by allowing your organs to function more easily.

4. It makes you look slimmer and younger. Good posture will instantly take off 3-5 lbs. in your appearance. It will make you look slimmer, younger and your clothes will look better.

5. Your voice will sound better. If you maintain good posture when you speak, and are careful not to let your chest "collapse" as you exhale, your diaphragm will open, making your voice sound better.

6. It helps your muscles, joints and spine. Good posture helps us keep bones and joints in correct alignment so that our muscles are used correctly, decreasing the abnormal wearing of joint surfaces that could result in degenerative arthritis and joint pain, letting muscles work more efficiently, allowing the body to use less energy and, therefore, preventing muscle fatigue, muscle strain, overuse disorders, and even back and muscular pain. **Back support is especially important for people who spend many hours sitting in an office chair or standing throughout the day.** Over time, the stress of poor posture can change the anatomical characteristics of the spine, leading to the possibility of constricted blood vessels and nerves.

7. It can change your frame of mind. When you are well, feeling happy and on top of things, posture tends to be upright and open. In contrast, people who are depressed and in chronic pain, often sit or stand slumped. Good posture in sitting and standing makes it easier to breathe fully and naturally, helping both relaxation and concentration, many Eastern practices such as yoga and tai-chi work on posture.

Recommendations

When you make a decision to work on your posture don't expect it to happen overnight but rest assured it will improve and you will see and feel the difference. You should probably do a 21-day slouching fast. I did it, and I literally stand 2 inches taller now. And because it only takes 21 days to form a habit, I stand straight without having to think about it now.

Sitting

- ☐ Align your back with the back of the chair. Avoid slouching or leaning forward, and Keep your shoulders straight.
- ☐ If you work a desk job, your arms should be at a 75- to 90-degree angle at the elbows. You may have to adjust the chair.
- ☐ Make sure your neck, back, and heels are all aligned.
- ☐ Keep both feet flat on the floor. If there's a problem reaching the floor comfortably, get a box to rest your feet on.
- ☐ Get up every once in a while. Sitting all day is bad for you.

Walking

- ☐ Keep the head up and eyes looking straight ahead. Avoid pushing your head forward.
- ☐ Keep shoulders properly aligned with the rest of the body.

Driving

- ☐ Sit with the back firmly against the seat for proper back support. The seat should be a proper distance from the pedals and steering wheel to avoid leaning forward or reaching.
- ☐ The headrest should support the middle of the head to keep it upright. Tilt the headrest forward if possible to make sure that the head-to-headrest distance is not more than four inches.

Carrying Objects

- ☐ Always bend at the knees, not the waist. Use the large leg and stomach muscles for lifting, not the lower back. If necessary, get a supportive belt to help maintain good posture while lifting.
- ☐ Keep large or heavy objects close to the chest when carrying them. Switch arms frequently if you are carrying something with only one arm.
- ☐ Keep backpacks and purses as light as possible, and balance the weight on both sides as much as possible, or alternate from side to side. When carrying a backpack, avoid leaning forward or rounding the shoulders. If the weight feels like too much, consider using a rolling backpack with wheels.

Sleeping

- ☐ Use a firm mattress for proper back support, but remember that individual preference is very important.
- ☐ Sleeping on the side will damage your posture after enough repetitions but keeping a relatively flat pillow placed between the legs will help keep the spine aligned and straight. Sleeping on your

back will help straighten your shoulders, and it is usually more comfortable for the back than sleeping on the stomach.

☐ Use a pillow to provide proper support and alignment for the head and shoulders. Consider putting a rolled-up towel under the neck and a pillow under the knees to better support the spine.

☐ If sleeping on the side,

Print this article and put it somewhere you can see it daily. It will remind you to check your posture.

Notes:

THAT'S JUST NASTY

BASIC HYGIENE AND SELF-MAINTENANCE

SH*TTIN OUT THE WINDOW
BY SUPREME UNDERSTANDING

Historically, Original people have always been very big on being clean. We were the ones who invented soap, bath houses, and even shampoo – all before anyone ever thought to say "cleanliness is next to godliness."[33] We've included hygiene in all of our religious and cultural traditions. Meanwhile, Europeans were historically pretty gross. From living in caves sealed with feces to bathing only once or twice a year (yes, a year!), when we came to Europe as the Moors, we had to teach them how to bathe! If you saw Robin Hood when it first came out, you'll notice that the Moorish brother is the one who has to teach Robin Hood and them to wash up. We also had to teach them about sanitation. We came from civilizations that had sewers and flushing toilets as early as 3500 BC.[34] But as late as the 1800s, Europeans used "chamber pots," which they poured out the window when they were done! Now imagine what's in the streets! But a lot of that was cleaned up by the huge rats and pigs they had running through the streets of Europe at the time. You can imagine the health complications. When Europeans came to North America, they brought a gang of diseases (most of which came from animals), as well as their standards of hygiene. Feenie Ziner, who wrote a biography of Tisquantum (better known as Squanto), recorded that Squanto, "...tried without success to teach them [the Pilgrims] to bathe." The Native people of Mexico would hold flowers to their noses when talking with the Spanish Conquistadors in an attempt to mask the odor they could smell through the ARMOR of the Spanish.

---

[33] That phrase actually doesn't appear in the Bible, as many believe. It was said by British preacher John Wesley, founder of the Methodist Church, in 1791. Wesley studied the Native Americans in Georgia, became a vegetarian, worked against the enslavement of Africans, and came to believe in the doctrine of Theosis (man becoming God).

[34] The most popular examples are those built by the Black people of ancient India, but there's also plenty of evidence from ancient Africa (visit www.BlackHistoryStudies.com for an article on this) as well as the Mayans (www.msnbc.msn.com/id/34575056) and other Original people

In fact, Queen Isabella of Spain – who once boasted that she had bathed only twice in her life, the first time when she was born and the second time the day of her marriage – upon hearing Columbus' reports on the frequency of bathing among the Native People issued an edict that stated in part, "They are not to bathe as frequently as hitherto." Everywhere you look among people of color, we have washed regularly, put "fruits and berries" in our hair and skin (remember "Coming to America"?), and kept up the highest standards of hygiene. And even when our homes were built from clay and straw, they were impeccably clean. Don't let those ancient ruins fool you. You gotta see a mock-up of how they looked BEFORE they became ruins. Or visit a tribal village today. Those little huts get SWEPT daily. In fact, we invented the broom too! But what on earth happened to us?

Think about the things we see in our communities nowadays:

- ❐ People with stinking, hot garbage breath, who love talking 'face to face'
- ❐ Wild, unkempt hair, sometimes containing lint, lice, and 4 month old weave.
- ❐ Yellow, buttery teeth and long dirty fingernails...on girls!
- ❐ Dude sagging their pants with doodoo stains on their draws
- ❐ People whose homes smell like urine even when nobody's peeing
- ❐ So many roaches you don't want to sit down on the couch
- ❐ So much more ratchetness and nastiness I don't want to describe it while I'm eating

What happened to us? Simple. We fell victim. Poverty and oppression changed our cultures drastically. Many of us are in plain survival mode, while others are just not tryin because we've lowered our standards for ourselves and each other. But **there's a reason why both the US Army and the Nation of Islam demand that their members be clean cut and spotless at all times. Think about the respect either of those groups commands.** Think about the respect you DON'T get when you look sloppy. And think about all the infections you're exposing yourself to when you don't keep your space (or yourself) spic and span. Forget yourself. Think about your children. Isn't it nice when they can lie on the floor because you know it's clean?

Whether it's keeping yourself from stinking or keeping your home in order, there are several BASIC things every one of us should be doing. And once you start doing them regularly, they're not difficult at all. Let's start with the basics.

> **Make your physical appearance a part of a healthy lifestyle. Freshen up what needs work. You'll look or at least smell much better.**

HOW TO NOT HAVE A ROTTEN FACE

FROM GHOSTFACE KILLAH'S AUDIOBOOK, THE WORLD ACCORDING TO PRETTY TONY

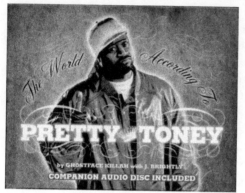

Crusty Eyes

Yeah, y'all niggas walkin around here with mad crust in ya eyes and sh*t, nigga. Make sure you clean that sh*t, man! Nobody wanna see ya little rotten-ass face, y'nahmean, with that white sh*t all in the corner of your eye, man! Get that up out of there, man, that's not nice, man, that's not a good look for you. You feel me? Get that sh*t up out of there. You too old for that sh*t, man! Y'all niggas actin like y'all five years old, man!

White Corners on Your Mouth

Yo, y'all niggas is foul, man. How you gonna let your man step outside, G, and have that little white sh*t in his mouth and sh*t, and he out here kickin it with y'all niggas like he just ate mad f*ckin corn flakes or somethin, man? Dried out milk around the side of his mouth like he stuck his tongue in a bottle of powder or somethin, man.

Food in Your Teeth

Y'all niggas gonna sit there, and see a nigga with food on his teeth or somethin, and not say nothin. Y'nahmean, you may have not seen this nigga in years...you gonna let him go ahead and go to church with that sh*t on his lips or on his teeth or...Y'nahmean, wherever the f*ck he goin and sh*t. You know what I'm sayin? Nigga goin to the fights with greens on his teeth...Let that nigga know, son! You know what I'm sayin? Stop frontin, man! That's not a nice thing to do, man, Y'nahmean?

Boogers in Your Nose

If it's me, son? And I got a f*cking booger in my nose or something like that, man, HOLLER AT THE BOY, man. Tell it, yo say, "Yo Tone, that's not looking real right right there, my nigga! Get that green kickball out your f*cking nose or somethin, nigga!" Y'nahmean? I'm gonna be, "Ohhhh, sh*t, word? Oh, alright, true, true...you got it, my dude!" Y'nahmean, that's what it is, "Good lookin, good lookin! Word up, there, I was about to just step to that bitch right there, son..." Y'nahmean? Word up, man, set me free, man! On some Martin Luther King sh*t, man! Stop playing, man, word up! I know what to do, man, it's Tone, man!

Take care of that rotten face and you won't get clowned on.

HOW TO KEEP YOUR JIBBS

BY C'BS ALIFE ALLAH

When your gums are breaking down that is because you have a whole bunch of bad bacteria growing like some fungus in your basement under a moldy rug. When that happens, your teeth don't have good soil to grow in and start their decay process. Now, this is how you can stop it.

First off – like yellow eyes, weak finger nails, and brittle hair – rugged gums and rotten teeth are symptomatic of your overall body's health. It basically means your body isn't fighting off what it needs to, thus bacteria is able to get a foothold. So one of the basic things that can assist with your mouth's health is making sure you reduce stress in your life, get some sleep, check what you're eating, and have some general exercise up in there.

Saliva and blood flow to the gums are the caretakers of your mouth. **Saliva keeps the area clean from bacteria and blood flow gets the nutrients to the gums and teeth.** Together they work to keep that grill healthy.

Take the 'temperature' of your mouth otherwise known as your pH. You can get litmus paper at a pharmacy. Before you eat spit on it and you can get a reading of your saliva's acidity level. If it's too acidic add more fruits and vegetables to your diet while cutting back on the grains and meats.

Chewing food breaks down your food, easing digestion and helping remove pieces of food from the mouth. It also makes sure that circulation is top notch throughout your gums.

Finally, get an irrigation device from your pharmacy. This is basically a device that pushes water under your gums like a hose reaching places where your brush and floss can't. Adding an antimicrobial rinse will disinfect whatever's beneath your gums.

All of the above is about taking *preventative* care, but if your teeth are already messed up, you'll have to get them taken care of by professionals, and *then* you can add on with proper care from that point on.

If bad bacteria can break down teeth imagine what they can do to the soft tissue in your body. Make sure everything is taken care of.

"Washing Up" is Not the Same as Bathing
BY SUPREME UNDERSTANDING

Bathing and Showering

It's amazing how we (Original people) had the first bath houses and impeccable standards of hygiene even in ancient times…and now some of us don't even know how to wipe our ass right. When I was in Japan, I learned the traditional way Japanese people bathe. **They don't just hop in the tub and wallow in their own filth like a pig.** They find the American style of bathing disgusting. **Instead, they take a cool shower where they scrub and rinse off, and THEN sit in a steaming hot tub.** That way, the entire family can share the same bath water, because the bath water is actually clean. Doesn't that make more sense than trying to clean yourself in a tub while you sit in whatever you cleaned off? **With some Epsom salt and some smell good in the room, a hot bath relieves aching muscles, improves your circulation, and helps you relax your mind.**

Got one more clip from Ghostface, his words of wisdom on showering:

> Y'all niggas that be f*ckin with that bird bath sh*t, thinkin y'all clean? Like you gonna go into the bathroom and just wash your nuts and wash your face, man? Y'nahmean? That's not cleaning yourself! Now I don't give a f*ck how much soap you put on your little bird-ass chest, nigga! Y'nahmean? It ain't workin, my nigga! Y'nahmean? Get your ass in a shower, son! Get between your toes, nigga! Wipe your ass, nigga! And you wipe your motherf*cking— when you get in the shower, nigga, for niggas who don't know how to take showers, wash your f*cking face first, man. THEN wash your nuts. Don't wash your nuts and then wash your face! You feel me? You goin backwards! Y'nahmean? Lotta y'all niggas don't even KNOW that sh*t! Y'nahmean?
>
> And scrub hard! Scrub your balls hard, nigga, scrub your little dirt off your ankles, nigga, that when you was a little kid you couldn't get 'em off and sh*t! Y'nahmean, sh*t kept stickin and— even though how hard you tried, nigga, get the— Y'nahmean? For y'all niggas that got that sh*t, man, y'all niggas ain't clean, man. Word up, man. And have a bitch get your back. Because your back is dirty, son. The back of your ass AND the back of your back! That's right, yeah, scrub that sh*t, nigga. Clean your ass with the best soap, nigga. The best soap from the heavens above, nigga. That's Dove.

As usual, Ghostface's advice on personal hygiene is on the money with what any hygienist would tell you…though perhaps not in the same language. But there's one point I disagree with. **Dove is definitely not the best soap out there.** Not only is it – like many other soaps – made with animal fat, but it's one of the few soaps on the market that might have pork in it.[35] But not only are there other soaps that don't have any cow fat in them, there are BETTER soaps out there. What do I recommend? There's so many choices, you can really pick what you like best, but here's some suggestions:

Dr. Bronner's Soap (any kind): This organic liquid soap is made without animal ingredients or harsh chemicals like Sodium Lauryl Sulfate. Because it's mild and safe, it also has a ton of other uses, including everyday body-washing, light cleaning, heavy-duty grease cutting jobs, shampoo, laundry, and even toothbrushing.

African Black Soap (any kind): Also known as "Dudu Osun" this soap, handmade from roasted plantain skins, is typically available in solid bars. For centuries, Ghanaians have used Black Soap to help relieve acne, oily skin, clear blemishes and various other skin issues. Africans have used this natural soap for bathing and washing their hair. In recent times, it's also been used for removing make-up. Black Soap will leave your skin soft, clear and smelling good. It contains no scents, preservatives OR chemicals. But there are now FAKE Black soaps on the market, mostly made in the USA. Fake Black soap is usually made from vegetable oil, with Black dye added. Real Black Soap is always brownish-black. The longer the plantain skins are roasted the darker the soap. But the soap is never completely black. Recently, people have been selling liquid forms of Black soap as well. Some of them are made from the same ingredients as real black soap, while others are not, so make sure you ask.

There's a ton of vegetable-based natural soaps that incorporate everything from peppermint oil to oatmeal (to relieve dry, itchy skin) available in most health food stores and even most large supermarkets. **And if you want to "buy Black" then Dudu Osun is your sure bet.** You can usually even buy it from the Black street vendors who sell oils and incense in the hood.

Make sure the way you bathe is not filthy itself. Buy soaps not made from animal fats, and put on a clean set of clothes after bathing!

---

[35] Some groups list Dove as questionable, but I suggest you contact the company directly if you want to research it further, since ingredients can change from year to year. Other animal ingredients to look out for in soap: Sodium Tallowate (from beef fat); Stearic Acid (from beef tallow); Lanolin Alcohol (from animal matter); and Oleic Acid (from beef or pork).

TEEFUS

BY C'BS ALIFE ALLAH

I rolled to the dentist once when I was young, and I was curious. You know how all of those commercials say something like 7 out of 10 dentist use such and such toothpaste. So of course I was curious as to what toothpaste he used. He said he uses…salt and baking soda. What? My father and mother. – they advocated the same thing. It made sense when I went to an Environmental Racism conference and one of the presenters said something to the degree of not using anything that your grandparents or great grandparents didn't use.

Maaaaan funk your commercial toothpaste. I remember when I first brought this idea up to people, they were talking about tooth decay from not brushing with the 'FDA' approved 'fluoride' toothpaste. Despite what they would have you to believe, ancient man didn't walk around toothless. **What prevents cavities** (did I mention that I only have one micro-cavity and I have only recently gone to the dentist. I haven't been in over 18 years) **is DENTAL care.** And there isn't any better dental care than Do-It-Yourself dental care.

For DIY toothpaste, get you some sea salt and baking soda. You miss the minty fresh smell/taste in your mouth? Grow mint in your house, It's one of the easier herbs to grow and chewing it will freshen up that breath right away.

Main thing, get that excess food out of your mouth. **After meals brush and floss.** Rinse with a nice DIY mouthwash or natural one. **The decaying bits of food in your mouth breaks down your teeth.**

Two, the MAIN SOURCE of tooth decay is eating all of those sugary, corn syrupy, refined sugar sweets and junk food. That's what is making all of those dentists rich. Plus drink more water. LOTS more water. I bet you if you do the above two things you will see an increased change in your dental health.

Also here's a list of things that jack your teeth up, from staining to weakening them:

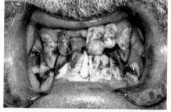

- ❏ smoking cigarettes (stains your teeth)
- ❏ cheese (sticks to the teeth and seeps into the gums)
- ❏ soda (weakens the teeth)
- ❏ gum (weakens the teeth because you're just chewing plastic)

Finally, do what a lot of people in indigenous cultures do. Chew on licorice root. Licorice strengthens the immune system, stimulates the adrenal gland, and is diuretic and laxative (in other words it keeps you regular). The roots contain glycyrrhizin, which is 50 times sweeter than sugar. You've seen the brothers chewing on those 'sticks' (hence the name "chewsticks") that have been dipped in various flavors such as peppermint. You shouldn't eat the part you're chewing, but you can definitely scrub your teeth with it and reduce plaque. Yup, you can use chewsticks to keep your teeth clean by chewing on the stem until it turns into a brush and begins to produce a bitter foam. Also, it increases saliva production in the mouth which reduces tooth decay. It has been used worldwide in this fashion. It was even found in the tomb of King Tut. Get with it.

DIY Toothpaste
Get sea salt, baking soda and peroxide. Dip your brush in a solution of ½ peroxide and ½ water. Next dip it in a mixture of ½ salt and ½ baking soda.

Eat whole foods and clean out any piece of food stuck between your teeth. Your breath will thank you as well.

WHEN GOLD GRILLS GO BAD
BY SUPREME UNDERSTANDING

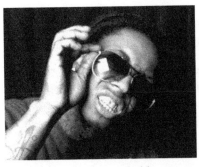

The "medical situation" that convinced a judge to postpone Lil Wayne's sentencing in 2010 was "a serious dental problem," according to Wayne's people. What could have been wrong with Lil Wayne's teeth? Plenty, if you consider the fact he's had a mouth full of gold teeth for over ten years now, probably put in by some hood dentist, and it's not a removable grill, which would have been recommended by any sensible dentist. Why? Because **if you can't get to your teeth, they're rotting under that gold shell.** And considering that he nearly lives on the road, his diet must be rough and proper dental hygiene's gotta be tough.

Following the news, Dr. Sherry Rudd speculated on the situation:

> He probably has a bad tooth, a tooth that's abscessed. With all of [gold and diamond material] in his mouth, it's going to be really difficult to get clean because of all of the different crevices. I don't know if they're bridges or if they are all individual. But if it's going to be two weeks [from surgery to recovery], then I don't think he's going to get them all off, because of the

potential damage. Without knowing what's exactly there, it's probably decayed and the decay got into the nerve, which causes the nerve to die.

According to TMZ, the postponement wasn't a DMX-style ruse to avoid prison. Weezy actually underwent marathon oral surgery, including a whopping eight root canals, several tooth implants and other repairs to his grill in one day. Wayne was reportedly in surgery for eight hours. Goddamn! While Original people (people of color) been modifying their teeth for over ten thousand years (literally – including gold and jewel-studded teeth in Ancient Egypt, China, Peru, etc.)…you definitely need to think twice before you put any metal in your mouth PERMANENTLY.

And we're not just talking about grills here. **Those fillings can be just as bad for you.** Except, instead of rotting your teeth, they might rot your brain!

Mercury in My Mouth?

Mercury is one of the most toxic substances known. Yet it's used in dental fillings, so you've probably got some in your mouth right now. For years, the dental industry has claimed that these "small amounts" of mercury are safe. But in 2008, the FDA finally issued a warning that the mercury used by dentists for fillings and other procedures may cause neurological harm (brain damage!) to children and pregnant women. Here are a few facts about the mercury in your mouth:

❏ Mercury from silver/amalgam fillings can permanently damage the brain, kidneys, and immune system of children.

❏ This mercury has been linked to Alzheimer's disease, gastrointestinal problems, sleep disturbances, concentration problems, memory disturbances, lack of initiative, restlessness, bleeding gums and other mouth disorders.

❏ The mercury release from fillings is absorbed primarily as highly toxic elemental mercury vapor. The type of mercury fillings that began to be used during the last couple of decades, non-gamma-2 (high copper), releases many times more mercury than the older style of amalgam fillings.

❏ Mercury absorption from fillings is 4 times higher than from fish consumption.

❏ Having gold teeth, platinum teeth, crowns, and even braces (anything containing other metals) can increase the release of mercury significantly.

❏ Chewing gum, grinding your teeth, and exposure to magnetic fields (including those from a computer monitor) can also increase the release of mercury significantly.

❏ The mercury builds up in your organs, and in your unborn child's organs. Mercury released from fillings builds up in your brain, pituitary, adrenals, and other parts of your body. Mercury from fillings in pregnant women also causes mercury accumulation in the brain, kidneys and liver of human fetuses (all of the areas tested). Studies have shown that mercury can be passed to infants from breast milk.

Obviously, not everybody gets outright and obviously sick from the mercury in their fillings. However, virtually everyone has mercury build up in their bodies from these fillings, and only time will tell how much damage this daily exposure is doing. If I were you, I'd have that stuff removed. You might find yourself "miraculously" feeling better afterwards. **A recent study found that proper removal of mercury amalgam fillings from 118 subjects showed an elimination or reduction of 80% of the classic mercury poisoning symptoms.** In many cases, it took 6 to 12 months after mercury amalgam removal for the symptoms to disappear. Keep in mind that Mercury amalgam fillings should be removed only by dentists with experience using the IOAMT mercury amalgam removal protocol. And while plastic isn't perfect, it appears that composite (plastic) fillings are a better (and definitely less toxic) replacement than metal (e.g., gold) fillings. Again, make sure you have a professional (preferably one who knows about the toxic mercury thing) put them in.[36]

> Did You Know?
> The Indus Valley Civilization has evidence of dentistry being practiced as far back as 7000 B.C. This early form of dentistry involved curing tooth related disorders with bow drills, probably operated by skilled bead craftsmen. These craftsmen apparently also added cosmetic touches, like gold caps and embedded jewels. Recent studies have shown that these ancient methods were reliable and effective. Similar examples of advanced dentistry in ancient times can be found in Egypt, Sumeria, and the Americas.

**If a metal filling can be removed, a mental one can as well.
Remove all sources of toxins from your life.**

WHEN SHARING IS BAD

15 THINGS YOU SHOULDN'T SHARE
BY SUPREME UNDERSTANDING

You learned a long time ago that part of being a good little boy or girl was whether you could share. And sharing really is fundamental as a social skill for children because sharing and collectivism are the foundation of "civilized" human society. So it's great if you can still 'play nice' and share as adults, but there are some things you simply should NOT be sharing, for your own sake. Here's the Top 14:

Toothbrushes. You can get everything from gum disease to blood-borne diseases, such as hepatitis B and C (and reportedly even HIV).

---

[36] For more information on non-toxic dentistry and a directory of Mercury-free dentists, visit www.talkinternational.com or www.holisticdentalnetwork.com

In fact, these things spread more easily via toothbrush than by tongue kissing. You can also pick up a respiratory illness, cold, or flu. Brush with your finger instead!

Deodorant. Not good. Forget the health risks – that's just plain nasty.

Contact Lenses. Why would you even do this? Apparently, people do it, but it's an easy way to get an eye infection...and those get nasty.

Bikini Bottoms. I didn't believe girls actually shared things like underwear and bathing suit bottoms, but apparently some do. And some people learn the hard way that this is how bacterial infections and even certain STDs can spread. Even if you're not trading undies, you can pick up bacteria or pubic lice just by trying on bikini bottoms at the store, because that little paper guard is for the clothing's protection, not yours. So always wear underwear. Clean ones. And make sure they're your own.

Clothes. Buying used clothes (whether they're "vintage" or from Goodwill) is a common way of getting scabies, which are eight-legged mites that burrow into your skin and cause intense itching and blisters. Same with getting secondhand clothes from yard sales, as well as sleeping on dirty, old sheets and pillows. Oh, and scabies are contagious.

Sex Partners. But I guess cross-contamination is exciting for some folks.

Drinks and Smokes. Passing the bottle, cup, or just about anything you put in your mouth (including cigarettes and – ahem – other things you smoke), is an easy way to share a respiratory infection, cold, flu, or even some nasty oral infection, including Herpes!

Hairbrushes. This is an easy way to spread lice, MRSA, ringworm fungus, and other infections. Same applies to sharing pillows with people.

Makeup. A two-year study found high levels of bacteria in the majority of skin, eye and lip makeup samples at drug and department stores. And your girlfriend's makeup kit ain't exactly fresh and clean either. All those germs and bacteria can spread quite easily from face to face. Sharing mascara, for example, is an easy way to pass on folliculitis or conjunctivitis, commonly known as pink eye. Sharing lipstick can spread oral herpes. You should also discard old makeup after about 6-8 months.

Shopping Carts. At least not without wiping them down with one of those disinfecting wipes. Fortunately, many supermarkets are beginning to provide those at the front door. I suggest you use em.

Microbiologist Chuck Gerba's cross-country survey found that up to **80 percent of carts in some cities have E. coli** on them, along with other bacteria and viruses that could lead to colds, flu and diarrhea. Another recent study showed that placing children in shopping carts put them at increased risk for Salmonella infections.

Public Touch Screens. Like those at the supermarket "self-check-out aisle" and ATM. Gerba's study also found that **25% of self-checkout touch-screens have E. coli** on them, as well as other more common bacteria and viruses. But several of the touch-screens also contained strains of methicillin-resistant Staphylococcus aureus (MRSA), a bacterium that is highly resistant to several antibiotics. MRSA can cause serious skin infections sometimes leading to death. ATM screens presented several risks as well, with indoor ATMs being worse offenders than those out in the sun. So take sanitizer.

Pens. Because most people put them in their mouths, personal pens tend to be coated with germs. As a result, you can pick up respiratory viruses, mouth infections, and more. Gerba's studies have shown that teenagers' pens carry the most bacteria. Carry your own pen!

Shaving Razors. If I've gotta explain the risks (think: blood) associated with this one, I don't know what to tell you. I guess I should also tell you not to share hypodermic needles with drug addicts.

Don't share anything that can get you sick. If its handled by everyone or used in unsanitary conditions, it's not for you.

USING PUBLIC BATHROOMS
BY QUEEN CIVILIZED ZAG

The Pros and Cons
Public bathrooms are convenient and accessible, offering changing tables, and Interesting graffiti. However, they can transmit streptococcus (a form of strep throat and meningitis), E.coli, hepatitis A, and staphylococcus (the virus behind food poisoning and a form of pneumonia). Not to mention the urine and fecal matter you CAN'T see on the doors, floors and handles.

A lot of people don't wipe down the changing tables when they change their children. So it's best to either put a changing pad, layer of paper towels, or blanket down AFTER you wipe it down yourself with an antibacterial wipe.

Recommendations
- ❐ Though the toilet seat is 'the cleanest part', because of strict cleaning, use the disposable seat covers and/or an extra layer of

tissues (for women...perfect that "balancing act" we all know and love)

☐ Always use a napkin or piece of tissue when touching any handles on the way in AND out of the stalls and the bathroom itself.

☐ Wash your hands before AND after you use the bathroom

☐ Close the toilet lid before you flush (even at home). Flushing can propel small drops of fecal matter over 20 feet beyond the toilet, landing on potentially every exposed surface. Researchers have found feces on faucets, sinks, counters, combs, brushes, and yes, toothbrushes. one gram of feces contains up to a million bacteria, ten million viruses, 100 worm eggs, and 1,000 parasitic cysts. (The average healthy adult expels about 450 grams – about a pound – of feces a day.)

☐ Public restrooms usually have some kind of ventilation system, but you may not be getting ANY air in your bathroom at home. Either get a ventilation system or open a window, because some intestinal virus can remain in the air after you defecate and flush, and cause infection in inhaled or swallowed.

☐ The filthiest areas are actually the floor, the flush handle and the doorknob, so use a tissue and keep your stuff off the floor. Also, if the toilet paper roll doesn't have a cover on it, don't use the first few sheets of toilet paper because they're probably contaminated from the last flush.

Avoid touching as much surface area as possible. Use paper towels to touch things if possible.

WASH YOUR HANDS!

Did you know a dog's tongue is cleaner than your hands? Hell, for most of us, a dog's butt is cleaner than our hands. Why? We don't wash, and when we do wash, we don't wash em right. As a result, we overexpose ourselves to germs that eventually get the best of us, giving us everything from strep throat to eye sties to food poisoning.

Follow these simple steps to properly wash your hands.

☐ Wet your hands with running water.

☐ Apply liquid, bar or powder soap.

☐ Lather well.

☐ This is the important part. Rub your hands vigorously for at least 20 seconds. Remember to scrub all surfaces, including the backs of your hands, wrists, between your fingers and under your fingernails.

☐ Rinse well.

☐ Dry your hands with a clean or disposable towel or air dryer.

☐ If possible, use your towel to turn off the faucet.

And that's it. That's all you gotta do to keep fecal bacteria from getting into your eyes the next time your rub em.

Always wash your hands before:

- ☐ Preparing food
- ☐ Eating
- ☐ Treating wounds or giving medicine
- ☐ Touching a sick or injured person
- ☐ Touching an infant or young child
- ☐ Engaging in sexual activity (you figure it out)
- ☐ Inserting or removing contact lenses

Always wash your hands after:

- ☐ Preparing food, especially meat, if you still eat that stuff
- ☐ Using the toilet
- ☐ Changing a diaper
- ☐ Touching an animal or animal toys, leashes or waste
- ☐ Blowing your nose, coughing or sneezing into your hands
- ☐ Treating wounds
- ☐ Touching a sick or injured person
- ☐ Shaking hands with weirdoes and riff raffs
- ☐ Handling garbage or something that could be contaminated, such as a cleaning rag or soiled shoes
- ☐ Handling chemicals or other irritants
- ☐ Of course, it's also important to wash your hands whenever they look dirty.
- ☐ Other Things To Wash
- ☐ Soda can tops (those cans get nasty between the warehouse and store)
- ☐ Fresh fruits and vegetables (for wax, pesticides, and dirt)
- ☐ Your Penis (especially before you have sex)
- ☐ Baby toys (before you let your child have them, and every few days after)
- ☐ Tupperware (before you use them, and in between uses)
- ☐ Tooth and hair brushes
- ☐ Remote controls, cell phones, headphones, etc...
- ☐ I'm sure you can come up with a few more on your own. Just think about where the germs and nasty stuff are. And wash it.

Think of everything you touch. By cleaning and scrubbing off the trash, you won't worry about it getting the best of you.

HAND SANITIZER VS. SOAP AND WATER?
WHAT'S THE DIFFERENCE?
BY QUEEN CIVILIZED ZAG

Antibacterial hand sanitizers are marketed as an effective way to "wash hands" when traditional soap and water are not available. These "waterless" products are particularly popular with parents and people who are on the go a lot. Manufacturers of hand sanitizers claim that the sanitizers kill 99.9% of germs. Based on the name and this claim, you'd assume that you're effectively "sanitizing" your hands and killing nearly all the germs. Recent research suggests that this is not the case.

How do hand sanitizers work?

Hand sanitizers work by stripping away the outer layer of oil on the skin. This also prevents bacteria present in the body from coming to the surface of the hand. However, not all of those bacteria are the ones that will make us sick. Not only that, but **research shows that hand sanitizers do not significantly reduce the number of bacteria** on the hand and in some cases may potentially increase the amount of bacteria on the hand.

How can the manufacturers make the 99.9 percent claim?

The manufacturers of the products test the products on inanimate surfaces hence they are able to derive the claims of 99.9% of bacteria killed. If the products were fully tested on hands, there would be different results.

Hand Sanitizers vs. Soap and Water

Interestingly enough, **the Food and Drug Administration** (in regards to proper procedures for food services) **recommends that hand sanitizers not be used in place of soap and water** but only as an alternative when there is no other option. What does that mean? It means, if you can, WASH YOUR HANDS with soap and water. It's just plain nasty to consider that some people are touching everything from garbage to snot and only using sanitizer, which doesn't even remove crud from your skin.

What about antibacterial soaps?

Research has shown that plain soaps are just as effective as antibacterial soaps in reducing bacteria-related illnesses. In fact, using **consumer antibacterial soap products may increase bacterial resistance to antibiotics in some bacteria.** These conclusions only apply to consumer antibacterial soaps and not to those used in hospitals or other clinical areas.

Can you overdo the hand-washing thing?

Yes. Other studies suggest that ultra-clean environments and the persistent use of antibacterial soaps and hand sanitizers may inhibit proper immune system development in children. This is because inflammatory systems require greater exposure to common germs for proper development. Meaning germs can make us stronger against germs. Children who grow up sheltered from all forms of germs tend to get sick more easily later in life.

How to Use Sanitizer

If you choose to use a commercially-prepared hand sanitizer, make sure the product contains at least 60% alcohol. Then follow these simple steps:

- ❏ Apply enough of the product to the palm of your hand to wet your hands completely.
- ❏ Rub your hands together, covering all surfaces, for up to 25 seconds or until they're dry.

If your hands are visibly dirty, however, wash with soap and water. Antimicrobial wipes or towelettes are another option, although they're not as effective as alcohol-based sanitizers.

If your hands are dirty, wash with soap and water. Antimicrobial wipes or towelettes are good, but alcohol-based sanitizers are better

---

FOOD POISONING

BY SUPREME UNDERSTANDING

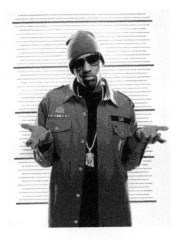

In September of 2009, Fabolous was rushed to the hospital after he believed he was poisoned. He was probably right, but this wasn't a James Bond movie. He probably had food poisoning. Every year, millions of people report illnesses that have been traced back to something they ate. **Many mistake the symptoms of food poisoning for stomach flu.** The most common sources of food poisoning are from E. coli and salmonella bacteria. And **the most common place to get food poisoning is when you eat out at places that don't take extra efforts to serve CLEAN** (and fresh) **food with CLEAN hands and CLEAN utensils.** Unfortunately, that's not too common...especially at fast food restaurants. Whiles there are tons of possibilities, including raw vegetables, mushrooms, and grains, don't get it twisted. **Over 90% of all food poisoning comes from meat.**

In the summer of 2010, at least 155 people in several states became ill from salmonella-tainted food served at Taco Bell restaurants. One of the first people to report symptoms was met with the typical indifferent response you'll get at most fast food spots…even the ones that routinely food-poison their customers. He told *The Consumerist* (www.consumerist.com):

> I just wanted to warn the store, and hopefully prevent somebody else having to go through what I did.
>
> As soon as I told them I had food poisoning, the manager immediately became defensive, spouting off their health inspection records and assuring me that their restaurant was clean – I guess nobody trained the manager that a dirty cooking area isn't the only vector for food poisoning. She also forcefully told me that nobody else had reported getting sick.
>
> The most ludicrous part was when after describing my symptoms (nausea, hourly vomiting, diarrhea), the manager tried to tell me that if you weren't used to eating their food, it could cause an adverse reaction. Yes, the manager tried to blame food poisoning symptoms on me not having the intestinal fortitude to handle Taco Bell!
>
> After that I figured it wasn't worth continuing the conversation. What a shame that the manager at the store seemed more interested in playing CYA than listen to somebody who was trying to help.

And food poisoning might be the least of your concerns. The week before this book went to print, health officials in Salt Lake City, Utah reported the possibility of Hepatitis A exposure at a Quizno's restaurant.

Symptoms

When you have food poisoning, it often feels like a severe case of the flu or a stomach virus. The typical symptoms include nausea, vomiting, stomach cramps and diarrhea. The symptoms normally occur within 6 to 48 hours of your consuming the contaminated food or drink.

You should seek medical attention if:

☐ Your symptoms last more than two days
☐ If a child under 3 years old is the one sick
☐ If you start running a fever
☐ If you get dizzy, collapse, or have difficulty breathing
☐ If your cramping pains last longer than 10 to 15 minutes

Other causes for concern include a swollen abdomen, skin or eyes turning yellow or serious dehydration.

Preventing Food Poisoning

The best way to avoid the most common cases of food poisoning is to prepare your own food and eat out less, especially at places with low prices and even lower standards of hygiene. But even then, you can still food poison yourself (and your family) if you're not careful. Here's some ways to avoid food poisoning at home:

☐ Be very careful to wash your hands and to clean any dishes or utensils when you are making or serving food.

- Promptly refrigerate any food you won't be eating right away.
- If you take care of young children, wash your hands often and dispose of diapers carefully so that bacteria can't spread to other surfaces or people.
- Always refrigerate fish well.
- Eat fruits and vegetables, many of which contain coumarins, a substance that helps stop the growth of E. coli. However, make sure you peel and wash them carefully before eating, especially if you're in another country.
- Eat foods rich in Vitamin A, which appears to help eliminate harmful bacteria from the body faster. People deficient in Vitamin A may be more prone to Salmonella infection.

Treating Food Poisoning

Even if you're OCD clean, there's still a chance you'll get food poisoning, especially if you eat out. Fortunately, many cases of food poisoning can be taken care of at home before symptoms worsen. Here are some steps to treat food poisoning, based on recommendations from health writer Nonna Joann:

Step One: Flush your system out with fluids. Drink coconut water to replace loss electrolytes. Avoid carbonated drinks, caffeinated drinks, and dairy products. Drink chamomile tea or ginger tea (to soothe your inflamed stomach or intestine). It's vital to stay hydrated.

Step Two: Apple cider vinegar is a purifier. It is effective in detoxifying various organs and it helps oxidation of the blood. It promotes digestion, assimilation and elimination. It neutralizes toxic substances taken into the body. Adults take 1 to 2 tablespoons organic apple cider vinegar several times a day, mixed into a glass of water (children should take less). It's most effective on an empty stomach (And it's an aphrodisiac).

Step Three: Eat dark toasted bread (though any bread can work). Bread will soak up the poison and diminish intestinal irritation. Activated charcoal is an effective (and inexpensive) treatment for food poisoning, but few of us have it on hand. You can get it at most health food stores.

Step Four: Take probiotics as they will help fight off potential infections and restore intestinal pH. Again, available at most health food stores.

Step Five: Most importantly, REST. Let your body have time to heal itself. As your body begins to heal, begin eating easily digested soft, bland foods. Broth, mild soup, bananas, yogurt, rice, and applesauce are good foods to introduce first.

Step Six: If you think the contaminated food came from a store or restaurant, tell the staff and your local health department.

Here are some more home remedies that can help:

- ☐ For nausea, eat a small amount of grated (or candied) ginger. Another remedy is to hold a clove of garlic between your teeth.
- ☐ Bittervine, a plant extract from a traditional Jamaican folk medicine, shows activity against several types of bacteria, including S. aureus and E. coli.
- ☐ Thyme oil, the essential oil of the herb thyme, kills the bacteria Salmonella typhimurium and works against S. aureus.
- ☐ Barberry, another herb may help ease symptoms in some people with food poisoning caused by E. coli and V. cholera.

Most food poisoning occurs at home. How safe is your kitchen? Visit the Baby Bites blog (www.babybites.info/2010/04/13/is-it-safe-to-eat) for a quick quiz.

Observe how clean a restaurant is before you order. Make sure your kitchen remains clean and keep some remedies handy just in case.

K.O. THE B.O.

C'BS ALIFE ALLAH

I got with an 'au natural' chick back in the day. I don't mean one of those 'back to the backwoods' types who swear off shaving their legs and underarms. This was a chica who just wasn't feeling putting a whole bunch of stuff on her body that had ingredients that seemed like they were out of a secret scientific experiment. She was the first person who I met that didn't use deodorant.

Now by the time she told me this fact, I had already sniffed her body up in various different ways, and she ain't NEVER smelled bad. So after hanging with her for a minute, she let me in on several open secrets. Now I ain't saying everyone should go and drop your deodorant. Cause frankly, there are a host of things that you need to do in order to go free of it. Yet there are some things that anyone can do to make sure that they're 'so fresh and so clean,' and this will help with your overall aroma.

- ☐ The most obvious is to wash your stankin ass! If you need to do it more than once a day just do it! Get around your under arms and your groin. These are the smelliest parts of your body. Biologically, these are the areas where your body produces pheromones to attract the opposite sex. Because we interfere with them so much (from what we put in our body and what we put on our body) they pump out some repulsive stuff nowadays known as B.O (Body Odor).

- Change your dirty ass clothes. More than once a day if necessary. That moist shirt or underwear is a breeding ground for bacteria. The bacteria getting caught up in your shady regions is producing that stank.
- Rock cotton. It absorbs perspiration and then it can evaporate more quickly.
- Watch what you are putting into your body. Some foods seek to exit the body via your pores. So be aware when you are overdoing it on fish, garlic, curry, tobacco, caffeine, alcohol, etc. Switch up your diet to fresh fruits (especially pineapple), and teas with vanilla extract.
- A lot of over the counter deodorants have metals such as aluminum in them that poison people's lymphatic system (which assists in your body's immunity). There has been a lot of research pointing to breast cancer in women rooted in those deodorants. Seek out some natural deodorants or sprinkle some baking soda on a lemon wedge and rub it up your underarms. It really works.
- If you're really stinking, throw a couple of cups of tomato juice in your bath water and soak for 15 minutes. As you may know, this is also the remedy when you get sprayed by a skunk.
- Now some body odor is actually a beacon to issues within the body like kidney disease, liver disease and other fungal growths. It also happens in adolescence due to the remix in hormone levels and sweat gland growth.
- Step your smell game up with oils vs. perfumes/colognes. They work with your body's natural smell vs. against it. You can also take supplements like Chlorophyll (deodorizer), B Vitamins (waste remover), Zinc (balances the body's natural metabolism), Magnesium (enhances Vitamins B and Zinc), Thyme and Lavender Oils (kill bacteria), Sage (in a tea reduces sweat gland activity)

Get to the root of the problem and don't just 'cover it up' cause you know people still smell the dog crap even when you spray lysol on it.

HOW TO KEEP YOUR BREATH FROM HUMMING
BY SUPREME UNDERSTANDING AND C'BS ALIFE ALLAH

Ghostface Killah, in his audiobook, *The World According to Pretty Tony,* rants:

I'm tellin' y'all, man, when y'all get up in the morning, man, don't just brush your teeth, man, scrub your tongue, man! Scrub that f*cking halitosis off that f*cking tongue of yours, man! Word up! This is real talk right here, man, Tony from New York, man! Scrub your tongue, man, that's where all your bad breath— your little f*cking corroded bacteria be runnin' around, tap dancing on y'all f*cking tongue at night, son! Word up! Y'nahmean, dried-up food, nigga! Niggas got that food tongue, man, wake up mouth smellin' like sh*t, son! Y'nahmean, 'cause it— it's all in your f*cking mouth, son! It's GROWIN' on that sh*t! Y'nahmean? Scrub that sh*t, son! Put some toothpaste on that sh*t, brush yo teeth and scrub your tongue, man! Scrub your lips and all that sh*t, man, I don't give a f*ck! Stick the toothpaste, the toothbrush down your f*cking throat if you have to, my nigga! Word up! Get that sh*t up off there, man! That's not nice. That's not a good look, son! Brush your f*cking teeth EVERY DAY, man, because your mouth, y'all might not care to smell it, but y'all sh*t is smellin' like MAD SH*T, son. Y'nahmean, brush your f*cking teeth, man, do it hard, man! Brush them sh*ts 'til your gums bleed, my nigga! Do somethin' man! Throw– Swallow a box of bakin' soda and peroxide, nigga! And throw a little bit–This how you do it. Brush your teeth, throw some Listerine in there too, at the same time, man! Your sh*t gonna be on fire, but it work!

That dude is hilarious. But his "advice" is actually sound. According to Karyn Chabot, D.Ay., LMT:

> Ancient indigenous cultures all practiced daily tongue scraping to remove toxins and increase their immunity. Using a tongue scraper has been shown to be more effective than a toothbrush, dental floss or mouthwash and it doesn't make one gag or dry the mouth in the way alcoholic mouth rinses can. This doesn't mean you should throw away your floss and toothbrush, but brushing your tongue with a toothbrush isn't nearly as effective as using a tongue scraper. The medical community once thought halitosis was attributed more to tooth decay or stomach problems but they now concur that bad breath is primarily caused by harmful tongue bacteria that isn't removed by brushing, flossing, or gargling alone. Bad breath is produced by toxic volatile sulphur compounds (VSCs) which the Journal of the American Dental Association (Sept., 2000) advises one remove with a tongue scraper.

Does your breath stink? Your significant other probably won't tell you. Neither will most of your friends. But chances are, you've had stank breath at some point in the past…and didn't find out until someone embarrassed you.

The reason you can't smell your own bad breath is because your oral cavity is connected to your nose by way of an opening in the back of our mouth (in the region of the "soft palate" of our tongue). Our noses tend to filter out and ignore background odors (or odors we've become desensitized to), so your nose filters out and ignores the quality of your own breath (and sometimes your own body odor, if you stink every day). This means that you might have total doodoo breath and not know it.

How Can You Tell If You Have A Breath Problem?

You can ask your dentist or hygienist at your next dental appointment. After all, evaluating oral conditions is part of their job.

If you really want an honest answer, and want to avoid asking an adult, try asking a child. As you know, the least inhibited and most honest responses come from children. But be warned, kids can say the cruelest things.

To know how the end of your tongue smells like lick your wrist, wait about five seconds till the saliva somewhat dries, and give that a whiff.

For a more accurate test, take a spoon, turn it upside down, and use it to scrape the very back portion of your tongue. The material that's been scrapped off usually is a thick whitish material. Now take a whiff of that. This is probably the way your breath smells to others.

What Causes Doo Doo Breath?

Dirty Tongue. As you can probably tell by now, for most people, the fundamental cause of bad breath is the coating that accumulates over the back of the tongue. **Bad breath is caused by the bacteria that live in this coating. The second most common cause of bad breath is bacteria accumulated elsewhere in your mouth** (like between your teeth, so make sure you floss). Clean your tongue before brushing your teeth with a solution of hydrogen peroxide and water, and clean your mouth by gargling baking soda in warm water. You can also substitute one squeezed lemon in water.

Food. Everyone knows that certain foods, like garlic and onions have a reputation for causing bad breath. But that stuff will resolve on its own in a day or so as your body completes the process of breaking down and utilizing, or else excreting, the offending molecules. **Drinking water will not only hydrate your mouth but will help keep the bacteria to a minimum.** You may have "ketone breath," a potential side effect of being on a low-carb diet, so after eating some bread, help yourself to some mint or parsley leafs, two traditional herbs that keep your breath fresh.

Smoking. I'm sure you've heard of "smoker's breath." Most of it is directly related to the tar, nicotine, and other foul smelling substances derived from tobacco's smoke that accumulates on a person's teeth and oral soft tissues (tongue, cheeks, gums, etc.). However, smoking can also destroy some stuff on the inside of your body that will eventually have funk pouring out of every hole in your body. Smoking also contributes to dry mouth and gum disease, both of which cause bad breath. Short of quitting smoking, there is no effective way to totally eliminate smoker's breath.

Dry Mouth. The reason your breath stinks in the morning is because saliva flow keeps your mouth fresh. This same souring effect happens to teachers, preachers, and anyone else whose mouth goes dry after speaking for a prolonged period of time. Additionally, people who breathe through their mouth, are fasting, or are under stress can get dry mouth. Some people have chronically dry mouths, or "xerostomia." Xerostomia can be a side effect of medications like antihistamines (allergy/cold medications), antidepressants, blood pressure agents, diuretics, narcotics, or anti-anxiety medications. Xerostomia can also come from the dehydration associated with old age. **Saliva is your best weapon against bad breath, by washing away food particles and bacteria, it eliminates odor.** Chewing gum stimulates saliva production, while mints on the other hand temporarily mask the odor. A recent study of the cinnamon-flavored gum **Big Red** found cinnamon to have breath-odor fighting abilities.

Sinus Problems. Upper respiratory infections and allergies can create a foul-smelling, foul-tasting, postnasal drip that ends up on the back of your tongue. What's worse, oral bacteria will feed upon this discharge and create their own smelly waste products. Plus you'll probably need to breathe through your mouth, which leads to funky dry mouth.

Other Factors. On rare occasions bad breath can signal larger problems. Medical problems associated with the respiratory (pulmonary or bronchial), hepatic (liver), renal (kidney), and gastrointestinal (stomach and intestine) systems. **Any active infections in a person's mouth, such as those associated with abscessed teeth or a partially erupted wisdom tooth can cause bad breath.** Teeth having extensive untreated decay can trap enough debris and bacteria that they become the source of foul odors. Your dentist can identify and treat these problematic dental conditions if they exist. Visit a doctor if they aren't able to find a cause for your bad breath.

Sometimes your words are only as fresh as your breath. You can't be a smooth talker with a foul smelling grill.

DIRTY MOUTH?

GUM DISEASE IS THE ORIGINAL GANGSTA GRILL
BY SUPREME UNDERSTANDING

Periodontal disease, or gum disease, is an infection of the tissues surrounding your teeth. When plaque develops, bacteria irritate the gums and cause them to swell. In the early stages, it's called gingivitis and only affects the gums. In more advanced phases, the disease is known as periodontitis. The bacteria go under your gum line, eventually attacking the tissues and bone around your teeth. That's when you start losing your teeth. And it's not rare. **Nearly 75% of American adults have some form of periodontal disease, according to the American Dental Hygienists' Association.** The symptoms can be so mild that you might not know you have it.

Warning Signs
❏ Gums that bleed easily

❏ Red, swollen, tender gums

- Gums that have pulled away from the teeth
- Persistent bad breath or bad taste
- Permanent teeth that are loose or separating
- Any change in the way your teeth fit together when you bite
- Any change in the fit of partial dentures

Risk Factors

You just might have doodoo breath because you literally have doodoo in your mouth. I'll explain. While there IS a medical condition called copremesis (which basically means you sh*t out of your mouth), there's something way more common, and it's a 50/50 chance I'm talking about you here. As you've read elsewhere, feces particles can spray when you flush the toilet with the lid up. They land on things like your toothbrush. This ain't rare or minor. **One study found 49% of used toothbrushes tested positive for bacteria from feces, while another lab found up to 100,000,000 colony-forming germ units on a single ordinary toothbrush.** Because the sharp tips of firm toothbrush bristles can cause tiny lacerations in your gums (which allow infections to enter the body), you don't want sh*t bacteria on your toothbrush. This is why dentists have recommended that a toothbrush be kept at least 6 feet away from a toilet (and washed regularly with hot water). I also recommend you close that lid when you flush. Then again, if your name is Filthy McNasty, the problem isn't that you're brushing too much...the problem is that you ain't brushin at all! Besides poor oral hygiene, several factors raise the risk of gum disease: smoking/tobacco use; genetics; stress; prescription medications; poor nutrition; diseases that affect multiple organs, such as diabetes; pregnancy and puberty; clenching or grinding teeth; crooked teeth; and defective or loose braces or other dental fittings.

> **Did You Know**
> Gum disease has also been linked to increased risk of Type 2 Diabetes and heart disease. The ADHA has reported that approximately 95% of Americans with diabetes also have periodontal disease. Harvard Medical School has linked chronically infected gums to coronary heart disease, and a University of Buffalo study of 1,372 people found that those with gum disease had triple the risk of heart attacks in a 10-year period.

Gum Disease and Premature Labor?

Gum disease can also complicate pregnancies. According to the AAP, expectant mothers with periodontal bacteria are seven times more likely to have a premature and low-birth-weight baby. The bacteria and the toxins from the periodontal disease enter the bloodstream and cause inflammation that triggers premature labor. As you probably know, the chances of survival depend on how early the baby arrives. At 24 weeks, a baby has about a 10% chance of survival. At 26 weeks, the chance increases to 55%, and at 28 weeks, it is 77%.

It's all connected: What you eat, what you do, and what you die from!

CAN YOU HEAR ME NOW? TREATING EAR INFECTIONS

BY C'BS ALIFE ALLAH

It can make a grown man cry. The ear drum is a tender organ and one of the few that is partially exposed to the air. When it gets infected, it can reduce most to a whimpering pile of mush. Children are very susceptible to ear infections because their ear canals are still developing and may be very small.

The nose, throat and ear are all connected. Often, when an infection starts in one section, if not dealt with immediately it'll spread to another. This is why a throat infection can become a head cold and an ear problem can signal an upcoming throat problem. Once a cold has developed, it can then go into the chest. The main reason an infection develops is not just because you 'catch' a cold, it's because your body's environment is in such a poor state that becomes unbalanced. It is similar to when food spoils that it molds and starts to smells. In the case of the human body if the body becomes too acidic (versus alkaline) then your body will be subject to disease. The breeding ground for an ear infection comes from fluid buildup in the ear canals/cavity that causes bacteria to flourish. This can either cause or become the cause of sinus infections.

When infants get an ear infection, many people rush to get antibiotics. Infants are developing, and antibiotics kill good and bad bacteria, which is why my doctor suggested not rushing to get antibiotics all the time (for a child or adult). The bad bacteria can eventually build up immunity against the antibiotics. Thus stronger and different types of antibiotics would have to be used. So it's important to know that there are alternative methods, especially with adults. As we've noted elsewhere, when emergency care is needed, do what is necessary. Don't risk a life in pursuit of an alternative method. At the same time, don't medicate every sniffle and ache.

Clear your Throat and Blow your Nose

Since the nose, throat and ear are connected, by making sure that your nasal cavity and throat aren't bacteria-friendly, you're also offsetting an ear infection. When your throat starts to get scratchy suck on half of a lemon every half hour or so and gargle with salt water 3 times a day after each meal. This will start to cut through all of the bacteria, mucus and fluid buildup in the throat and even upper lungs. It might be best to attack any infection from all angles to stop it from migrating use a *neti pot* (mentioned in detail in our article on asthma) to clear everything that finds its way into the nasal cavity.

The second thing is that, sometimes, if you don't treat an infection in one area quick enough it will just migrate. You might just have to attack from all areas in order for it not to migrate. In order to keep the nasal cavity clear one should indulge in the Indian practice of using a *neti pot*.

Use a Natural Antibiotic

If you have a grandma you already know a couple of the remedies for an ear infection. Basically you want to kill the bacteria that are in the cavity. The easiest way is to apply a natural antibiotic directly to the infection via some type of oil. **The two types of oils that can be used for this are tea tree oil or sweet oil** (which you can buy from any corner store, which is just olive oil). In order to increase the power of sweet oil you can infuse it with garlic (put some garlic cloves in it and let it sit for a few hours. **garlic has incredible anti-fungal and anti-biotic properties.** Some old timers actually stick cloves of garlic in the outer ear). What you want to do is gently warm this oil and place a few drops in the ear and let it sit. Keep applying it several times a day. This is useful only on the onset of the infection. If it is to the point that you cannot even stand the infection, has spread too far into the inner ear. **In addition to the two oils you can use a few drops of hydrogen peroxide.**

Stay Clean

Finally, it's important to have good hygiene. Your earwax is actually a barrier that blocks germs and bacteria from getting in. **While you don't want to have excess earwax** (which is a sign of a health problem in itself)**, you actually don't need a daily Q-tip in there either.** You can actually rupture (bust) your eardrum, as Supreme Understanding once did. It'll heal on its own, but it will teach you not to dig so deep and leave your ears defenseless against any threats. And while those threats can come from other places inside your system, they can also come straight from things you put inside your ear. For example, **wearing headphones for just an hour will increase the bacteria in your ear by 700 times.** So just imagine what wearing that Bluetooth headpiece (which you probably don't clean) all day will do.

A Quick Note on Noise Control

There's other ways to ruin your ears. 26 million adults in the US have high-frequency loss caused by exposure to loud noises, also known as noise-induced hearing loss. So what's safe and what's too loud? This could help:

Safe Range (in dB)				Risk Range				Injury Range		
30	45	60	70	85	95	100	110	120	140	165
A quiet library	Hum of a refrigerator	Normal conversation	Washing machine	Heavy city traffic	Motorcycle	Top volume on iPod	Rap concert	Ambulance siren	Jet taking off	Shot-gun blast

The best way to attack an infection is from multiple angles, giving it no room to grow.

Notes:

WOMEN'S HEALTH

SOMETHING FOR THE LADIES

It's a documented fact: Being Black in America is bad for a woman's health. In the acclaimed documentary, *Unnatural Causes*, a critical examination of health care disparities in the U.S., Dr. Richard Davis states, **"There's something about growing up as a Black female in the United States that's not good for your childbearing health."** According to the "weathering" hypothesis first described by Dr. Arline Geronimus, the poor health conditions (and gradual health deterioration) experienced by Black women is linked to the cumulative impact of repeated experiences with racism, adversity, and marginalization. Meaning Black women are "reproducing" suffering, both physical and mental. Something's gotta change. So this chapter addresses some of the specific issues women need to be aware of, in addition to the stuff we're covering throughout the rest of the book.

Life is continued through the womb of our women. If our women aren't healthy, our entire future will suffer from it.

PROTECT YOUR FERTILE SOIL
BY EBONI JOY ASIATIC EARTH
ORIGINALLY PUBLISHED IN THE 14TH DEGREE AND BEYOND

The Original woman's womb is the healthy fertile soil of the planet Earth, where God, the Original man, plants the seeds of life. And so it is important that the womb remains free of any toxins that may destroy her fertility, so that God and Earth may continue to build up our nation by reproducing healthy fruit from her soil.

I am writing this because women are not being informed about the dangers of something most of us use; tampons. I am taking a class this month and I have been learning a lot about biology and women, including much about feminine hygiene. **Recently, we have learned that tampons are actually dangerous** (for other reasons than TSS). I'll tell you this, after learning about this in our class, most of the females wound up feeling angry and upset with the tampon industry, and I for one, am going to do something about it. To start, I want to inform everyone I can.

Here is the scoop: Tampons contain two things that are potentially harmful: Rayon (for absorbency), and dioxin (a chemical used in bleaching the products). The tampon industry is convinced that we, as women, need bleached white products – in order to view the product as pure and clean. The problem here is that the dioxin produced in the bleaching process can lead to very harmful problems for a woman. Dioxin is potentially carcinogenic (cancer-associated) and is toxic to immune and reproductive systems. It has also been linked to endometriosis and lower sperm counts for men – for both it breaks down the immune system. Last September the Environmental Protection Agency (EPA) reported that there really is no set "acceptable" level of exposure to dioxin, given that it is cumulative and slow to disintegrate. The real danger comes from repeated contact. (Karen Houppert "Pulling the Plug on the Tampon Industry"). I'd say using about 4 – 5 tampons a day, five days a month, for 38 menstruating years is "repeated contact," wouldn't you? Rayon contributes to the danger of tampons and dioxin because it is a highly absorbent substance. Therefore, when fibers from the tampons are left behind in the vagina (as usually occurs), it creates a breeding ground for the dioxin. It also stays in a lot longer than it would with just cotton tampons. This is also the reason why TSS (toxic shock syndrome) occurs.

What are the Alternatives?

Using feminine hygiene products that aren't bleached and that are all cotton. Other feminine hygiene products (pads/napkins) contain dioxin as well, but they are not nearly as dangerous since they are not in direct contact with the vagina. The pads/napkins need to stop being bleached, but obviously tampons are the most dangerous. So, what can you do if you can't give up using tampons? Use tampons that are made from 100% cotton, and that are UNBLEACHED. Unfortunately, there are very, very few companies that make these safe tampons. They are usually only found in health food stores. Countries all over the world (Sweden, Germany, British Columbia, etc.) have demanded a switch to this safe tampon, while the U.S. has decided to keep us in the dark about it. **In 1989, activists in England mounted a campaign against chlorine bleaching. Six weeks and 50,000 letters later, the makers of sanitary products switched to oxygen bleaching** (one of the green methods available).

What TO DO NOW: Tell People. Everyone. Inform them. Let's do something about it! Please write to companies: Tampax, Tambrands, Playtex, O.B., Kotex. Call the 800 numbers listed on the boxes. Let them know that we demand a safe product – ALL COTTON UNBLEACHED TAMPONS.

I urge you to consistently check the labels of the sanitary pads or tampons that you are going to buy and see whether you spot any of the familiar signs stated in this information. It is no wonder so many women in the world suffer from cervical cancer and womb tumors.

Start or support an already existing campaign against bleached tampons. Write or call companies demanding an alternative!

KEEP YOUR KITTY RIGHT
BY SCIHONOR DEVOTION

When Things Go Wrong

Yeast Infections are one of the most common reasons that women consult health professionals. But they're not that hard to treat or prevent. These infections are the result of an overgrowth of a fungus called Candida albicans. The most common symptom is itching of the internal and external genitalia and a white discharge that can be thick and just pretty gross to describe. Severe yeast infections can lead to inflammation of the vaginal tissue and subsequent redness, swelling and even bleeding.

Other Conditions

Before you treat what you think is a yeast infection, confirm that it is actually yeast, not Bacterial Vaginosis, Noninfectious Vaginitis, or Trichomoniasis.

Bacterial Vaginosis happens when the harmful bacteria and beneficial bacteria in the vagina are off balance and produces a foul-smelling, gray, fishy smelling discharge. It can be spread through sexual intercourse, and is common in women who douche with commercial brand douches or use an IUD birth control device.

Noninfectious Vaginitis irritates the skin around the vagina and is most often found in women who use spermicidal, douches, perfumed soaps, bubble baths, feminine hygiene sprays, wipes and other products to keep their vaginas "fresh." Some women experience Noninfection Vaginitis when going through menopause due to low estrogen levels.

Trichomoniasis, often just called Trick/Trich, is a sexually transmitted disease caused by a parasite. Like yeast, it can be found in both men and women but is often unnoticed in men. Women will see yellowish-greeny discharge that can look like ice cream froth. **People who have trick have a higher risk of getting other Sexually Transmitted Diseases** (STD's) like gonorrhea, syphilis and chlamydia. If you have any of the symptoms of the above diseases or have a fever, chills, nausea, vomiting, abdominal or back pain, bloody discharge, or difficult or increased urination, you probably have more than just a yeast infection and may need to be treated medically.

Untreated yeast infections and vaginal disorders can lead to premature delivery and low birth weight babies in pregnant women. It can also lead to the scarring of the fallopian tubes and cause infertility under the name of PID or Pelvic Inflammatory Disease. As with all treatment of any ailment, weigh and judge and plan your steps before you take action.

How to Get it Right

❐ Many doctors prescribe pills and creams, but a diet low in fats, sugars, and refined foods is important to avoid vaginal yeast infections. Avoid eating too many starches (like bread) which turn to sugar, this also includes sodas, beer, wine, hard alcohol, artificial sweeteners and dairy. Cow's milk creates mucus and promotes allergic reactions in the vagina. Hydrogenated and partially hydrogenated oils stimulate yeast growth, use flax, coconut, olive or even safflower oil.

☐ Lactobacillus Acidophilus, often just called acidophilus, is a friendly bacterium that prevents the overgrowth of unfriendly bacteria and candida. Acidophilus produces lactic acid, which acts like a natural antibiotic. You can get it in yogurt or in the form of capsules or powder. It can also be administered intra-vaginally. If you take antibiotics for something, be sure to take probiotics after your treatment to keep the healthy bacteria alive and active. Avoid commercial douches that have artificial scents. They wash away helpful mucus and bacteria in our vaginas that is needed to maintain good function. Douching can negatively affect the natural pH balance of your vagina (and other things that keep it healthy), so it's really only meant to be used to straighten things out when they're "not going right."

☐ There are tea tree suppositories that can be inserted vaginally and will help to fight the yeast. It can also be diluted with water and made into a douche by mixing 1 teaspoon of tea tree oil and 2 cups of water. Douching with that twice a day may help with the infection. Many doctors of natural medicine recommend garlic for treatment of yeast infections. You can eat cloves of garlic, or insert a clove vaginally. Cinnamon essential oil contains agents believed to be responsible for the oils medicinal effects. The vapors are extremely potent antifungal compounds.

☐ Since Yeast Infections are usually accompanied by an itch, making a paste to apply to the itchy areas may help. Mix 10 drops of tea tree oil in 2 tablespoons of aloe vera gel or vitamin E oil and make a paste. Then apply this mixture to the itchy areas. This can be used for men too when they have a yeast itch but they must also take further action to rid themselves of the yeast.

☐ Avoid petroleum-based vaginal lubricant. If your coochie is as healthy as she should be after these suggestions, you probably won't need help from outside lubricants. Often, yeast infections can be passed through sexual transmission so treat your partner as well. Avoid wearing tight clothing, especially synthetic fabric, and keep your panties cotton. It will allow your body to breathe. Wearing loose-fitting pants and jeans is another good idea.

☐ Wipe from front to back after using the bathroom. For some reason, I think either many of us missed that lesson growing up, or our mothers didn't teach us how to clean ourselves. After you bathe, be sure to dry yourself properly. A moist environment is not good for maintaining a healthy vagina.

Follow the above recommendations to keep the womb feeling right.

THE IMPORTANCE OF PAP SMEARS AND MAMMOGRAMS

BY TAMIKA HOGAN

Pap Smears

A pap test is administered by taking a sample of cells from the cervix using a wooden scraper or swab. The cells are placed on a slide and sent to a laboratory for testing of abnormalities. **Despite recent medical professionals suggesting that women limit how many pap smears they get, there is still a critical need for Black women to get tested regularly.** Pap smears should be done at least once a year and are used to aid in the early detection of cervical cancer. According to the American Cancer Society, Black women have a 50% higher mortality rate from cervical cancer than all other groups of women.

It's important for Black women to talk to their doctors about cervical cancer (especially if there is a family history), to understand the test, start screening as young as 18 (definitely before 21 and/or as soon as the woman becomes sexually active), and to keep getting tested until the age of 70 or older.

An abnormal pap smear does not automatically mean that the woman has cervical cancer but the test should be repeated and further examinations should be administered to rule out or confirm cervical cancer. Other examinations include colposcopies (known as biopsies where tissues are taken from the cervix and examined closely under a microscope). Women who have had a total hysterectomy do not need to have pap smears.

Cervical cancer is highly preventable. When tested regularly, you have the privilege of early detection and treatment. Those who do not have pap smears regularly have a higher risk factor in developing this form of cancer. Other risk factors associated with cervical cancer include having multiple sexual partners, HIV infection, HPV infection, and smoking.

Mammograms

A mammogram is a test used as a screening tool to detect early breast cancer in women experiencing no symptoms and to diagnose breast disease in women experiencing symptoms such as a lump, pain or nipple discharge. The test involves screening whereby compressing the breast to the smallest and flattest form so that tissues can be visualized. An x-ray of the breast is then taken and can detect even the smallest of lumps or abnormalities. The x-rays are taken from various different positions and usually take about 30 minutes.

New health guidelines also suggest that women wait until they are 50 to get a mammogram and limit the test to once every two years. This is because a mammogram itself presents a cancer risk because of the technology used. However, there are safer alternatives, like thermography and digital mammography, which you can ask your doctor about.

It is a fact that Black women are more likely to have a mastectomy than other women. While it is true that doctors tend to overprescribe such procedures based on race and income (as with amputations for Black diabetics), this is also due to not getting tested early enough.[37] Early intervention and detection is key to the survival of Black women who have breast cancer. Get tested!

Don't hesitate. Talk to your doctor about which exams are best for you. Ask them about thermography and digital mammography.

PLEASE MASTER SELF (PMS)
BY EARTH EM'MAYA JEWEL

Whether we call it a period, a cycle, our "time," our "gift" or our "curse," once a month and primarily in a 28 day cycle, women bleed. Some of us have heavy bleeding and others have a light steady flow and still others, with the proper diet, only experience a light spotting for the duration. Whatever your personal experience is, oftentimes it's preceded by an onslaught of inexplicable symptoms that some of us don't even associate with our cycles. Fatigue, backache, depression and panic attacks are just some of the symptoms that can occur before the actual bleeding begins. Some women experience debilitating stomach cramps, others have uncontrollable crying spells, migraines, fluid retention, constipation, and irritability.

PMS is a disorder characterized by a set of hormonal changes that trigger disruptive symptoms in a significant number of women for up to two weeks prior to menstruation. Of the estimated 40 million sufferers in the US, more than 5 million require medical treatment for marked mood and behavioral changes. Tension, lack of coordination, decreased work or social performance and altered sex drive are all emotional and behavioral changes that may occur during the two weeks that proceed a woman's cycle.

---

[37] Another reason is because many Black women do not have the finances to support treatment, but many healthcare providers of low income Black families will pay for a Mastectomy. Plainly stated, Black women are more underinsured than white and Hispanic women.

So, no, you are not bipolar!

Painful joints, backache, headache, heart palpitations and weight gain are also common. These are natural occurrences as the womb prepares to purge itself of harmful toxins that have accumulated in the body. Often symptoms tend to taper off with menstruation and women remain symptom-free until the two weeks or so prior to the next menstrual period. Over 150 symptoms have been attributed to PMS. But symptoms may vary from month to month and there may even be symptom-free months. **No woman presents all of the symptoms and some women are lucky enough to not have any!**

However if you do feel that you suffer from PMS here are some ways to lessen the symptoms:

❏ Eat a low-fat, vegetarian diet that includes legumes, whole grains, fruits, vegetables, nuts, seeds, and yogurt. This keeps hormones in check and therefore many PMS symptoms at bay. Consuming more fiber from these sources helps to flush excess hormones from the body. Eating magnesium-rich foods like peanut butter, lima beans, kale, and nuts, has been found to reduce the bloating, weight gain, and breast tenderness, while calcium rich sources like spinach and broccoli can cut food cravings and mood swings, most likely because calcium enhances the brain's processing of serotonin.

❏ Avoid refined carbohydrates and sugar-filled foods because they disrupt blood-sugar levels causing fatigue and mood swings. Coffee can also make things worse, along with sodium which contributes to bloating and breast tenderness, while non-organic dairy products and meats contain hormones that can cause inflammation and thus worsen cramps and bloating.

The majority of PMS symptoms are the result of an imbalance in hormones. Women with mild or moderate symptoms may get enough relief from changes in diet and lifestyle alone. Regular aerobic exercise for twenty minutes at least three times a week may also be helpful. Though there haven't been many scientific studies done on herbal treatments, dandelion, borage seed oil and black cohosh may be helpful. It is very important to check with your physician before taking any of these products as they should be avoided by women on certain medicines and with certain health conditions.

It is also important to understand that it may take a few months of trying one of these changes before you notice any improvement. Start at least a week or two before your period and do it each month to ensure you get the benefits.

Making sure you cycle consists of whole foods, exercise, and emotional well-being will leave less room for "errors."

MENOPAUSE

DON'T WORRY, YOUR LIFE IS NOT ON PAUSE
BY SCIHONOR DEVOTION

Menopause is the time in which a woman's menstruation and ability to reproduce begin to go away, usually between the ages of 45 and 55, but can happen early or prematurely if the woman has had a hysterectomy. Because a woman produces less estrogen at this time, she'll experience symptoms. **Did you know that in Chinese medicine a woman's placenta is encapsulated and often given to her during her menopausal time to help balance her hormones and manage other symptoms that she may be experiencing?** Well, when you think about it most mammals do eat there placentas after giving birth and it seems they have good reason to do so. Some symptoms are:

- Hot flashes
- Depression
- Moodiness and irritability
- Insomnia
- Poor memory
- Irregular periods
- Urinary or vaginal infections
- Vaginal dryness
- Fatigue
- Weight gain
- Night sweats
- Dry thin hair and dry skin
- Incontinence
- Increased hair growth on face, chest and stomach
- Pain during sex due to thinner vaginal walls and dryness

Dietary adjustments always affect symptoms. Follow the nutrition guidelines from the previous article. Some foods that have plant-like estrogen that can help ease symptoms are:

- Garlic
- Alfalfa
- Oats
- Pomegranate
- Soy beans
- Wheat and sprouts

Exercises like bike riding, swimming, running or even walking may help. Try meditation, deep breathing and sex to reduce stress.

Herbs:

- Valerian and skull cap- Tension and anxiety
- Senna – Laxative
- Shepherds purse, Yarrow, Golden seal – Heavy bleeding
- Dandelions roots- Liver cleansing; reducing the risk of cell changes like growths in the breasts
- Black Cohosh – Balances hormones, night sweats, and hot flashes
- Ginkgo Biloba – Memory and concentration
- Cramp Bark – Antispasmodic
- Dong Quai – Hot flashes and vaginal dryness
- Motherwort – Vaginal wall sensitivity

❏ Dandelion Leaves – Water retention	❏ Ginseng – Balance hormones

Essential Oils:

❏ Sage – Hormonal balance	❏ Ylang Ylang – Aphrodisiac

Vitamins and Minerals:

❏ B Complex – Anxiety and moodiness	❏ Zinc, magnesium, vitamin E, vitamin E – Painful menstruation
❏ Vitamin E, Acidophilus – Tender breasts	❏ Magnesium – Insomnia
❏ Vitamin C – Constipation	❏ Vitamin E Capsules – Pierce capsule and put in vagina to help with lubrication
❏ Vitamin A, Iron, Zinc – Heavy flow	

The above recommendations should decrease symptoms.

UTERINE FIBROIDS
BY QUEEN CIVILIZED ZAG

Fibroid tumors are non-cancerous growths that appear on the muscular wall of the uterus and consist of dense, fibrous tissue, nourished and sustained by a series of blood vessels. They are the most common tumors of the female genital tract. They have other names like leiomyoma, leiomyomata, or myoma and range in size from microscopic to almost filling the entire abdominal cavity making you look up to 5 months pregnant. Uterine fibroids can affect women of all ages, but are most common in women ages 40 to 50.

See below for the three different types of uterine fibroids

Intramural Uterine Fibroids. These are located in the wall of the uterus and are the most common type of fibroids. They cause uterine enlargement, pelvic pain, heavy menstrual bleeding, back pain, and pressure.

Submucosal Uterine Fibroids. Located inside the lining of the uterus, they 'face' inward causing heavy bleeding and heavy, prolonged periods.

Subserosal Uterine Fibroids. Located outside the lining of the uterus 'facing' outward, they have less of an effect on your period, but may cause back pain or pressure. They can grow on a stalk attached to the uterus, in which case it is called 'pendunculated' and can cause severe pelvic pain.

Fibroid Symptoms
Although fibroids are not cancerous, uterine fibroids can cause problems, depending on size, location and number of fibroids. Symptoms include:

- Pelvic pain and pressure
- Excessive bleeding, including prolonged periods and passage of clots, which can lead to anemia.
- Abdominal swelling
- Pressure on the bladder, leading to frequent urination
- Pressure on the bowel, leading to constipation and bloating
- Infertility

Even though fibroids are common, most don't cause symptoms. However, they still may require treatment.

Why do I Have Them?

No one knows. Some doctors have pointed to lack of exercise, poor diet, and even the overuse of latex condoms as contributing factors. **Fibroids affect 40% of American women over 35 years old, and have a higher rate of incidence among African Americans than any other group.** In fact, African American women have three times more cases than Caucasian women. Additionally, fibroids tend to be larger and occur at an earlier age in African Americans. Fibroids can grow very large during pregnancy, when estrogen levels are high, and can shrink back down after pregnancy. They usually improve in menopause, when estrogen levels decrease.

Finding Out if you Have Fibroids

You can get an ultrasound from your gynecologist which can determine the presence of fibroids. MRI's (Magnetic Resonance Imaging) are the most used and can determine if fibroids can be treated and if there are any other issues.

Uterine Fibroid Treatment

Non-Surgical Options. Uterine artery embolization (UAE), also called uterine fibroid embolization (UFE) is an endovascular procedure, meaning it is done through the arterial system. It is non-surgical and minimally invasive. It does not require general anesthesia-the groin is numbed and the patient is sedated, but still conscious enough to respond to a question.

Recovery time after uterine fibroid embolization is usually an over-night stay in the hospital, mostly to monitor pain.

Surgical Options. Uterine fibroids can be treated with surgery, including hysterectomy, which removes the entire uterus, and myomectomy, which only removes the fibroids. Both are major surgeries requiring 4 days in the hospital and a 6-week recovery period. Myomectomy can preserve fertility, but carries the risk of recurrence, since most women have multiple fibroids and it's impossible to cut them all out.

Always talk to your doctor about the least invasive means to remove uterine fibroids.

CAN A BRA INCREASE MY RISK OF BREAST CANCER?

BY TAMIKA HOGAN

Bras have been worn in different ways all over the world since the 1400's. Indigenous people of the world were not exposed to these luxuries and did not care much to have their breasts lifted, supported or enlarged. In many areas of the world, this practice of wearing a bra is still non-existent. In this society that we live in today, most women wear bras, especially us sisters, in that we tend to have bigger breasts than some other groups of people.

So how is wearing a bra associated to the risks of developing breast cancer, you may wonder? The breasts contain mammary lymphatic tissues which rely heavily on circulation. When the breasts are restricted inside of a bra, the movement and circulation is lowered. When this happens, there is low oxygen content (known as anoxia) which leads to fibrosis. Fibrosis, a development of excess body fiber, is linked to increased risks of cancer. Not to mention that **the restriction of breast movement and airflow prevents the breast from excreting dangerous cancer-causing chemicals.**

There is a MYTH that underwire bras are no good and can cause breast cancer. This has not been studied much and the few studies that have been conducted are inconclusive in backing this myth from any factual standpoint. The underwire is used as support, to decrease the discomfort and sometimes pain caused to a woman's back from carrying unsupported large breasts.

With that being said, here are a few bra tips:

- ❑ Limit wearing a bra to half a day (12 hours at most).
- ❑ Make sure the bra is the right size. Bra size is measured around the torso (under the breasts) AND the cup size (so you can be wide with a small cup - eg. 36 A cup).
- ❑ If you have fat coming from between your armpits and where the bra begins or the top of your breasts are squeezing out of the top of the bra then it DOES NOT FIT YOU. Get a new one that does.

- ❏ Don't make the straps too tight around your shoulders or torso because that can increase pressure and strain which can also increase discomfort.
- ❏ Do NOT buy cheap bras from cheap stores (most of those cheap bras are made with the Polyester. And after one wash won't fit anymore, so why waste your time and money just invest in a good bra.
- ❏ Make sure you wear a cotton bra or a bra that has cotton inside of the cup to allow for the circulation of air (most satin bras are satin on the outside for show but have cotton inside of the cup).
- ❏ If you wash your bra and it's still dingy – throw it away. It's called dirt and it's not coming out. Buy a new one.
- ❏ Lastly, if you're going to go bra-less, wear a shirt that doesn't show everything. Don't walk around like you're about to enter a wet t-shirt contest.

You don't have to burn your bras but as with everything in life, don't over-do it. Let your skin and body feel free and breathe in some air.

FIGHTING BACK ON BACKACHES
BY QUEEN VICTORIOUS LANASIA EARTH

As Original women, we often find ourselves battling back pain on a daily. Usually this is because of pregnancy, being overweight, having big breasts, or even because of the way we handle stress and manage daily physical activities.

The back is a complex structure of muscles, bone and elastic tissue and is known as the life of the bone of the body. The spine is made of 24 blocks of bone piled one on top of the other. Sandwiched between these bony blocks are cushions of cartilage and elastic tissues called intervertebral discs. The vertebral discs act as shock absorbers for the back. Mobility would be impossible without these discs. But your back needs proper care to stay pain-free and fully functional. Backaches are increasingly common because they generally result from sedentary living habits and hazardous work patterns. The psychological conditions associated with emotional stress can bring about muscle spasms, including those in our back.

How do you know if you have a back problem?
In most cases, the pain is felt either in the middle or lower back. It may spread to both sides of the waist and hips, with acute pain. In cases of acute pain, it may even have you bedridden.

Acute or chronic illnesses like kidney or prostate problems, female disorders, influenza and arthritis, may lead to back pain.

Other causes include stress, subluxations (dysfunctional blocks of vertebral joints in your spine), dysfunctional organs, inflammation from allergies, improper lifting of weights, and even emotional problems.[38]

Poor posture, especially improper sitting posture, can lead to back pain. (See "Bad Posture Does More than Make You Look Lame") Shoes with high heels place a tremendous strain on your back and other muscles of your body. (See "Heels are Sex…but Bad for your Feet") Sleeping on too soft of a mattress, which results in an improper back and neck posture, can also cause tension, headaches, and pain in your upper and lower back.

Treatment

Drugs prescribed to relieve pain or relax muscles in backache disorders do not cure common back problems. These can become habit forming and may actually perpetuate the disease in case of excessive intake.

True treatment of backaches comes with maintaining a good diet, proper exercise, and modification of daily activities. The most important of these is exercise, which improves the supply of nutrients to spinal discs, thereby delaying the process of deterioration that comes with age and eventually affects everybody. Safe exercises include walking, swimming and bicycling (making sure your back is upright on the bike). Also, excess weight greatly increases the stress on soft back tissues. **Those with sedentary occupations should take a break and stand up every hour.** Soft-cushioned seats should be avoided and one's position should be changed as often. **Sleep on a firm mattress on your side with knees bent at right angles to the torso.** Do not let your mattress sag in the middle, place a board under the mattress if needed, to prevent it. **You should take care never to bend from the waist down to lift any object** but instead should squat close to the object, bending the knees but keeping the back straight and then stand up slowly.

Neck tension arising from long hours at the desk or behind the wheel of the car can be relieved rotating your head, allowing it to drop forward and backward and turning it to the right and left as far as possible several times. These exercises help to loosen up tight neck muscles which might be blocking blood supply to your brain, making

---

[38] In fact, there's an entire school of alternative medicine dedicated to the energy blockages associated with emotions and stress, which are thought to manifest themselves as acute pain occurring along the paths the energy (sometimes called "Chi") normally takes. For those who find this approach too mystical, it's important to know that the chi meridians overlap with the nervous system, and the nervous system in most certainly one that depends on thought and energy.

you less of a zombie at work.

It's all about alignment. When sleeping, sitting, or moving make sure you aren't in a position that adds stress to your spine.

HEELS ARE SEXY...BUT BAD FOR YOUR FEET
BY SUPREME UNDERSTANDING

There's a reason doctors tell you not to wear heels when you're pregnant, not only are you at greater risk for twisting your ankle, you can give yourself all kinds of foot problems like "pump bumps" and bunions. And heels might help your butt stick out, but they're also bad for your back. In *What the Yuck: The Freaky and Fabulous Truth about your Body*, Dr. Roshini Raj lists the following foot problems commonly caused by unhealthy footwear:

Pump Bump, an enlargement of the bone in the back of your heel, caused by shoes with a stiff back. This irritates the back of your foot and causes inflammation and swelling.

Morton's Neuroma, an abnormal growth of nerve tissue between the third and fourth toe that can cause pain and burning in the toes and foot, caused by too-tight or pointy-toed shoes which force your toes together.

Hammertoe, a condition where the toes bend up at the joint (instead of down), also caused by narrow shoes.

Blisters, which are pockets of raised skin filled with fluid, caused by friction from poor-fitting or too-tight shoes.

We're not saying never wear heels. Just don't overdo it. **Most foot doctors recommend wearing heels for less than 3 hours at a time.** It's on you to figure out how to budget that time! Oh, and high heels aren't the only bad guys. Wedges are better than stilettos, but still not the best choice for people with knee problems. Mules give you zero ankle support (greater risk of "rolling" your ankle...it hurts), and can cause toe and upper foot pain. Flip-flops are surprisingly almost as bad as 6-inch stilettos! They provide no arch or ankle support and force you to crunch your toes to keep em on when you walk, which can cause cramps and other problems. Dr. Raj says they're okay for short-terms use, but not as your daily wear. Ballet flats don't provide any support either, and no padding for the bottom of your feet, which can lead to sore heels or inflammation. So what's left? Actually plenty, so long as it's – as Dr. Raj says – "One with cushioning, support, and gobs of room for your toes. And for everyday use, try to keep the heel below one inch (nights out are a different story!)."

It's about moderation. There's no reason you should have high heels when running errands, keep a pair of sneakers in the car if need be.

NO MORE STRETCH MARKS
BY DR. KANIKA JAMILA

What Causes Stretch Marks?

Stretch marks are caused by rapid weight gain and loss. Women abhor stretch marks on the stomach due to pregnancy and try many methods of preventing and diminishing the appearance of them. Men are not exempt to this one as they are with cellulite. Though women are at the top of the list with complaints men experience rapid weight gain and loss as well. **The effectiveness of totally getting rid of stretch marks is based on the proper skin care that stabilizes collagen and elasticity in the skin.** Celebs undergo procedures such as laser scar removal and even surgical tummy tucks to get rid of these scars. The laser resurfacing method is usually done by a cosmetic surgeon or dermatologist.

Hydration is important to prevent stretch marks. Most people are dehydrated due to consumption of high sugar content in the drinks and lack of proper water intake. Most of us need more than eight glasses of water a day. We need to drink half our weight in ounces per day. Also, we use skin lotions and creams that deprive oxygen and moisture from the skin. I cannot say it enough, but petroleum based products damage the skin. RNA also known as Ribonucleic acid; involved in the replication of cells, is an ingredient in effective treatments that penetrate deep into the skin tissues. **Skin care products that contain RNA help to renew the skin and ultimately diminish and even remove stretch marks.** This is true for any type of scar repair treatment; not just stretch mark treatment.

Body Wraps

As a preventative measure for weight gain and loss it is a good tool to use measures such as body wraps and hydrating, cell regenerating products to prevent the stretch marks. **These methods are also effective in inch loss and cellulite reduction.** A good body wrap that I have seen to be effective is a contouring wrap. This wrap is an internal cleansing treatment that can be done on a weekly basis. The niacin (vitamin B3) in the wrap cream is complemented with the benefits of avocado, aloe vera, glycerin, garlic, and cinnamon. This helps to increase blood circulation, hydrate the tissue, and promote inch loss. **Though body wraps are not recommended during** pregnancy, shortly after pregnancy they make the perfect treatment to shrink the skin of the stomach, buttocks, hips, and thighs back to normal in a short period of time. I recommend not using body wraps that involve sweating or intensive exercise in a sweat suit for inch loss. These wraps may be called herbal wraps. This promotes dehydration due to the loss of water through sweat but also is not the best types of wrap to get more long term inch loss. Steam treatments are better at hydrating the skin but water consumption must be increased after wards. The water weight returns rapidly just as the inch loss. **Good body wraps contain inch loss over a period of days as the lymphatic system has been activated and will continue to cleanse for up to 72 hours.** These treatments are best performed in a spa by an experienced skin care specialist or esthetician.

Topical Creams

After stretch marks have become lighter in color they are harder to get rid of and need more invasive procedures to fade the scars. They can be diminished at this stage but not removed. It's best to treat in early stages of scarring when the stretch marks are darker in color. Many women apply cocoa butter, Shea butter, vitamin e, and other oils to effected areas during pregnancy. It is good practice to apply these ingredients to the affected areas during the full length of the pregnancy or any time the skin will be stretched once or twice daily. Vitamin a, sesame oil, cinnamon, and eucalyptus oils are also good ingredients to look for in stretch mark repair creams. These ingredients are rich in essential fatty acids promoting tissue repair and most effective when used together to hydrate, increase circulation, and repair cells.

There are many products that claim to get rid of stretch marks. The key is consistent usage of topical creams that provide hydration and circulation to the skin and contain RNA or collagen builders like vitamin A, E and C.

Avoid or prepare for rapid weight loss by always staying hydrated. Use body wraps and creams when stretch marks first appear.

Notes:

CLEAN HOUSE

YOUR HOME SHOULD BE YOUR HEAVEN

HOW TO KEEP A HOME IN THE HOOD
BY SCIHONOR DEVOTION

L et's keep it real. Some of us look good on the outside and – if you're reading this book, I have an idea that you want to be healthy on the inside – but honestly, some of us are living in filth at home!

It doesn't matter if you live in the projects, on a farm, in the suburbs, in a studio apartment, or in a huge house. **Filth is filth no matter where you are, and no matter where you are, you can practice basic refinement.**

Even the children can get involved. Some of us were taught as a child how to keep our homes and some were not. Please do not make the mistake of not teaching your child how to maintain their space. **Children can be guided on when and how to take care of certain age appropriate household chores.** If they get into the habit as a child, their partner/spouse won't complain about them later in life. Also, cleaning often will prevent your workload from piling up and becoming a huge mess. If you yourself were not taught proper housecleaning, please look at friends and family who are good examples and be inspired by their good habits and organization.

Safety

Keeping your home safe is the first thing to focus on. This means to make sure all drugs (legal and illegal) are not in the reach of children. This includes anything made from chemicals, especially cleaning supplies (such as bleach, ammonia, alcohol, peroxide, Ajax, etc.), vitamins, supplements, topical creams, etc. All cleaning supplies should be placed out of reach or in a sealed container that they can't get to. I have a friend whose son drank some cleaning supplies that he was keeping in a Snapple bottle. Needless to say, the boy had major health problems as a result and was eating through a tube for a while. Fortunately, he is better now.

If you have weapons, please be sure to keep them out of children's reach, yet make sure that if you need be, they are easily accessible to you. You can buy gun cases or safes to keep them out of the way. Having a home alarm, or extra locks, is not a bad idea in terms of an extra precaution to keep your family safe. It may even minimize the need for a gun under the pillow.

Oh, and I can't forget to remind you to make sure that you have working smoke alarms, carbon monoxide detectors, and fire extinguishers that everyone in the home knows how to use. Also, if you live in a building above the 1st floor, make sure your building owners have sufficient window guards. Trust me; I've heard too many fatal stories.

Germs, Germs, Everywhere

A dirty home can cause illness. Bacteria will grow wherever there is dirt and moisture. **Allergens such as dust can irritate you and your family, especially if you have asthma or another respiratory illness.** Shoes can be left at the door and replaced with slippers if necessary. This is especially great if you have children who are often on the floors.

I don't advocate dragging germs from the outside into your home. Just think about it…Look at where you live. You may be stepping on all kinds of sh*t.

The Bathroom – How can you clean yourself if the room is filthy?

There is nothing more horrific than going into a bathroom (public or private) that is wet. Wetness is a breeding ground for germs. **Strive to keep your bathroom dry to prevent germs from taking over and make sure you keep that toilet lid closed before flushing!**

Now, some people tend to cover their toothbrushes so that in case someone breaks the "close the toilet rule," their brush will be protected, if you have roaches, it is not a choice at all. Cover it! Either way, **I recommend disinfecting your brush weekly with peroxide and changing your brush at least once each month.**

Clean the flush handle, faucets, light switches and doorknobs daily, if possible. Bar soup should be avoided and replaced with "pump" soap. It's more sanitary. The garbage should be taken out often and the can should be cleaned before placing a new bag. Towels and washcloths should be changed at least once a week. **If you have males in the home, you may want to reconsider those toilet cover sets or the rugs that hug the bottom of the can.** If you must keep a plunger in your bathroom, please be sure to place it in some sort of container (bowl, flower pot, etc.). Please don't just allow it to sit on the floor next to the toilet after you've just plunged who knows what!

The Kitchen – How can you turn the light off on THAT?

Each night, a routine should be practiced that includes packing away uneaten food into the fridge, wiping countertops, the stovetop, the oven (if there was a spill in it), the dining table, sweeping floors, mopping up any spills (especially if you have pests/insects), tying the garbage, washing the dishes, and then disinfecting the sink and faucets. **Your refrigerator should be cleaned at least every two weeks.** I usually clean mine before I bring my groceries home after big shopping twice a month.

Meat should not be leaking in the fridge and should go directly from your refrigerator to the sink. **If you do use your countertops and sink for meat preparation, be sure to disinfect them properly.** Cutting boards should be scrubbed with hot soapy water after each use and soaked weekly in a mixture of peroxide, salt and vinegar.

The Bedroom – Heaven or Hell?

My bedroom is my heaven. This is where I go when I want to decompress and really relax. **Your bedroom will have a major impact on how you feel emotionally when entering it.** When I have laundry piled up on my bed that needs to be folded, I strive to quickly get rid of them. I love my bed and have rules for it. No, I'm not talking about having "Hospital Corners" although that would be nice. I'm talking about not allowing dirty "street clothes" on my bed so I don't end up in the hospital. I can't even imagine someone riding on the New York City's 2 train and then sitting or climbing in my bed with the same clothes on. That is just disgusting! And, how do people even think it's OK to get in bed with shoes on? That's just nasty! When I get in bed, I want to know that everything in it is clean, including my sheets. Sheets should be changed weekly.

Especially children's sheets, which will minimize their risk of parasites that many children have that their parents don't even know about. Also, if you are a drooler, or have a cold or other respiratory problems, your pillow cases should be changed often. **Just keep it simple and change the whole sheet set weekly.** Oh, and If you have multiple "partners," please change the sheets before you switch up, for their sake.

Getting Rid of Clutter

Your home should be a sacred, safe place, and a refuge from utter chaos. Yes, even in the hood! That being said, how can you strive to escape chaos by coming home to chaos? Now I know that many of you scholars reading this have hundreds of books, research and other knowledge all over your homes, however, in order for our homes to feel like a temple, you will have to organize. Our CDs, DVDs, books, computer station, important documents and paperwork, bills, mail, etc. should all have a place. **And I wouldn't recommend just tossing important mail in the dumpster. You never know who lurks around them and what they may be looking for.** Documents should be shredded as soon as we deem something unnecessary to keep. Mail should not pile up but should be sorted through each day, and each item should be put in its' correct place. Keeping a folder or some sort of organizer for current and paid bills is a good idea. Important documents such as passports, life insurance, health insurance, mortgage papers, rental receipts, public assistance documents, school information, social security cards, etc. should be stored somewhere, preferably in a safe. **Copies of important documents should also be put into your emergency supply kit.** Remember Katrina, when people were separated from their children and other family? Well, an emergency kit should be put together and each member of the family should have a "go" bag. These bags should be placed where they are easily accessible, yet out of the way.

Anyway, getting rid of clutter means that you may have to part with things that you may not want to. Trust me, getting rid of it will make you feel so much better. There are a few questions that you can ask yourself to help decide if you should toss it or keep it. These questions can be applied in any room of your home. They can actually be used in any area of the physical body as well, but that's a whole notha' article. They are…

☐ Why do I need this? If you can't answer that then it most likely needs to go, however, just to make sure, move to question #2.

☐ Have I ever used this and will I really ever use this? If not, get rid of it. You can give it away or just donate it to an organization, library, etc.

☐ Am I saving this for someone? If so, give it to them. Mail it if you won't be seeing them anytime soon or have them pick it up. If they want it, they will come get it. Give them a time period. If they miss it, the item goes out.

☐ Is this sentimental? This is where I get weak. I love sentimental items. Almost everything is sentimental to me. If someone gives me a journal, I don't write in it. If I get lotion, I only use a little bit as to try to save it for as long as possible. Point is, Use it! What's the point of having it just take up space? It was a gift, Enjoy it! If you are a collector, find a space for your collection in a reasonable amount of space.

☐ Am I making excuses for it? Be honest with yourself. If you are making excuses, just get rid of it.

❑ What's the worst thing that could happen if I don't have it anymore? Most likely, it's not that bad. You'll see. (For more, see "Let it Go")

Organizing is key. Notice how peaceful your home will become once everything is in its proper place, the mind and body are no different.

CLEAN HOUSE
WHAT TO USE (AND WHAT NOT TO) TO CLEAN YOUR HOME
BY LETITIA SALAZAR

We all know that we aren't supposed to drink bleach. However, bleach and its various shelf companions are toxic beyond ingestion. Skin exposure, fume inhalation and toxic residues are also hazardous. **Our chemically laden, store bought cleaners are poisons to our home environment.** Chemicals are not easily broken down; instead they bind to our cells and are stored in adipose (fat), joints and connective tissues, etc...for years.

Environmental chemical agents play a role in long term health decline. Bleach, toilet bowl cleaners, window cleaners, floor cleaners, disinfectants and air fresheners all have damaging effects on the respiratory, nervous, immune and digestive systems, as well as, the skin and eyes. Synthetic chemicals aggravate and contribute to conditions like asthma, bronchitis, migraines, auto-immune diseases, allergies, arthritis, and so on. You can find known carcinogens or toxic preservatives such as formaldehyde in common cleaners we have come to depend on. **To add insult to injury, most of these synthetic compounds are extremely inexpensive to produce and we pay high mark ups.**

The **occasional** use of chlorine bleach, ammonia, disinfectants, fabric softeners, detergents, abrasives and all-purpose cleansers are not of major concern to our health. However, if used **regularly** and **in combination** while cleaning these practices increase the danger they pose to our health. Their use should be limited to the occasional outbreaks of the plague, body fluid clean-ups and aberrant refrigerator morphology. Most of the time, **everyday cleaning can be**

accomplished with safe, simple and inexpensive homemade products.

Here is a beginner's list of natural, safe, inexpensive ingredients you can put together in just a few minutes. Next time you make up your grocery list consider some of these alternatives. The options are infinite. **You can concoct cleaning products of your own that are economical, safe, effective and pleasant.** I have given you a few ideas to get you started, but there is a ton of websites and literature available to those who really want to take this practice to new and creative levels in their homes.

Baking Soda

Baking soda is, in short, fantastic! At approximately a $1 a box, it is easily the most affordable of your natural cleaners. It is useful in so many ways, this serves as only a brief introduction.

Scouring agent: A wonderful replacement for Ajax, Comet and other scouring powders. Shake directly on surfaces (bath tubs, sinks, toilets, countertops) and scrub away. Use for brushing teeth, facial scrub, removing grease from pots and pans, laundry detergent, polishing chrome, removing crayon marks, dishwashing (by hand or in dishwashing machine), etc.

Deodorizer: For ages it has been kept in refrigerators to minimize food odors, but it can be used in shoes, litter boxes, carpets, upholstery, deodorant, cleaning your coffee pot, trash cans, etc.

Baking soda is just Sodium bicarbonate, a naturally occurring salt. Its use has been traced back to ancient Egyptians who used natron, a combination of sodium compounds including sodium bicarbonate, as soap. It is a safe, natural chemical compound that can be combined safely with solvents such as water and vinegar for many uses.

All-purpose spray: Add ¼ cup baking soda to 1 quart of water in a large spray bottle. Shake until dissolved. Store for use on various household surfaces and for washing fruits and vegetables prior to consumption.

Keep dry powder baking soda handy as your go-to abrasive (scrubbing agent) and deodorizer. Add 1 tsp of lemon juice to ¼ cup baking soda and use for scrubbing away bathroom/kitchen scum. Use with a liquid castile soap (such as, Dr. Bronner's) for good measure.

Carpet deodorizer: Add Lavender flowers to 1 cup of baking soda. Shake directly onto the carpet, allow sitting and vacuuming up.

Ant repellent: Blend equal parts baking soda and table salt, shake around the areas where the ants are coming in to discourage entry.

Drain cleaner: Use equal parts baking soda and white vinegar. Pour baking soda directly into your drain, follow by pouring the white vinegar into the drain. Allow to sit in the drain for about 15 minutes. It will bubble enthusiastically. Rinse with boiling water. (Caution: Don't use this technique if you have recently used a chemical drain cleaner)

When using baking soda, remember to rinse thoroughly.

Vinegar

White vinegar, like baking soda, is simple and inexpensive. It also has a wide array of uses. Vinegar is derived from the fermentation process of a variety of plant products. Vinegar is acidic, it can cut through oils, odors and germs.

Disinfectant: Kills germs. Great for bathrooms and kitchens. It can be a great alternative to bleach or Lysol during cold and flu season. Use a vinegar solution to clean toys and play areas, handles, doorknobs, light switches and whatever else you can think of. I spray my vinegar cleanser on the countertops, kitchen table, wipe it clean and have full confidence that I and my family will be able to sit right down with food or homework without fear that we'll be consuming harmful fumes. It is great for cleaning vegetables prior to consumption.

Deodorizer: If you are like me and find satisfaction with that clean "smell" that comes from the lingering aroma of cleansers, then you too may enjoy vinegar. It has a very mild but reassuring scent that lets you know that even though you are finished cleaning, it is still working on your behalf. Trash cans, refrigerators, sinks, drains, animal accidents on the floor (specifically indicated for hardwoods) – I use it for mopping floors, regularly.

Please note: Although, safe, vinegar is acidic. It should be diluted for most uses, unless a recipe specifically indicates otherwise and even then, trust your own comfort level for dilution. It is not advisable to use on marble surfaces.

Handy cleaning solution: Add ¼ cup white vinegar to 1 quart of water. Keep in a readily accessible spray bottle for use as needed. When cleaning your bathtub, spray on the entire surface then shake baking soda onto the damp surface and scrub.

Laundry soap: Mix 1/8 cup liquid soap, 1 tablespoon washing soda (also known as Sodium carbonate, which is close to baking soda, but not the same thing, though typically sold on the same store shelf), and ¼ cup vinegar.

Dryer Sheets: You need 2 cups vinegar, an essential oil of choice (lavender, lemon, etc.), and some rags. Combine vinegar and essential oil into a large jar and shake well. Fill the jar with rags and add 1 rag to your dryer load.

Other Essentials

Liquid Soap/Castile soap: A great surfactant that does not contain sulfates (lathering agents). It's a great addition to your homemade cleaning recipes, but can be used as is for the household or on the body.

Oxygen bleach: An effective alternative to chlorine bleach. Oxygen bleach is safer and more environmentally friendly than chlorine bleach. It removes stains and whitens. Powder oxygen bleaches are either sodium percarbonate or sodium perborate. Liquid oxygen bleach is also known as hydrogen peroxide. Both powder and liquid forms can be added to the laundry or used for a wide range of cleaning jobs common and tough.

Lemon juice: An effective mild acid. Useful for breaking up mineral deposits, soap scum and disinfecting. Removes stains and polishes surfaces (woods and metals). Leaves a pleasant, healthy fragrance behind.

Essential Oils

These are the lipid constituents of plants that have been isolated for concentrated applications. Essential oils can be used to add non-perfume fragrances to your blends and have the added benefit of being therapeutic.

Citrus oils: Lemon, orange, mandarin, and grapefruit are anti-microbial and mood elevating. They will add "lightness" to the atmosphere of your home.

Flower oils: Such as, lavender, rose, jasmine, vanilla and chamomile provide a relaxing energy.

Mint oils: Peppermint and spearmint will add anti-viral therapies while giving an energy lift.

Tree/bush oils: Tea tree, spruce, rosemary, frankincense and pine oil are also anti-microbial. They invigorate and stimulate the respiratory system making your home "breathable."

Of course, essential oils have innumerable applications and therapeutic benefits. Try one at a time and then try them in combination. They can be used on surfaces all around the home and in the laundry. For these purposes, any of the brands sold in your local health foods market will work fine.

Recommended Reading

Many of the following books can be found used on Amazon.com for as little as $0.01: *Clean & Green* by Annie Berthold-Bond; *The Nontoxic Baby* by Natural Choices; *Dan's Practical Guide to Least Toxic Home Pest Control* by Dan Stein; *Home Safe Home: Protecting Yourself and Your Family from Everyday Toxics and Harmful Household Products in the Home* by Debra Dadd; and *The Healthy Home: An Attic-To-Basement Guide to Toxin-Free Living* by Linda Hunter

---

Transition away from toxic chemicals into natural alternatives. Get the support from everyone in the household. Share this article.

DON'T LET THE BED BUGS BITE

BY SCIHONOR DEVOTION

You can find almost anything in the hood. But what you will almost inevitably find in the hood are bugs and bugs do bite. There are bugs all over but some can harm us more than others. Did you know that roaches can bite? Well, they can. Be sure that you and your children go to bed with clean faces because you can actually get bitten by a roach if you happen to have crumbs on your face!

Bed Bugs

Even though I grew up hearing that bedtime rhyme, "Good night, sleep tight, don't let the bed bugs bite," I didn't know that bed bugs were actually real live insects. For some reason, I thought they were as real as the Tooth Fairy or Santa Claus. Years into

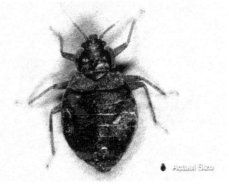

♦ Actual Size

my adulthood, come to find out these suckers are real. And they are literally suckers too.

Bed bugs have been a huge issue in big cities lately. They're usually reddish brown in color and have flat oval-shaped bodies. They are about 4-5 millimeters long (size of a pin's head). Their babies are usually translucent or light tan in color. They live off a host's blood and usually feed off of you during the night time hours while you are resting. They pierce the skin and inject saliva into your skin. Bed bug bites are often small, red marks. They are often found in a row, which is sometimes called the breakfast, lunch and dinner row, since they've probably bitten you three different times. Sometimes, you may not even know that you are being bitten. **Some people have allergic reactions.** It's rare, but can happen. If you experience shortness of breath, wheezing, chest pains, difficulty swallowing, a swollen tongue or lips, dizziness, itchy rashes or fever, it may be an allergic reaction.

It's possible for human diseases to be transmitted but it has not yet been totally established. These bugs hide in seams, cracks and crevices in mattresses, box springs, couches, bed frames, baseboards, furniture, wall paper, curtains, and even clutter. They stay close to the host, so they are usually in the bedrooms. Bed bugs can be picked up and brought home from hotels, dorms, apartments, hospitals, buses, movie theaters, etc. They are easily transported through clothing, bags, and even used furniture. So before you bring that nice dresser that you found on the curb home, remember that it may just be out there because it is infested with bed bugs. Inspect your home. Check the borders of your mattresses and box springs for dark spots which are actually the feces of the bed bugs. I have heard of people doing all kinds of things to prevent or rid their homes of bed bugs.

- ❑ Some people put bowls of water under all four of their bed rails. This will often catch and drown the bugs.
- ❑ Go to bed with your skin covered
- ❑ Get rid of clutter and seal holes and cracks
- ❑ Wash everything that can be washed in hot water. Then dry on high heat.
- ❑ Steam clean everything that can't not be washed in the washing machine
- ❑ Put your mattress and box spring in plastic covers made for mattresses and cover the zipper with duct tape once it's closed.
- ❑ Call an exterminator. They have both chemical insecticides and organic insecticides which include Eucalyptus and Peppermint essential oils.
- ❑ Spray your furniture and floor borders with alcohol in a spray bottle.

Dust Mites

Dust mites live in warm, moist places like mattresses, couches, pillows and carpets. They cannot be seen with the naked eye and live off of dead skin cells (also called dander) of humans and pets. Sometimes, people can actually have an allergic reaction to the waste dropping from the mites and may experience sneezing, itching, watery eyes and may even contribute to lifelong illnesses in children into their adulthood like asthma, eczema and hay fever. To avoid these possibilities, vacuum, wash your sheets and pillows at least once a week in hot water, and just strive to keep a clean home.

Head Lice

Head lice are parasites usually found in children's hair. Because of the way they attach themselves to fine or wavy hair, they are rarely found on those of us with a coarser texture of hair.[39] Full-grown adults are approximately the size of a sesame seed. The color of head lice tends to match the hair color of their human hosts, ranging from pale tan to dark brown. They are slow feeders and cling tightly to head hair while feeding. **They can be transferred from person to person by having direct and indirect contact.** So, you can get it if you try on a hat that a lice infected head had on, or a scarf, or a headrest in the movie theater, or in a bed, coat, carpet, hair supplies like combs, brushes and barrettes, and even off of teddy bears.

Pubic Lice

Pubic lice is a whole notha kind of lice and is usually spread through sexual contact, but not always. "Crabs" as they are often called, can be passed through bedding, clothing, towels, and anything that may be shared that is soft like fabric. So, if your partner says they got crabs from a toilet seat, you can go ahead and knock them over the head, because they're probably lying. (Crabs can't live away from a host for too long, because they live off of blood and their bodies are not equipped to hang out on smooth surfaces like toilet seats.) Anyway, crabs can even live in your eyebrows, facial hair, under your arms, or wherever course hair is.

There are a few things you can do if you have head lice, body lice, or crabs:

- ❏ Scratch the heck out of the area because it will itch like hell. (Just joking. Don't do that)
- ❏ Get an over the counter remedy from the local pharmacy.
- ❏ Know that cutting your hair probably won't help since they may have even laid eggs on your head or skin.
- ❏ For those who don't want to use an over the counter remedy, make something at home. Here's a recipe: 5 tsp Carrier Oil (Olive Oil or Coconut Oil), 5 drops of each essential oil – Tea Tree, Rosemary, Lavender and Eucalyptus, and about 3 oz. Peppermint Castile or Tea Tree Castile Soap
- ❏ Wash with this solution and use a "nit" comb which can be bought at the local pharmacy and rinse with vinegar or apple cider vinegar at least 2 times a day for a week. You may begin to see results after the second day.

---

[39] However, I've read that even the lice in Africa has been "Africanized" like the African Killer Bees and are able to attach to coarse hair easier than the lice in other continents.

- While you are bathing in oils and vinegar, like a potato chip, be sure to wash all of the clothing that you've worn or used like bedding in hot water and dry on high.
- Also, there may be things that you cannot wash like teddy bears. Bag them up in plastic bags and keep it sealed for at least two weeks.
- Be sure to vacuum mattresses, couches, chairs, rugs, floors, car seats, and anything else that you may have been in contact with that they may be living in. Then be sure to get rid of the vacuum bag.

Mosquitoes

If you get bitten by a mosquito, pour some vinegar, apple cider vinegar or lemon juice directly on it. This will help reduce the irritation. You can also make a paste of baking soda and water and dab it right on the bite site.[40] Mosquitoes like stagnant water. Stay away from it. Better yet, clean it up, so they have no water to live near. **Mosquitoes don't like camphor and citronella. Burn candles with these scents, burn the essential oils, or even wear them to keep these bugs away.**

Bees

When bees sting, they leave their stinger inside your skin, which releases venom. If you get stung by a bee, don't squeeze the area where the stinger is, because it will aggravate the venom sac left in your body. Instead, take a straight edge like a credit card and scrape the stinger away from your skin. Wash the area with soap and water and apply a cold pack for about 20 minutes. You can also pour some vinegar, apple cider vinegar, or lemon or lime juice directly on it. For wasp stings, you can cut an onion in half and place the open face of the onion directly on the sting site. If you begin to feel nausea, dizziness, stomach cramps, diarrhea, itching all over, hives or wheezing, you may be and need to go to a hospital fast.

Spiders

Spider bites are another issue to look out for. Two poisonous spiders to specifically look out for are the Black Widow and Brown Recluse. Black Widows are usually found in the southern states of the United States. The Southern Black Widow has the red hour glass shape on its belly, while the Northern Black Widow can have red, yellow or white marks on its body. If you get bitten by a Black Widow, within 15

---

[40] Fortunately, mosquitoes don't usually kill people here in the United States as they often do in many countries. While it isn't a concern here, you should know about malaria, simply because it's a preventable illness that kills millions, 90% of whom live in Africa. You can learn more about how you can help prevent these deaths at www.MalariaNoMore.org

minutes, you will feel her wrath. Her venom attacks the nervous system. You will get stiff muscles, vomit, sweat profusely, and have respiratory difficulties and dizziness.

The Brown Recluse, sometimes referred to as the Fiddle Back because of a violin shaped mark on its back, is usually found in the Midwestern and Southeastern states. If you get bitten by one, it may take between 4 and 8 hours to see its bite mark. Its bite may eventually turn into a blister type area. You will feel itching, nausea, vomiting, fever and muscle pain.

Here's a few things you can do to keep spiders out of your home:

- ☐ Get rid of clutter in attics, basements and garages.
- ☐ Clean your home thoroughly, regularly.
- ☐ Make sure your screens are tight fitting.
- ☐ If necessary, get an exterminator.

Ticks

Lyme Disease is carried by the Deer Tick. These things are often found in tall grass and often bite people in their ankles and legs. **If a tick bites you, use tweezers to pull it straight out.** Don't twist and turn it since that will irritate it even more. **Don't burst the tick either. Its goo can still spread infection.** Within 7-10 days, a rash will appear at the bite site. You may experience fever, muscle pain, joint aches, and swollen lymph glands. Lyme disease can get worse if it's not treated.

Keep things extra clean at home, wear appropriate amounts of clothing, and be mindful of little bites on your skin.

AIR OUT YOUR DIRTY LAUNDRY
BY SCIHONOR DEVOTION

Plenty of times, I have walked into a Laundromat and seen people putting their dirty clothes on the counter tops or in the clothing carts, either to get them from the car to the washing machine or to sort out the different colors. **I've seen people put clothes with vomit or sneakers with sh*t on them in washing machines.** I've even seen children in the carts. My suggestion would be to get a good ol' washing board to use at home. Just joking…

- ☐ Sort and fold your clothes at home.
- ☐ Add Eucalyptus, Lavender and/or Tea Tree to your soap. If you don't have any of that stuff, put a little ammonia in the soap just to kill some germs.

- Whatever you decided to add to your soap, take a little of that and mix it with some water in a spray bottle to clean out the machine, dryer, carts and countertops before you use them.
- Also, if you have to use the clothes carts, line them with a plastic bag or even your laundry bag if you have nothing else to use.
- Lastly, be careful with those scented detergents and dryer sheets. They may smell good but everything that smells good ain't always good for you. (See "Clean House")

Make sure what you use to clean your clothes is clean itself!

THE DANGERS OF HAVING PETS IN THE HOME

BY TAMIKA HOGAN

Having pets can be good for adults and children alike. The benefits can include companionship, affection, teaching responsibility (and caretaking) to children, feeling protected, and the relationship that is formed and shared with the pet. **Historically, people kept their pets outdoors** (in their natural environment), **rather than allowing them to share the same beds and bathwater, as many pet-owners do now.** We can't expect to reverse a trend in the way people now relate to their "animal friends" but we can try to help keep you safe if you choose to keep your pet in the home.

> **Did you Know?**
> Dogs are responsible for almost 5 million bites each year? About half a million of those bites need medical attention and about half of those who get bitten are children. Some are even killed. All dogs don't have the same temperament that maybe your neighbor's poochie has. So, don't approach a strange dog. If you're approached, don't run and scream. Stand still and it may just sniff you or lick you. Ewww. If you get knocked down by the dog and you don't have a weapon, don't worry about how you look. Just roll up into a ball and stay still like a little b*tch. But seriously though, I'm serious. Don't ever challenge a dog by staring at it in the eye. You don't wanna have a Boondocks-type "n*gga moment"

Many of us don't know that there are many dangers surrounding having pets in the home, threating the health of people who co-exist with these pets. **There are many diseases and infections known as Zoonotic Diseases** (also as Zoonoses) **that are transmittable to humans.**

Humans who have compromised immune systems (Asthmatics, Bronchitis, people who have autoimmune diseases such as HIV/AIDS, cancer patients, organ transplant recipients) **need to be very careful of not contracting pet carrying humanly contagious diseases.** African Americans are statistically the most vulnerable and afflicted by the ailments listed below, so we need to be extra careful with pets in our home and around our children. **Additionally, young children, infants, and pregnant women are at a great risk of**

being affected by these diseases.

Just like humans, pets carry germs. Some illnesses, common among house pets, that can be transmitted to humans include distemper, canine parvovirus, rabies, ringworm, flea and tick diseases, Lymohocytic choriomeningitis (LCM), and heartworms, just to name a few out of the hundreds known.

When Playful Scratches and Bites go Wrong

Distemper is a paramyxovirus, which appears to be very similar to the paramyxovirus that causes measles in humans. In cats and dogs, distemper can affect a wide range of organs including the skin, brain, eyes, and intestinal and respiratory tracts. The virus is transmitted through the air through coughing by infected animals and also through body secretion such as urine. It mostly affects animals less than 6 months of age.

Distemper is contagious to human's when/if the human is bitten or scratched by the infected animal. It is highly contagious to other animals that may be around and can be fatal. Almost all pet owners have been "playfully" bitten or scratched by their pet. So take precaution by getting your pet vaccinated and keeping the pet from other animals that may be infected.

Canine Parvovirus is Common

Canine Parvovirus is another disease that can be spread from pets to humans and is the most commonly spread disease in the United States. It is a highly contagious disease that is characterized by diarrhea that is oftentimes bloody. **Any contact with feces containing the virus can cause the disease to spread. The virus is known to survive on inanimate objects such as clothing, food pans, and cage floors. This virus can remain in these locations for up to 5 months or more in certain conditions.** Insects and rodents can serve as vessels for transmission of this virus. The symptoms of "parvo" include vomiting, diarrhea, dehydration, dark/bloody feces and in severe cases, lowered white blood cell counts. While these symptoms sound familiar to other infectious diseases that pets carry, parvo is mostly diagnosed through a test for specific enzymes in the feces.

Parvoviruses are more contagious to other animals than they are to humans; however, there is a strain of the parvovirus that is harmful to young children. **Parvovirus B19 virus causes Erythema infectiosum** (Fifth disease) **in children, especially those between the ages of 5 and 15.** Fifth disease typically produces a distinctive red rash on the face that makes the child appear to have a "slapped cheek." The rash then spreads to the trunk, arms, and legs. Fifth disease is actually just a viral illness that most kids recover from quickly and without complications (or so they say), there are no studies on long term or re-occurring bouts of fifth disease to date.

When cleaning an infected area, gloves and masks should be used as well as a bleach solution on all bedding, dishes, kennel floors and other materials that may have been contaminated. An infected canine is treated with intravenous fluids, antibiotics, antiserums against endotoxins and/or corticosteroids (if the animal is in shock).

You Don't Want Heartworms

Heartworms can affect dogs and cats and like the other diseases, can be transmitted to humans. They are located in the right side of the animals' heart and the large blood vessels connecting the heart to the lungs (Similar to the hookworm that attaches itself to another major organ, but the hookworm typically comes from ingesting pork and other undercooked meats). **Heartworms are contracted to animals through mosquitoes that have bitten infected animals.** Infected animals can live up to 7 years and can have several hundred heartworms in their hearts and vessels.

Heartworms can migrate to the lungs where the larvae can block vessels causing an infarction (an area of dead tissue caused by the blocking of blood circulation). At the site of the infarction, a nodule develops which can be seen through radiographs. The human may or may not show any signs of infection and in most cases the nodules have to be surgically removed. So how does that work for Black people with no health insurance or for those who do NOT have regular check-ups? **Many people walk around carrying this disease until it affects some other part of their body or causes some other illness. Eventually the person dies from one or the other.**

Also, other types of worms, like hookworms and ringworms, can be transmitted through the skin and can even penetrate through your feet if you walk barefoot. These worms are present in dogs, cats, other pets, as well as the animals that humans eat for food.

Lymphocytic choriomeningitis is a Big Word for Rat Nastiness

For those of you who like rodents (rats, mice, hamsters) as pets – the diseases they carry are airborne and are highly contagious to humans. One disease is known as Lymphocytic choriomeningitis (LCM). It is a contagious viral disease that is transmitted by inhaling infectious airborne particles of rodent urine, feces, saliva, or ingesting food contaminated with the virus.

Cat Litter can Kill...Really.

For the cat lovers, your cat may be the carrier of a parasite causing toxoplasmosis. It is usually transmitted through contact with their feces (cleaning cat litter boxes) as well as eating raw or undercooked meat. **Toxoplasmosis can cause miscarriage, birth defects and premature births** (which is why pregnant women are instructed NOT to clean cat litter boxes during pregnancy). Let's not even talk about the folks who have a rodent infestation in their home and decides that getting a cat is the best way to get rid of that rodent infestation. So now they have a pet cat that eats mice and they have to clean the cats' feces out of the litter box. So they would actually be doing more harm to their family than they know.

Don't Sniff the Pee

The smell of pet urine in the home can be both physically and emotionally harmful. And the urine of female dogs is worst to children and adults than male dog's urine, due to the higher content of ammonia.

If your home is too small to receive adequate ventilation, inhalation can burn the lungs and the throat. This is more dangerous for an infant, who still has developing organs which the smell of ammonia can affect negatively. The foul smell of urine can also trigger headaches in humans. Even after you believe that you have cleaned up the urine, if there is any trace of the smell, there may be mold growing where the urine was. Mold can attract harmful bacteria that are dangerous to humans. **For those of you who are allergic to pet dander, the smell of pet urine can also trigger one's allergies.**

Don't Get Freaky With Animals...Even if You Stop at "First Base"

So now you want to kiss a dog or cat in the mouth. This same dog or cat that grooms himself, his offspring, the floor, underwear (female dogs will lick human female's underwear if there are any signs of blood from menstruation), and anything else with its MOUTH. That is just disgusting. **No human should be kissing any animals on the mouth, especially not the French kissing we typically see among "pet lovers."**

Let me not forget to mention that dogs with folded faces (or smushed-in faces) such as Sharpeis, Pugs, and Boston Terriers, can have bacterial infections accumulating in their lip folds, which by the way can be transmitted to humans. Kissing these types of dogs in the mouth can cause the human to contract that infection which results in a very nasty and re-occurring skin rash on their MOUTH! Then they kiss their spouse, kids, mother, etc. That's just NASTY! If you need any more encouragement, just keep in mind that **dogs and cats can even carry the herpes simplex virus.**

The Problem with Chemical Cleaners

Other toxic and harmful situations that humans risk by having pets in the home are the vast array of toxic chemicals that are used in products that protect the animals from infections and diseases. These toxic chemicals are also in other common cleaning products (See "Be Clean").

Most of these products contain "organophosphate insecticides" (OPs). **OPs are dangerous and affect the brain and the nervous system.** Some even contain cancer-causing poisons. In large doses or heavy exposure, these OPs can kill animals and humans alike. The most common OPs are chlorpyrifos, dichlorvos, phosmet, naled, tetrachlorvinphos, diazinon and malathion and they are the most active ingredients in dozens of pet products and pesticides. If your dog or cat has a Hartz collar, you're being poisoned, slowly but surely.

The EPA is still working on assessing the risks associated with these products and cannot legally prohibit their sales. Their focus has been on the two most significant risks: risks from poisoning and risks from long-term effects on the brain and the nervous system. The only resolution at this point is to use safer alternatives. They have products on the market that include insect growth regulators (IGRs), which are not pesticides but chemicals that arrest the growth and the development of young fleas. Doesn't sound as poisonous, but doesn't sound healthy either. Another EPA suggestion – frequent washing and combing of the pet and vacuuming carpets and furniture which can bring a mild flea infestation under control. A MILD FLEA INFESTATION huh? Again, that doesn't sound healthy.

So you decide. Is keeping a pet in the home harmful to you and your family? Are you taking the right precautions to safeguard you, your family and your pet? Or is having that pet indoors even worth all of these risks?

Every person, place, or thing has its proper place in your life. How close to your heart will you keep your pet?

---

11 THINGS NOT TO GET FROM THE DOLLAR STORE

BY KING DIVINE ALLAH

There are many things you can buy from the dollar store that are great bargains, like wastebaskets, party decorations, and even some basic tools. But **when dealing with things you put on your body or in**

your system, you may want to rethink going cheap. It won't do you any justice saving money on products that may cause more harm than good.

Olive/Vegetable Oil: I don't care if the bottle says extra virgin olive oil and has pictures of olives on the label it's not pure olive oil, as a matter of fact its 94% soybean oil (which is probably fake soy beans – GMO's) and 6% olive oil. Vegetable oil is no exemption. After it has been processed it resembles cellulose or plastic more than oil. (See "Oils Are Not Health Foods")

Household cleaners: Products such as oven cleaner, all-purpose cleaners, detergents, furniture polish etc.

Soap: Dollar store soap is usually made of animal fat full of synthetic hormones, coloring, and chemicals. (See "Washing Up is Not the Same as Bathing")

Juice: All dollar store juices are either juices that are from concentrate or juices that are loaded with synthetic sweeteners (High Fructose Corn Syrup) and food coloring. Some of these juices actually have more sugar than sodas and full of synthetic colors and "natural flavors." (See "Beetle Juice")

Deodorant: Many deodorants are anti-perspirants, meaning they stop your underarms from sweating. The problem with that is that your body doesn't sweat just to cool you down; sweating also eliminates liquid toxins from your body. Deodorant containing benzoic and chlorate hydrate can actually prevent this elimination leading to kidney disorders. (See "K.O. The B.O")

Meat: Meat from the dollar store more than likely is the worst part of the meat that you can get from a hormone-pumped animal, whose living condition probably made its health deteriorate. Look at the package it has ingredients like mechanically separated meat (chicken, pork, and beef). This sh*t looks like some nasty ass pink grayish paste. It is made up of the bones, hooves, immature sex glands and left over tissue. All they do is strip the animal of the higher quality cuts and put this carcass at high temperature through a sieve.

Toothpaste: Some dollar stores sell expired and foreign non-ADA standard formulations of toothpaste, and because some of these products are foreign, manufacturers don't have to go by the same rules and regulation as American Companies do.

Vitamins: According to a 2004 *Consumer Reports* study of multi-vitamins, some of the nutrients listed on the label were missing from half of the 18 dollar store brands tested and other vitamins didn't dissolve fast enough to be absorbed by the body. They recommend sticking to the tried and true mainstream brands sold in pharmacies. Not only do the dollar store versions serve no purpose, some contain animal fat and harmful food colorings.

Medicine: Like vitamins, dollar store medicine is old and outdated. This is a waste of money because when medicine is out of date it loses its potency. So if you take them you will feel little to no effect from the meds.

Condoms and Pregnancy Tests: I know that they now have condoms and pregnancy tests at the dollar store, but I still would not suggest that you buy them. Think about it, why someone would want to spend $1.00 on a pack of condoms or a no named pregnancy test when you can get these items for free at your local health clinic. It's one thing to get a bargain at the dollar store but it's another thing when you have resources that provide these needed items free of charge. Take advantage.

Some dollar store products aren't as effective or safe as you may think. Sometimes, cheaper isn't better.

Notes:

APPENDIX

In the following pages, you'll find tons of resources to help you along your journey, including helpful guides to vitamins, minerals, nutritional deficiencies, and animal ingredients, and dozens of other things you'll want to use, possibly just to show off how smart you are. Whatever works for you.

THE ESSENTIAL VITAMIN GUIDE

"God, in His infinite wisdom, neglected nothing and if we would eat our food without trying to improve, change or refine it, thereby destroying its life-giving elements, it would meet all requirements of the body." – Jethro Kloss

Food provides our body with the fuel it needs to function. And because our body is so complex and multi-layered, there are different things we need from the food we eat. It's more than just calories and carbohydrates for energy, vitamins and minerals keep every system in our bodies fine-tuned and healthy. Nothing wrong with good flavor, but flavor without nutrition is like the wagon without the horse (or a fresh paint job without the car, for you modern folks who never heard of folk sayings).

What are Vitamins?

"The human body heals itself and nutrition provides the resources to accomplish the task." – Roger Williams Ph.D.

Vitamins are organic substances which help change the food we eat into skin, muscles, nerves, and other parts of our bodies which a basic, balanced diet provides. Certain vitamins lacking in our diet causes deficiency diseases. On the same note, vitamins in excess of what the body needs may actually produce illness rather than increase health and wellbeing. Many scientific studies have shown that a high dietary intake of vitamins is associated with health and a low dietary intake of vitamins is associated with disease. Unfortunately, many of the vitamins in our foods are often rendered inactive before we get a chance to consume them. Loss of vitamin content occurs in food products because of all the methods used to "treat" our food before it gets to us, including: overheating, processing, preservation, pasteurization, irradiation, and genetic modification. Thus, the best sources for vitamins are found in raw and fresh fruits and vegetables, the peels of fruits and vegetables (and the outer covering of some grains), and the hearts of many grains, seeds, and fruits. It's also clear that the nutrients in food work best in conjunction with each other, rather than isolated in supplements.

"Nutrition can be compared with a chain in which all essential items are separate links. We know what happens if one link of a chain is weak or is missing. The whole chain falls apart." – Patrick Wright, Ph.D.

Our bodies need at least 13 vitamins to function, which fall into two specific vitamin groups:

Fat-soluble (stored in the body's fatty tissue and the liver)	Water soluble (not stored so they must be taken into the body every day)	
Vitamin A	Vitamin B1	Vitamin B7
Vitamin D	Vitamin B2	Vitamin B9
Vitamin E	Vitamin B3	Vitamin B12
Vitamin K	Vitamin B5	Vitamin C
	Vitamin B6	

Vitamin A (Retinol in animal foods/Beta-carotene in plant foods)

Functions: Helps you see normally in the dark, promotes the growth and health of all body cells and tissues, and protects against infection by keeping healthy the skin and tissues in the mouth, stomach, intestines and respiratory and uro-genital tract.

Deficiency problems: Night blindness and other eye problems; dry, scaly skin, problems with reproduction, poor growth.

Food sources: Beta-carotene can be found in brightly colored fruits and vegetables such as apricots, pumpkins, and carrots, as well as leafy green vegetables, squash and melon.

Excess amounts: Can lead to birth defects, headaches, vomiting, double vision, hair loss, bone abnormalities and liver damage.

Vitamin B1 (Thiamin)

Functions: Converts bloods sugar into energy, and is involved in key metabolism. Promotes growth and is a tonic for the nerves. There is some evidence that vitamin B1 may help to improve IQ/ memory and it may help to control diabetes.

Deficiency problems: Alcoholics are frequently low in thiamin and suffer fatigue, weak muscles and nerve damage as a result. Depression, irritability, withdrawal, and schizoid tendencies can also be symptoms of deficiency.

Food sources: Whole grains, potatoes, nuts and legumes. Legumes include beans, lentils, peas, and peanuts.

Excess amounts: In very high doses (usually only possible with supplements), excessive thiamin can be toxic. But excessive natural intake of thiamin is expelled in the urine.

Vitamin B2 (Riboflavin)

Functions: Helps all body cells produce energy. Riboflavin is an antioxidant, also involved in the production of red blood cells and maintaining a healthy heart.

Deficiency problems: Severely malnourished people may suffer eye disorders (such as cataracts), dry and flaky skin, and a sore red tongue.

Food sources: Milk and other dairy products (particularly yogurt), whole grain products, eggs, green leafy vegetables, nuts, mushrooms, leafy green vegetables and yeast extracts.

Excess amounts: No known toxicity.

Vitamin B3 (Niacin)

Functions: Helps the body use sugars and fatty acids, and helps all body cells produce energy. It also helps enzymes function in the body, aids the nervous system, helps digestion, and maintains healthy skin.

Deficiency problems: Symptoms include diarrhea, mental disorientation (including anxiety, confusion, fatigue, and depression) and skin problems.

Food sources: Some niacin is produced in the body. Foods high in protein, such as peanut butter and legumes, whole grains, nuts and yeast extracts are also usually good sources.

Excess amounts: Excessive intake of nicotinic acid (a form of niacin), which usually only occurs with supplements, may cause flushed (reddish, itchy) skin, liver damage, stomach ulcers and high blood sugar.

Vitamin B5 (Pantothenic Acid)

Functions: Helps all body cells produce energy by helping metabolize protein, fat and carbohydrate in food. It also aids in healing wounds, fights infections, strengthens the immune system and helps build cells.

Deficiency problems: Rare in healthy people who eat a balanced diet.

Food sources: All vegetables and many other foods, including whole grain cereals, oats, eggs, dried fruits and nuts.

Excess amounts: May cause occasional diarrhea and water retention.

Vitamin B6 (Pyridoxine)

Functions: Helps the body make proteins, which are then used to make body cells. It's required for the functioning of more than 60 enzymes, aids the nervous system, protects against certain types of cancer, and helps produce other body chemicals such as insulin, hemoglobin and antibodies to fight infection.

Deficiency problems: Depression, nausea, mental convulsions in infants and greasy, flaky skin.

Food sources: Legumes, eggs, whole grains, nuts, yeast extract, soybeans and bananas.

Excess amounts: Can cause nerve damage.

Vitamin B7 (Biotin)

Functions: Helps all body cells produce energy. It also helps metabolize protein, fat and carbohydrates in food.

Deficiency problems: Heart abnormalities, appetite loss, fatigue, depression and dry skin.

Food sources: Peanuts and peanut butter, almonds, eggs, yeast breads and cereals.

Excess amounts: No known toxicity.

Vitamin B9 (Folate, Folacin or Folic Acid)

Functions: Plays an essential role in the metabolism of sugar, the manufacture of antibodies, the normal function of the nervous system, red blood cell formation in bone marrow, and for the normal production of DNA and RNA, which determines hereditary patterns.

Deficiency problems: Impaired cell division and growth, a type of anemia, and, during the first trimester of pregnancy, increased risk of delivering a baby with neural tube defects including spina bifida.

Food sources: Brewer's yeast, green leafy vegetables, oranges, bananas, red fruits, nuts, avocado, and whole grains.

Excess amounts: May interfere with medications and cause convulsions in people with epilepsy. It can also mask vitamin B12 deficiencies, which can lead to permanent nerve damage.

Vitamin B12 (Cobalamin)

Functions: Forms and regenerates red blood cells, serves in cells as a part of many body chemicals, helps the body use fatty acids and some amino acids, increases energy, improves concentration and maintains nervous system.

Deficiency problems: Anemia, fatigue, nerve damage, a smooth tongue, very sensitive skin. B12 deficiencies may be hidden when extra folate is taken to treat or prevent anemia. Strict vegans who eat no animal byproducts (and their infants) are the most likely to develop vitamin B12 deficiencies.

Food sources: Plant products do not contain B12. Non-vegans can get it from eggs, dairy, and strict vegans can use some yeasts and fortified foods.

Excess amounts: No known toxicity.

Vitamin C (Ascorbic Acid)

Functions: Helps the body absorb plant-based iron, vital for healthy skin, bones, muscles, healing and protection from viruses, toxins, drugs, infections and allergies. Necessary for cholesterol metabolism.

Deficiency problems: Scurvy, a disease that causes loose teeth, bleeding, swollen gums, and improper wound healing. Rare in the United States.

Food sources: Citrus fruits and many other fruits and vegetables, including berries, melons, peppers, leafy herbs and many dark-green leafy vegetables, potatoes and tomatoes.

Excess amounts: May cause kidney stones, gout, diarrhea and stomach cramps in excess

Vitamin D (Calciferol)

Functions: Promotes the absorption of calcium and phosphorus and helps deposit these minerals in bones and teeth to make them strong.

Deficiency problems: Greater risk of osteoporosis and osteomalacia (softening of bones). Children can develop rickets or defective bone growth.

Food sources: Vitamin D is known as the "sunshine" vitamin, because your body can produce it after sunlight or ultraviolet light hits the skin. Food sources include cheese, eggs, and some fish (such as salmon).

Excess amounts: Can lead to kidney stones or damage, weak muscles and bones, excessive bleeding and other problems. Excessive amounts usually come from supplements, not food or overexposure to sunlight.

Vitamin E (Tocopherol)

Functions: An antioxidant essential for absorption of iron and metabolism of essential fatty acids, protection of the circulatory system and cells, and slowing the aging process. May have a possible role in protecting against illnesses such as heart disease and some types of cancer.

Deficiency problems: Nervous system problems. Deficiencies are very rare, as vitamin E is abundant in foods. Premature, very low birth weight babies and people who do not absorb fat normally may have deficiency problems.

Food sources: Nuts, seeds, eggs, whole grains, unrefined oils, leafy vegetables, avocados and soybeans.

Excess amounts: May interfere with vitamin K action and enhance the effect of some anticoagulant drugs.

Vitamin K

Functions: Vitamin K, also known as Phylloquinone or Phytomenadione from vegetable sources (and Menaquinone or Menatetrenone from animal sources), helps blood to clot and stop bleeding.

Deficiency problems: Thin blood that does not adequately coagulate.

Food sources: Intestinal bacteria produce some of the vitamin K you need. The best food sources include green leafy vegetables such as kale, parsley, spinach and broccoli. Smaller amounts are found in milk and other dairy products, eggs, whole grains, molasses, fruits and other vegetables.

Excess amounts: No known toxicity.

Recommendations

Vitamins can be lost from foods during preparation, cooking, or storage. To prevent loss of vitamins:

- ☐ Serve fruits and vegetables raw whenever possible.
- ☐ Steam, boil, or simmer foods in a very small amount of water, or microwave them for the shortest time possible.
- ☐ When you boil vegetables, use the water (which contains a lot of the nutrients) to make a vegetable juice or broth.
- ☐ Cook potatoes in their skins. Be sure to wash the dirt off the outside.
- ☐ Refrigerate prepared juices and store them for no more than 2 to 3 days.
- ☐ Store cut, raw fruits and vegetables in an airtight container and refrigerate–do not soak or store in water. Vitamin C will be dissolved in the water.

THE ESSENTIAL MINERAL GUIDE

Dietary minerals are the chemical elements required by living organisms, other than the four common elements found in our cells (carbon, hydrogen, nitrogen, and oxygen). The trace minerals group includes over 50 chemical elements, all of which can be found in our bodies, but all of which are not essential to our health. Scientists group these minerals into three categories:

- ❑ The essential trace minerals. These are required in the diet for full health, and when the intake is insufficient, symptoms of deficiency will arise.
- ❑ The toxic trace minerals. The term is used for minerals that cause health problems even at levels that may be encountered normally in the environment. With these, the greater danger is getting too much instead of too little. This category changes from time to time, but generally includes aluminum, arsenic, cadmium, lead, mercury, and tin. Actually, too much of ANY nutrient can be toxic; how much is too much depends on the nutrient.
- ❑ Everything else. These are all the other minerals that are present in the body but are not essential in our diet or particularly toxic.

Like vitamins, minerals can also be lost from food due to processing and cooking. And just as with vitamins (except perhaps more so), minerals have been called a double-edged sword because too much of a mineral can be just as harmful as not enough. Malnutrition is the number one cause for mineral deficiencies. But mineral deficiencies can also be caused by anemia, cancer, colitis, constipation, convulsions, diabetes, dysentery, eczema, heart disease, intestinal diseases, menstruation disorders, paralysis, infantile paralysis, rickets, scurvy, tuberculosis, tumors and skin eruptions.

Our bodies need at least 15 minerals to function:

Calcium	Phosphorus	Magnesium	Chromium
Copper	Fluoride	Iodine	Iron
Manganese	Molybdenum	Selenium	Zinc
Chloride	Potassium	Sodium	Nickel*

Calcium

Functions: Calcium builds bones, in length and strength, and helps slow the rate of bone loss as you age. It helps muscles contract, plays a role in normal nervous system function, and helps blood clotting and blood pressure regulation. It's necessary for the body to metabolize iron and absorb vitamin B12, to keep the heart beating and for the release of neurotransmitters in the brain and reduces the risk of cardiovascular disease in postmenopausal women.

Deficiency problems: Affects bone density and increases the risk of osteoporosis.

Food sources: besides milk, other good sources include dark green leafy vegetables, nuts, root vegetables, broccoli and tofu.

Excess amounts: Too much calcium over a prolonged period can cause constipation, kidney stones and poor kidney function. It may also interfere with the absorption of other minerals, such as iron and zinc. But excess amounts are only consumed via supplements.

Phosphorus

Functions: Phosphorus helps body cells produce energy and acts as a main regulator of energy metabolism in body organs. It is a major component of bones and teeth, and makes up part of DNA and RNA.

Deficiency problems: Rare, but symptoms include bone loss, weakness, loss of appetite and pain.

Food sources: Protein-rich foods are the best sources. Legumes and nuts rank next. Bread and baked goods also contain phosphorus.

Excess amounts: Too much phosphorus may lower calcium levels in the blood and increase bone loss if calcium intake is low.

Magnesium

Functions: Repairs and maintains body cells; required for hormonal activity; required for most body processes, including energy production, the action of our muscles as well as proper bone development and growth.

Deficiency problems: Lack of magnesium absorption can lead to irregular heartbeat, nausea, weakness and mental derangement. Magnesium deficiency has also been linked to asthma.

Food sources: Magnesium is found in all foods in varying amounts. Legumes, nuts, whole grains, brown rice, soybeans, brewer's yeast, bitter chocolate and green vegetables are good sources.

Excess amounts: Too much magnesium can cause nausea, vomiting, low blood pressure and heart problems. Excess amounts from food are unlikely to cause harm, unless kidney disease prevents magnesium from being excreted.

Chromium

Functions: Chromium works with insulin to help the body use glucose (blood sugar).

Deficiency problems: Symptoms may resemble diabetes, including impaired glucose tolerance and nerve damage.

Food sources: Good sources include whole grains, brewer's yeast, molasses, mushrooms, eggs, cheese, and nuts.

Excess amounts: The effects of too much chromium are still being studied.

Copper

Functions: Copper is needed for the absorption, storage, and metabolism of iron. Copper helps make hemoglobin, which carries oxygen in the blood. It's also a part of many body enzymes and helps all body cells produce energy.

Deficiency problems: Rare, except from genetic problems or consuming too much zinc, which can hinder copper absorption. The symptoms of a copper deficiency are similar to iron-deficiency anemia.

Food sources: Unless you like eating liver, I'd say you can get enough from nuts and seeds. Cooking in copper pots also increases the copper content of foods.

Excess amounts: Too much copper can cause nausea, vomiting, diarrhea, coma and liver damage.

Fluoride

Functions: Fluoride helps harden tooth enamel, protecting teeth from decay. It may also protect against osteoporosis by strengthening bones.

Deficiency problems: Causes weak tooth enamel.

Food sources: Tea (especially if made with fluoridated water) and fish with edible bones, such as canned salmon. Many communities add fluoride to the water supply.

Excess amounts: Too much fluoride can mottle or stain otherwise healthy teeth. It can also lead to brittle bones, increasing the frequency of bone fractures.

Iodine

Functions: Iodine is part of thyroxin (thyroid hormone), which regulates the body's rate of energy use.

Deficiency problems: Interferes with thyroxin production, slowing the rate at which the body burns energy. Symptoms include weight gain and goiter (enlarged thyroid gland). Use of iodized salt has virtually eliminated iodine deficiency as a cause of goiter in the United States.

Food sources: Found naturally in saltwater fish and foods grown near coastal areas. Iodine is added to table salt.

Excess amounts: Too much iodine may also cause goiter, but not at levels usually consumed in the United States.

Iron

Functions: Iron is an essential part of hemoglobin, which carries oxygen to body cells.

Deficiency problems: Anemia, fatigue and infections. Deficiencies are more common among women with regular menstrual periods.

Food sources: Dark chocolate, molasses, dark green leafy vegetables.

Excess amounts: Adult iron supplements can be harmful to children, but naturally occurring iron (from food) is not likely to do much harm beyond causing constipation.

Manganese

Functions: Manganese is part of many body enzymes. It's necessary for the functioning of the brain; proper metabolism and normal functioning of the thyroid gland.

Deficiency problems: Rare.

Food sources: Whole grain products, nuts, root vegetables, brown rice, legumes, tea, and some fruits and vegetables, such as pineapple, kale and strawberries.

Excess amounts: Consuming harmful levels of manganese from food is very rare.

Molybdenum

Functions: Molybdenum works with riboflavin to incorporate iron into hemoglobin for red blood cells. It is also part of many body enzymes.

Deficiency problems: Rare with a normal diet.

Food sources: Milk, legumes, breads and grain products.

Selenium

Functions: Selenium works as an antioxidant with vitamin E to protect body cells from damage that may lead to cancer, heart disease and other health problems. It also aids cell growth. Selenium also improves liver function, maintains healthy eyes and eyesight, maintains healthy skin and hair, and may impede the aging process.

Deficiency problems: May affect the heart and immune system.

Food sources: Whole grains, nuts, seeds, brown rice and legumes contain selenium, but the amount can depend on the type of soil in which they were grown.

Excess amounts: Toxic in large doses, usually only possible with supplements.

Zinc

Functions: Zinc is essential for growth. It promotes cell reproduction, tissue growth, repair and wound healing. It forms part of more than 70 body enzymes and helps the body use carbohydrate, protein and fat. Zinc is also an excellent immune booster. Allergies have also responded to zinc.

Deficiency problems: Birth defects and retarded growth during childhood. Appetite loss, decreased sense of taste and smell, skin changes and reduced resistance to infection are also symptoms.

Food sources: Sunflower seeds, peanuts, whole grains, and soybeans are good sources.

Excess amounts: Excess zinc intake comes from supplements and can cause gastrointestinal irritation, vomiting, reduced HDL ("good") cholesterol levels and can interfere with copper absorption and immune function.

Chloride

Functions: Chloride helps regulate fluids in and out of body cells. It forms part of stomach acid to help digest food and absorb nutrients. It also helps transmit nerve impulses.

Deficiency problems: Rare, as chloride is found in table salt. Heavy, persistent sweating, chronic diarrhea or vomiting, trauma or kidney disease may cause deficiencies.

Food sources: Sea salt, seaweed, rye, tomatoes, lettuce, celery, and olives.

Excess amounts: Excess chloride may be linked to high blood pressure in chloride-sensitive people, but more study is needed.

Potassium

Functions: Potassium helps regulate fluids and mineral balance in and out of body cells. It also helps maintain normal blood pressure, water balance, the proper synthesis of protein, as well as nerve and muscle function.

Deficiency problems: Prolonged vomiting, diarrhea, laxative use or kidney problems can result in deficiencies of potassium. Symptoms include weakness, appetite loss, nausea and fatigue.

Food sources: Fruits and vegetables will give you all you need. Particularly good sources include apricots, avocados, bananas, cantaloupe, honeydew, kiwi, oranges, prunes, strawberries, potatoes, tomatoes, dried fruits, leafy green vegetables, nuts, and molasses.

Excess amounts: Excess potassium is usually excreted. If this doesn't happen, as in people with some types of kidney disease, heart problems or ulceration of the small intestine can occur.

Sodium

Functions: Sodium helps regulate movement of fluids in and out of body cells. It also helps transmit nerve impulses, regulate blood pressure and relax muscles.

Deficiency problems: Unlikely, except with chronic diarrhea, vomiting or kidney problems. Symptoms include nausea, dizziness and muscle cramps.

Food sources: Processed foods account for about 75% of the sodium we eat. Another 25% comes from table salt. Only a small amount occurs naturally in food.

Excess amounts: Healthy people excrete excess sodium, but some kidney diseases interfere with sodium excretion, leading to fluid retention and swelling. Sodium-sensitive people may experience high blood pressure eating a daily diet that contains high levels of sodium.

Note:

Meat, liver and seafood are often considered good sources of minerals like iron, zinc and selenium, but then you have to worry about what else they contain. Fortunately, nuts, seeds, and dark green vegetables typically contain enough of such minerals, so that if you're eating a healthy diet (which requires a significant amount of such foods), you don't have to worry about missing out on essential minerals, even if your diet is "missing" meat.

SYMPTOMS OF NUTRITIONAL DEFICIENCIES

Modern medicine tends to treat each symptom individually, whereas a nutritionist or naturopathic doctor looks for the underlying cause of symptoms. Many common symptoms are caused by deficiencies of vitamins and minerals. Further information on all the following vitamins and minerals can be found in The Essential Vitamin and Mineral Guide.

Do you have chronic fatigue syndrome? You could be deficient in MOLYBDENUM or MAGNESIUM.[41]

Is your child disruptive and aggressive? They may have a deficiency of ZINC, IRON, VITAMIN B6, or PROTEIN.[42]

---

[41] The evidence suggests CFS is a progressive immune disorder which affects all body organs and systems. The three major symptoms of CFS are: (1) disabling fatigue; (2) persistent muscle and joint pain; and (3) brain fog, irritability and depression. CFS appears to be a man-made ailment produced by problems in nutrition and lifestyle. People who tried molybdenum for CFS reported significant improvements. People with CFS usually have low red blood cell magnesium levels. A recent study in the UK concluded that 80% of CFS patients receiving magnesium reported "significantly improved energy levels, better emotional state, and less pain."

[42] Deficiencies in for zinc, iron, B vitamins and protein, exhibit a 41% increase in aggressive behavior by the age of 8, and by the age of 17 there is violent and antisocial behavior in 51%. And Zinc is the single most common deficiency in the American population, with an estimated 80% of the whole population at risk. Among adolescent males, Iron deficiency has also been shown to be directly associated with aggressive behavior. In fact, a recent study found juvenile prisoners were nearly twice as Iron deficient as their non-incarcerated

Do your children have behavioral and learning problems? They may be deficient in ZINC, MAGNESIUM, VITAMIN B6 and ESSENTIAL FATTY ACIDS.[43]

Are you forgetful? You may have a deficiency of B VITAMINS and ESSENTIAL FATTY ACIDS.[44]

Do you produce excess ear wax? You may be deficient in ESSENTIAL FATTY ACIDS. [45]

Do you have tinnitus (ringing in the ears) or other hearing problems? You may have a dietary deficiency or a blood disorder.[46]

---

peers. Vitamin B6 is essential for the synthesis or metabolism of practically all the neurotransmitters (chemicals which help to transmit messages in the nervous system). A deficiency of vitamin B6 causes symptoms such as tiredness, nervousness, irritability, depression and insomnia. So it's not surprising that this deficiency can cause behavioral changes resulting in aggressive behavior. Finally, Protein is made up of amino acids, some of which are important in affecting mood and behavior.

[43] Children with low blood levels of essential Omega-3 fatty acids, have a greater tendency to have problems with behavior, learning and health consistent with attention deficit hyperactivity disorder (ADHD). Studies have indicated that symptoms associated with a deficiency in EFAS are exhibited to a greater extent in children with ADHD. Those symptoms include thirst, frequent urination and dry skin and hair. Some researchers were able to pinpoint Omega-3s as the fatty acids that may be associated with the unique behavior and learning problems in children with ADHD. Other research suggests that some children with ADHD have lowered levels of magnesium. In a recent trial study, ADHD children with low magnesium were given magnesium for six months and had a significant decrease in hyperactive behavior, compared with other magnesium-deficient ADHD children who did not receive magnesium.

[44] Memory deteriorates naturally with aging, but not to the extent we are seeing among many people today. Memory loss is often more related to poor nutrition and other abuses than to an onset of Alzheimer's disease. Other factors can include the side effects of various medications and other medical conditions such as depression, anxiety, alcohol abuse, drug abuse, certain brain conditions (e.g. stroke or brain tumors), insufficient supply of necessary nutrients to the brain, high cholesterol and triglycerides, insufficient nutrients to make relevant neurotransmitters, free radical damage caused by oxidation, menopause, allergies, stress, thyroid disorders, hypoglycaemia and poor circulation to the brain. Through avoidance of many of these factors and with proper diet and nutrition, your memory should remain good until well into old age. And by old age, we mean 85, not 58.

[45] Unless you actually have a troublesome ear infection, excess ear wax is a classic symptom of deficiency in EFAs. We need to get our EFAs from food, not fat and oil because they are usually damaged when processed.. EFAs include (A) the Omega-6 fatty acids, and (B) the Omega-3 fatty acids. EFAs are needed for many physiologic processes, including maintaining the integrity of the skin and the structure of cell membranes, as well as some functions of the brain and retina. Notably, because of air pollution, people in big cities produce more ear wax.

[46] Tinnitus is the medical term for ringing in the ears. Symptoms may include hearing buzzing, roaring, ringing, whistling, or hissing sounds. These sounds can be intermittent, continuous, or pulsing. Some causative factors include iron deficiency, Magnesium deficiency, Vitamin A deficiency, Vitamin B12 deficiency (especially tinnitus), Vitamin D deficiency, Zinc deficiency (especially tinnitus), and excessive fat in the diet. Zinc supplements have been used to treat people who had both tinnitus and age-related hearing

Do you forgt your dreams? You may be deficient in VITAMIN B6.[47]

Do you have Insomnia? You may have a B VITAMIN or MINERAL DEFICIENCY.[48]

Do you crave Butter? You probably have a deficiency in SODIUM.[49]

Do you crave sugar, have blood sugar swings, or low blood sugar? You may be deficient in CHROMIUM. You may also have an intolerance to carbohydrates or suffer from gut fermentation syndrome.[50]

Do you crunch ice cubes or crave lettuce? You could be IRON deficient.[51]

Do you have shaky hands? You could be deficient in MAGNESIUM and VITAMIN B1.[52]

---

loss, though it only appears to be helpful in people who are zinc deficient to begin with. Researchers have discovered that Magnesium is key in preventing noise-induced hearing loss.

[47] Vitamin B6 aids in the formation of several neurotransmitters, essential in dreaming, and is therefore an essential nutrient in the regulation of mental processes and possibly mood. Why do you have vivid dreams after eating cheese? Because cheese is a very good source of Vitamin B6. It also contains morphine-like compounds and phenylethylamine, triggering a reaction in the brain that mimics Ecstasy and amphetamines. That's why pill-poppers develop a craving for cheese and pizzas as they are coming down from the drug-induced high. What are these substances doing there? It is thought that the mood changing substances in mother's milk produce a calming effect on the infant and, in fact, may be responsible for the mother-infant bond.

[48] Insomnia is either transitory (short term) or chronic (longer lasting). Deficiencies in certain vitamins, minerals, amino acids and enzymes may disrupt your sleep. Deficiencies in calcium, magnesium, B vitamins, folic acid and melatonin may keep you from sleeping altogether. (See, "Sleep –The Cousin Of Death?")

[49] Butter contains salt, and it has been documented that people who crave butter do so because of the salt it contains. We have an uncanny knack of knowing just how much sodium we need, and should always add salt 'to taste.'

[50] Mostly, sugar craving is a metabolic dysfunction that may be due to imbalance of sugar and insulin. Chromium has a major effect on controlling the sugar balance in the body, and is deficient in our diet because refining foods removes the chromium. So if you crave sugar you're probably deficient in chromium, and scientists advise that you're probably heading for diabetes or insulin intolerance.

[51] Many iron-deficient patients develop pica, an unusual craving for specific foods (ice cubes, lettuce, etc.) that are often not even rich in iron. Iron deficiency is the most common nutritional disorder in the world. Overall, it is the most vulnerable, the poorest and the least educated who are disproportionately affected by iron deficiency.

[52] Early symptoms of magnesium deficiency can include fatigue, anorexia, irritability, insomnia, and muscle tremors or twitching. People only slightly deficient in magnesium become irritable, high-strung, sensitive to noise, hyperexcitable, apprehensive, and belligerent. If the deficiency is more severe, or prolonged, they may develop twitching, tremors, irregular pulse, insomnia, muscle weakness, jerkiness, and leg and foot cramps; their hands may shake so badly that their writing becomes illegible. If magnesium is severely deficient, the brain is particularly affected. Clouded thinking, confusion, disorientation, marked depression, and even terrifying hallucinations can occur. Improvement is usually

Do you have white spots on your fingernails? You may have a deficiency in ZINC.[53]

Do you suffer from soft or brittle nails? You may be deficient in MINERALS.[54]

Do you have yellow palms? You may have excessive BETA CAROTENE intake.[55]

Do you have rough bumps on your upper arms? You may be deficient in ESSENTIAL FATTY ACIDS.[56]

Do you bleed easily? You may be deficient in VITAMIN C OR VITAMIN K.[57]

---

dramatic within hours after magnesium is taken. If your shaking or trembling has been present for less than 2 years, it may be caused by temporary conditions such as: increased anxiety or stress; certain medications; caffeine excess or caffeine withdrawal, excess alcohol or drug withdrawal. Long-term shaking or trembling could also be caused by conditions such as endocrine imbalances, electrolyte imbalances, or hormonal imbalances. Every cell of the body requires vitamin B1 to form the fuel the body runs on–adenosine triphosphate (ATP). Nerve cells require vitamin B1 in order to function normally. Deficiency can cause tremors. A decline in vitamin B1 levels occurs with age, irrespective of medical condition, but deficiency is most commonly found in alcoholics, people with poor absorption conditions, and those eating a very poor diet.

[53] Those unsightly little spots are often mistaken for a calcium deficiency, when in fact, they're more likely due to inadequate intake or absorption of zinc. The signs and symptoms of zinc deficiency include anorexia, growth retardation, delayed sexual maturation, hypogonadism and hypospermia, alopecia, immune disorders, dermatitis, night blindness, impaired taste (hypogeusia), and impaired wound healing.

[54] Brittle nails are characterized by splitting or breaking at the nail tip. The nail can also appear as thin, shiny, dry or translucent. The nails can reveal much about a person's general internal health, so nail abnormalities in either the fingers or toes can indicate an underlying disorder. Brittle nails are often caused by a deficiency in minerals and can even lead to an urge to bite your nails. (See, "PH Balance: A Matter Of Minerals")

[55] 15-20 milligrams is the most beta carotene an adult should consume in one day. Although beta carotene is not toxic for the average person who doesn't smoke or drink heavily, excess can cause nausea, loose stools, bruising, joint pain, and a yellow/orange coloring on hands and feet. With regards to carrots, yes you can eat so many of them that your skin will turn yellow. One 7½" carrot has 2025 RE of vitamin A, which is 203% of your RDI. So if you eat more than 3 carrots in a day, you have probably saturated your body's ability to store vitamin A over a short time and so it is showing up as an orange tint on your skin.

[56] Keratosis pilaris (KP) is a very common genetic follicular disease that is manifested by the appearance of rough bumps on the skin and hence colloquially referred to as "chicken skin." Primarily, it appears on the back and outer sides of the upper arms, but can also occur on thighs and buttocks or any body part except palms or soles.

[57] This can present itself as bleeding from gums when cleaning your teeth, frequent nosebleeds, and excess bleeding from minor injuries. In the 1700's, Surgeon James Lind proved that citrus fruit (rich in Vitamin C) cures scurvy, symptoms of which include bleeding gums, loose teeth and hemorrhaging. Vitamin C is an antioxidant vitamin important in forming collagen, a protein that gives structure to bones, cartilage, muscle, and blood vessels. Vitamin C also aids in the absorption of iron, and helps maintain capillaries, bones, and teeth. Vitamin K results in a tendency for spontaneous bleeding or in prolonged

Do you have greasy, reddish, scaly skin on your face and sides of your nose? You may be deficient in VITAMIN B2.[58]

Do you have Eczema? You probably have an ALLERGY.[59]

Do you suffer from scaly red skin round the eyes, nose, mouth and genitals? You may be deficient in BIOTIN.[60]

Do you suffer from burning feet or heels? You may have a deficiency in VITAMIN B5.[61]

Do you often have cold hands and feet? You might have a deficiency in MAGNESIUM.[62]

Do you have tender calf muscles? You may be deficient in MAGNESIUM.[63]

Do you have a white coating on your tongue? You might be DEHYDRATED or you could have a YEAST INFECTION.

Do you have a swollen tongue? You may have a FOOD INTOLERANCE.

Do you have a smooth tongue that is painful and sore? You may be deficient in FOLIC ACID.[64]

---

and excessive bleeding with trauma or injury. Without the vitamin, even a small cut would cause continuous bleeding in the body instead of clotting automatically.

[58] Vitamin B2 (otherwise called Riboflavin) is not stored in the human body for any period of time and it is therefore important to include a regular dietary. It is essential for converting carbohydrate into energy, normal tissue respiration, and for healthy mucous membranes. Signs of deficiency include: Cracks in skin at corner of mouth; soreness of lips, mouth and tongue; scaling of skin around nose, mouth, scrotum, forehead, ears and scalp; heightened sensitivity to light; conjunctivitis and watering of eyes; and anemia

[59] Eczema often gets worse at night, because the skin gets moist in bed, and surface allergens turn into a concentrated liquid that aggravates even more.

[60] One of the few ways you can end up lacking biotin is by eating raw egg whites on a regular basis. Avidin is a protein found in egg whites, which binds biotin and prevents its absorption. Cooking egg white doesn't produce this same problem, however.

[61] Known as "the anti-stress vitamin", B5 (Pantothenic Acid) is required by all cells in the body and is concentrated in the organs. A deficiency of pantothenic acid may cause fatigue, headache, nausea, sleep problems abdominal discomfort, and tingling in the hands or feet.

[62] Magnesium is the fourth most abundant mineral in the body and is essential to good health. When one sweats, significant amounts of magnesium and potassium are lost. While most athletes have been conditioned to drink a potassium rich drink after sweating, very few have been educated on the dangers of a magnesium deficiency. Magnesium may be the most under-recognized electrolyte disorder in the U.S. While most physicians know how vital potassium is for normal heartbeat, magnesium is an entirely different story, and many doctors don't even check for it.

[63] Research shows that in prehistoric times, we ate equal amounts of the two vitamins. But now, with an average of ten times more calcium than magnesium in our current diet, it's not surprising we have widespread magnesium deficiency in modern times.

[64] Folic acid is a B vitamin that is an essential nutrient for proper growth and development.

Do you have trouble swallowing? You could be deficient in MAGNESIUM.[65]

Do you suffer from constant mouth ulcers? You may be deficient in IRON, FOLIC ACID and VITAMIN B12.[66]

Do you have dry eyes? You may be deficient in VITAMIN A.[67]

Do you rub your eyes? You could have a stress-related or sleep-related problem.[68]

Do you have a crease on the end of your nose? You probably have an ALLERGY.[69]

Do you have poor sense of smell and taste? You may be deficient in

---

It may reduce a woman's risk of having a baby with a neural tube defect (NTD) when consumed before conception and during the early weeks of pregnancy. It is estimated that 88 per cent of all North Americans suffer from a folic acid deficiency. Folic acid is the synthetic form of the vitamin Folate that is used in supplements and fortified foods.

[65] If you have throat spasms set off by eating, yawning or talking, and have been experiencing weight loss, you may have a condition caused by low magnesium. Trembling and spasms (neuromuscular hyperexcitability) throughout the body are often a feature of low magnesium.

[66] The mouth is remarkably good at healing, so recurrent mouth ulcers last for only 1-2 weeks. But a few weeks later, it happens again. Recurrent mouth ulcers are often due to anemia or shortage of iron, folate or vitamin B12. A few women find that mouth ulcers are more likely before their periods, so hormones might have an influence as well.

[67] Globally, 3 million children suffer clinical Vitamin A deficiency, to the point of major eye damage and xerophthalmia. An estimated 140-250 million children under age 5 are at risk of sub-clinical Vitamin A deficiency, mainly in Asia and Africa. Long known to be a principle cause of childhood blindness (250,000-500,000 children lose their sight each year), Vitamin A deficiency is now recognized as a major contributing factor in an estimated 1-3 million child deaths each year. And it would be ridiculously cheap to fix the problem. A 2 cent dosage of vitamin A every 4-6 months could protect against blindness and have several other positive impacts on the health of young children.

[68] When you rub your eyes, it stimulates the ocularcardio reflex, which means rubbing your eye (ocular) actually affects your heart (cardio). This stimulation lowers heart rate, so we rub our eyes in order to slow ourselves down to prepare to sleep. This technique is used in martial arts, massage, hypnotism, and is a method of disabling violent prisoners and patients. This can be a calming feeling, and may be one reason why stressed people sometimes rub their eyes and face with their hands, especially after a stressful telephone call, meeting or confrontation. On the other hand, many people with eye rubbing problems have dry eyes that can be associated with an allergy. The more inflamed the tissue gets, the more it itches – this is called the itch/scratch/itch cycle that doesn't stop until damage has been done.

[69] The most sensitive part of your body to allergens is the nose, because 2,000 gallons of air pass through this tiny passageway every day. Congestion or inflammation of the nose (rhinitis), sinuses (sinusitis), and throat (pharyngitis) may be due to airborne irritants and allergens; however, food allergy may be the undiagnosed cause of these common problems. In infants and young children, nose congestion may present as mouth-breathing, sniffing, snuffling, snorting or snoring, and nose rubbing. This habitual nose rubbing normally has you pushing your nose up with the palm of your hand until a crease develops across the skin of your nose.

ZINC.[70]

Do you get a blocked nose after drinking red wine or eating fruit? You may be deficient in MOLYBDENUM.[71]

Do you have poor sensory systems? You may have a deficiency in VITAMIN B12, B1 and MAGNESIUM.[72]

Do you have premature grey hair? You may be deficient in PARA-AMINO BENZOIC ACID.[73]

Are you experiencing hair loss? You may be deficient in BIOTIN. You may also be deficient in ESSENTIAL FATTY ACIDS and ZINC, since these are also associated with excessive hair loss.[74]

Do you have hemorrhoids? You may have a deficiency of FIBER in your diet.

Do you experience poor healing? You may be deficient in MAGNESIUM, ZINC and EFAs.

Do you have Arthritis? You almost certainly have a BORON and SULPHUR deficiency.[75]

---

[70] Zinc deficiency suppresses taste and smell and leads to loss of appetite. However, Zinc can fix that pretty quickly. On the other hand, if you don't smell things as well as you once did on a long-term basis, it could be your age, a smoking habit, a drug habit, a head injury, a job that exposes you to strong odors, or even certain prescription drugs. As smell slips away, your sense of taste may suffer, since the two senses are so closely related that if you hold your nose when you bite an onion it won't taste any different from an apple.

[71] Sulfur-containing compounds called sulphites are used as preservatives in wines and as coating for many non-organic fruits and vegetables in the grocery. Molybdenum helps convert potentially harmful sulphites into taurine, a beneficial amino acid. Without molybdenum, the sulfites remain, causing congestion or wheezing.

[72] Vitamin B12 deficiency symptoms, like those of many other treatable health conditions, can be virtually identical to senile dementia symptoms and Alzheimer's symptoms. Correcting the deficiency can help those afflicted resume full and normal lives. Vitamin B1 (thiamin) deficiency can lead to brain abnormalities primarily in alcoholics.

[73] PABA or para-amino benzoic acid is one of the nutrients the body uses to make the anti-stress B vitamins, especially vitamin B5 which has, in turn, been linked with slowing down the rate of both greying and hair loss. You need to remember though that the trials which suggest this welcome benefit are small and only worked when prematurely greying hair was the result of either stress or a nutritional deficiency that the PABA could correct.

[74] But male pattern baldness (MPB) could be a warning sign for even bigger problems. MPB can be related to prostate problems in many older men. An Australian study found that men with bald spots at the top of their heads (vertex baldness) were one and a half times more likely to have prostate cancer than those without bald spots. However, no link was made between frontal baldness (receding hairline) and prostate cancer.

[75] In Australia, arthritis affects less than 1% of the population, and very few animals get arthritis, because there is more boron in the soil, and more boron in the water than in the Western world. In Israel there is even less arthritis, and guess what, the soil is rich in boron. Arthritis and its close relative osteoporosis affect about 30% of all people today. Sulphur is the fourth most plentiful mineral in the body, and can be found in almost every cell. Our

Do you suffer from osteoporosis? You may be deficient in MAGNESIUM and BORON.[76]

Do you suffer from high blood pressure? You may be deficient in MAGNESIUM.[77]

Do you frequently catch colds and other respiratory infections? You may be deficient in VITAMIN C and ZINC.[78]

Have you experienced infertility, miscarriage or premature labor? You or your partner may be deficient in ZINC.[79]

Do you or your family have a history of cancer? You may be deficient in SELENIUM.[80]

Have you had, or are you prone to heart attack? You may be deficient in VITAMIN E.[81]

---

skin, hair and nails all have a high sulphur content – if you've ever burned your hair or skin, that nasty smell was the sulphur burning!

[76] Osteoporosis is nothing more than brittle bones, or a loss of bone mass or bone density. Osteoporosis is really caused by only three things. They are: 1) diet, 2) physical exercise, and 3) lack of exposure to natural sunlight. Why? Bones are not just made up of calcium. In order to make healthy bones, we need the whole spectrum of vitamins, minerals, essential fatty acids and trace elements.

[77] A four-year study involving over 30,000 health professionals found that a lower risk of hypertension was associated with dietary patterns that provided more magnesium, potassium, and dietary fiber.

[78] Reviews of the research conducted on the use of Vitamin C over the past 20 years conclude that, in general, large doses of vitamin C have been found to decrease the duration and severity of colds, though not necessarily how many colds you have. Sufficient zinc is also essential in maintaining immune system functions.

[79] Three additional functions of zinc have been discovered apart from its important antioxidant one: (1) Zinc is important in the structure that encases tightly-wound DNA in the sperm nucleus; (2) Zinc keeps the sperm "calm" until they hit the female reproductive tract, which dilutes the zinc, acting like a mineral turbo charge that sends the sperm speeding towards their goal; and (3) By the time many sperm reach the egg they are no longer capable of penetrating it. This is because they used up the enzymes they'd need on the way. This is linked with a zinc deficiency.

[80] Our bodies need selenium, an antioxidant that may help control cell damage that can lead to cancer. In a study of 1,300 men and women, men who had taken selenium for 6½ years had approximately 60% fewer new cases of prostate cancer than men who took the placebo. Recently research on human cancer genes has found that foods that contain the mineral selenium and plant-based chemical sulforaphane in combination may have a 13 times greater ability to protect against cancer than when the food compounds are used separately. Vitamin E, like selenium, is an antioxidant, which might help control cell damage that can lead to cancer. In a 1998 study of 29,100 male smokers in Finland; men who took vitamin E to prevent lung cancer had 32% fewer new cases of prostate cancer than men who took the placebo. Studies have suggested that vitamin E also decreases the risk of Alzheimer's when taken with vitamin C, and protects against Parkinson's disease.

[81] Vitamin E may help prevent or delay coronary heart disease by limiting the oxidation of LDL-cholesterol and prevent the formation of blood clots, which could lead to a heart attack.

Do you experience Carpal tunnel syndrome? You may be deficient in VITAMIN B6.[82]

Are you over 60 years of age? You may be deficient in VITAMINS and MINERALS, especially the B VITAMINS and HYDROCHLORIC ACID.

Do you get chronic infections? You may be deficient in SELENIUM.[83]

ANIMAL DERIVED INGREDIENT LIST

Companies use animal ingredients because they're cheaper, not better. Slaughterhouses (and other industries involving animals) have to get rid of their leftovers, so they might as well make a profit in the process. Rendering plants process the bodies of millions of tons of dead animals every year, transforming decaying flesh and bones into profitable animal ingredients.

Some animal ingredients don't wind up in the final product but are used in the manufacturing process. For example, in the production of some refined sugars, bone char is used to whiten the sugar. And in some wines and beers, isinglass (from the swim bladders of fish) is used as a "clearing" agent.

The following list of animal ingredients (and alternatives) can help you avoid the many (often hard to detect) animal ingredients in food, cosmetics, and other products. This list is not all-inclusive. There are thousands of technical and patented names for ingredient variations. Not only that, but many ingredients can come from an animal, vegetable, or even synthetic source. In fact, some of the items listed below are commonly being made from synthetic (chemical) sources

---

[82] Symptoms of CTS include recurrent numbness, tingling, weakness, or pain in one or both hands in a location defined by the median nerve, which is compressed as it passes through the carpal tunnel in the wrist. Symptoms are usually worse at night and after prolonged use of the hands. Studies have found vitamin B6 deficiency to be common in people with CTS. Increased intake of vitamin B6 has reportedly relieved the symptoms of CTS in many cases.

[83] It is an established fact that viruses readily mutate in selenium deficient hosts and is more virulent, as shown in Selenium-deficient mice where viruses caused greater morbidity and mortality. In China, a vast area of selenium-deficient people was stricken with Keshan's disease and gastric cancer until the villagers were instructed to take extra selenium, after which both illnesses abated. Throughout Africa, it is claimed that HIV affects over 30-40% of the various populations. These populations are also selenium deficient. However, Senegal, a little country on the west African coast, apparently has an HIV incidence of about 1%. The population has the same sexual habits as its neighbors. The only difference is that Senegal lies on top of an old seabed and the soil has a very high mineral content including selenium. I understand that the Senegalese have some of the highest blood selenium levels in the world. Maybe it could be worthwhile if everyone took some extra selenium. As the renowned 19th century French physiologist Claude Bernard stated: "Le terrain c'est tout et le microbe n'est rien." ("The answer lies in the internal environment [you] and the microbe is nothing!")

nowadays. Adding to the confusion over whether an ingredient is of animal origin is the fact that many companies have removed the word "animal" from their ingredient labels to avoid putting off consumers. For example, rather than use the term "hydrolyzed animal protein," companies may use another term such as "hydrolyzed collagen." If you have questions regarding ingredients in a product, call or write the manufacturer. Many companies are used to responding to questions like this, so you can expect an accurate reply.

Adrenaline. Hormone from adrenal glands of hogs, cattle, and sheep. In medicine. Alternatives: synthetics.

Alanine. (See Amino Acids.)

Albumen. In eggs, milk, muscles, blood, and many vegetable tissues and fluids. In cosmetics, albumen is usually derived from egg whites and used as a coagulating agent. May cause allergic reaction. In cakes, cookies, candies, etc. Egg whites sometimes used in "clearing" wines. Derivative: Albumin.

Albumin. (See Albumen.)

Alcloxa. (See Allantoin.)

Aldioxa. (See Allantoin.)

Aliphatic Alcohol. (See Lanolin and Vitamin A.)

Allantoin. Uric acid from cows, most mammals. Also in many plants (especially comfrey). In cosmetics (especially creams and lotions) and used in treatment of wounds and ulcers. Derivatives: Alcloxa, Aldioxa. Alternatives: extract of comfrey root, synthetics.

Alligator Skin. (See Leather.)

Alpha-Hydroxy Acids. Any one of several acids used as an exfoliant and in anti-wrinkle products. Lactic acid may be animal-derived (see Lactic Acid). Alternatives: glycolic acid, citric acid, and salicylic acid are plant- or fruit-derived.

Ambergris. From whale intestines. Used as a fixative in making perfumes and as a flavoring in foods and beverages. Alternatives: synthetic or vegetable fixatives.

Amino Acids. The building blocks of protein in all animals and plants. In cosmetics, vitamins, supplements, shampoos, etc. Alternatives: synthetics, plant sources.

Aminosuccinate Acid. (See Aspartic Acid.)

Angora (Rabbit or goat hair).

Animal Fats and Oils. In foods, cosmetics, etc. Highly allergenic. Alternatives: olive oil, wheat germ oil, coconut oil, flaxseed oil, almond oil, safflower oil, etc.

Animal Hair. In some blankets, mattresses, brushes, furniture, etc. Alternatives: vegetable and synthetic fibers.

Arachidonic Acid. A liquid unsaturated fatty acid that is found in liver, brain, glands, and fat of animals and humans. Generally isolated from animal liver. Used in companion animal food for nutrition and in skin creams and lotions to soothe eczema and rashes. Alternatives: synthetics, aloe vera, tea tree oil, calendula ointment.

Arachidyl Proprionate. A wax that can be from animal fat. Alternatives: peanut or vegetable oil.

Aspartic Acid. Aminosuccinate Acid. Can be animal or plant source (e.g., molasses). Sometimes synthesized for commercial purposes.

Bee Pollen.

Beeswax.

Benzoic Acid. In almost all vertebrates and in berries. Used as a preservative in mouthwashes, deodorants, creams, aftershave lotions, etc. Alternatives: cranberries, gum benzoin (tincture) from the aromatic balsamic resin from trees grown in China, Sumatra, Thailand, and Cambodia.

Beta Carotene. (See Carotene.)

Biotin. Vitamin H. Vitamin B Factor. In every living cell and in larger amounts in milk and yeast. Used as a texturizer in cosmetics, shampoos, and creams. Alternatives: plant sources.

Blood. From any slaughtered animal. Used as adhesive in plywood, also found in cheese-making, foam rubber, intravenous feedings, and medicines. Possibly in foods such as lecithin. Alternatives: synthetics, plant sources.

Boar Bristles. Hair from wild or captive hogs. In "natural" toothbrushes and bath and shaving brushes. Alternatives: vegetable fibers, nylon, the peelu branch or peelu gum (Asian, available in the U.S.; its juice replaces toothpaste).

Bone Char. Animal bone ash. Used in bone china and often to make sugar white. Serves as the charcoal used in aquarium filters. Alternatives: synthetic tribasic calcium phosphate.

Bone Meal. Crushed or ground animal bones. In some fertilizers. In some vitamins and supplements as a source of calcium. In some tooth paste. Alternatives: plant mulch, vegetable compost, dolomite, clay, vegetarian vitamins.

Bonito. Dried flakes from fish. Frequently used in Japanese cooking.

Calciferol. (See Vitamin D.)

Calfskin. (See Leather.)

Caprylamine Oxide. (See Caprylic Acid.)

Capryl Betaine. (See Caprylic Acid.)

Caprylic Acid. A liquid fatty acid from cow's or goat's milk. Also from palm and coconut oil, other plant oils. In perfumes, soaps. Derivatives: Caprylic Triglyceride, Caprylamine Oxide, Capryl Betaine. Alternatives: plant sources.

Caprylic Triglyceride. (See Caprylic Acid.)

Carbamide. (See Urea.)

Carmine. Cochineal. Carminic Acid. Red pigment from the crushed female cochineal insect. Used in cosmetics, shampoos, red apple sauce, and other foods (including red lollipops and food coloring). May cause allergic reaction. Alternatives: beet juice (used in powders, rouges, shampoos; no known toxicity).

Carminic Acid. (See Carmine.)

Casein. Caseinate. Sodium Caseinate. Milk protein. In "non-dairy" creamers, soy cheese, many cosmetics, hair preparations, beauty masks. Alternatives: soy protein, soy milk, and other vegetable milks.

Caseinate. (See Casein.)

Cashmere.

Castor. Castoreum. Creamy substance with strong odor from muskrat and beaver genitals. Used as a fixative in perfume and incense. Sometimes labeled as "natural flavorings." Alternatives: synthetics, plant castor oil.

Castoreum. (See Castor.)

Catgut. Tough string from the intestines of sheep, horses, etc. Used for surgical sutures. Also for stringing tennis rackets and musical instruments, etc. Alternatives: nylon and other synthetic fibers.

Cera Flava. (See Beeswax.)

Cerebrosides. Fatty acids and sugars found in the covering of nerves. May include tissue from brain.

Cetyl Alcohol. Wax found in spermaceti from sperm whales or dolphins. Alternatives: Vegetable cetyl alcohol (e.g., coconut), synthetic spermaceti.

Cetyl Palmitate. (See Spermaceti.)

Chitosan. A fiber derived from crustacean shells. Used as a lipid binder in diet products, in hair, oral and skin care products, antiperspirants, and deodorants. Alternatives: raspberries, yams, legumes, dried apricots, and many other fruits and vegetables.

Cholesterin. (See Lanolin.)

Cholesterol. A steroid alcohol in all animal fats and oils, nervous tissue, egg yolk, and blood. Can be derived from lanolin. In cosmetics, eye creams, shampoos, etc. Alternatives:

solid complex alcohols (sterols) from plant sources.

Choline Bitartrate. (See Lecithin.)

Civet. Unctuous secretion painfully scraped from a gland very near the genital organs of civet cats. Used as a fixative in perfumes. Alternatives: (See alternatives to Musk.).

Cochineal. (See Carmine.)

Cod Liver Oil. (See Marine Oil.)

Collagen. Fibrous protein in vertebrates. Usually derived from animal tissue. Can't affect the skin's own collagen. An allergen. Alternatives: soy protein, almond oil, amla oil (see alternative to Keratin), etc.

Corticosteroid. (See Cortisone.)

Cortisone. Corticosteroid. Hormone from adrenal glands. Widely used in medicine. Alternatives: synthetics.

Cysteine, L-Form. An amino acid from hair which can come from animals, like from duck feather. Used in hair-care products and creams, in some bakery products, and in wound-healing formulations. Alternatives: plant sources.

Cystine. An amino acid found in urine and horsehair. Used as a nutritional supplement and in emollients. Alternatives: plant sources.

Dexpanthenol. (See Panthenol.)

Diglycerides. (See Monoglycerides and Glycerin.)

Dimethyl Stearamine. (See Stearic Acid.)

Down. (See Feathers.)

Duodenum Substances. From the digestive tracts of cows and pigs. Added to some vitamin tablets. In some medicines. Alternatives: vegetarian vitamins, synthetics.

Egg Protein. In shampoos, skin preparations, etc. Alternatives: plant proteins.

Elastin. Protein found in the neck ligaments and aortas of cows. Similar to collagen. Alternatives: synthetics, protein from plant tissues.

Emu Oil. From flightless ratite birds native to Australia and now factory farmed. Used in cosmetics and creams. Alternatives: vegetable and plant oils.

Ergocalciferol. (See Vitamin D.)

Ergosterol. (See Vitamin D.)

Estradiol. (See Estrogen.)

Estrogen. Estradiol. Female hormones from pregnant mares? urine. Considered a drug. Can have harmful systemic effects if used by children. Used for reproductive problems and in birth control pills and Premarin, a menopausal drug. In creams, perfumes, and lotions. Has a negligible effect in the creams as a skin restorative; simple vegetable-source emollients are considered better. Alternatives: oral contraceptives and menopausal drugs based on synthetic steroids or phytoestrogens (from plants, especially palm-kernel oil). Menopausal symptoms can also be treated with diet and herbs.

Fats. (See Animal Fats.)

Fatty Acids. Can be one or any mixture of liquid and solid acids such as caprylic, lauric, myristic, oleic, palmitic, and stearic. Used in bubble baths, lipsticks, soap, detergents, cosmetics, food. Alternatives: vegetable-derived acids, soy lecithin, safflower oil, bitter almond oil, sunflower oil, etc.

Feathers. From exploited and slaughtered birds. Used whole as ornaments or ground up in shampoos. (See Keratin.)

Fish Liver Oil. Used in vitamins and supplements. In milk fortified with vitamin D. Alternatives: yeast extract ergosterol and exposure of skin to sunshine.

Fish Oil. (See Marine Oil.) Fish oil can also be from marine mammals. Used in soap-making.

Fish Scales. Used in shimmery makeups. Alternatives: mica, rayon, synthetic pearl.

Fur. Obtained from animals (usually mink, foxes, or rabbits) cruelly trapped in steel-jaw leghold traps or raised in intensive confinement on fur "farms." Alternatives: synthetics. (See Sable Brushes.)

Gel. (See Gelatin.)

Gelatin. Gel. Protein obtained by boiling skin, tendons, ligaments, and/or bones with water. From cows and pigs. Used in shampoos, face masks, and other cosmetics. Used as a thickener for fruit gelatins and puddings (e.g., "Jello"). In candies, marshmallows, cakes, ice cream, yogurts. On photographic film and in vitamins as a coating and as capsules. Sometimes used to assist in "clearing" wines. Alternatives: carrageen (carrageenan, Irish moss), seaweeds (algin, agar-agar, kelp– used in jellies, plastics, medicine), pectin from fruits, dextrins, locust bean gum, cotton gum, silica gel.

Glucose Tyrosinase. (See Tyrosine.)

Glycerides. (See Glycerin.)

Glycerin. Glycerol. A byproduct of soap manufacture (normally uses animal fat). In cosmetics, foods, mouthwashes, chewing gum, toothpastes, soaps, ointments, medicines, lubricants, transmission and brake fluid, and plastics. Derivatives: Glycerides, Glyceryls, Glycreth-26, Polyglycerol. Alternatives: vegetable glycerin–a byproduct of vegetable oil soap. Derivatives of seaweed, petroleum.

Glycerol. (See Glycerin.)

Glyceryls. (See Glycerin.)

Glycreth-26. (See Glycerin.)

Guanine. Pearl Essence. Obtained from scales of fish. Constituent of ribonucleic acid and deoxyribonucleic acid and found in all animal and plant tissues. In shampoo, nail polish, other cosmetics. Alternatives: leguminous plants, synthetic pearl, or aluminum and bronze particles.

Hide Glue. Same as gelatin but of a cruder impure form. Alternatives: dextrins and synthetic petrochemical-based adhesives. (See Gelatin.)

Honey.

Honeycomb. (See Beeswax.)

Horsehair. (See Animal Hair.)

Hyaluronic Acid. A protein found in umbilical cords and the fluids around the joints. Used in cosmetics. Alternatives: plant oils.

Hydrocortisone. (See Cortisone.)

Hydrolyzed Animal Protein. In cosmetics, especially shampoo and hair treatments. Alternatives: soy protein, other vegetable proteins, amla oil (see alternatives to Keratin).

Imidazolidinyl Urea. (See Urea.)

Insulin. From hog pancreas. Used by millions of diabetics daily. Alternatives: synthetics, vegetarian diet and nutritional supplements, human insulin grown in a lab.

Isinglass. A form of gelatin prepared from the internal membranes of fish bladders. Sometimes used in "clearing" or filtering of wines and in foods. Alternatives: bentonite clay, "Japanese isinglass," agar-agar (see alternatives to Gelatin), mica, a mineral used in cosmetics.

Isopropyl Lanolate. (See Lanolin.)

Isopropyl Myristate. (See Myristic Acid.)

Isopropyl Palmitate. Complex mixtures of isomers of stearic acid and palmitic acid. (See Stearic Acid.)

Keratin. Protein from the ground-up horns, hooves, feathers, quills, and hair of various animals. In hair rinses, shampoos, permanent wave solutions. Alternatives: almond oil, soy protein, amla oil (from the fruit of an Indian tree), human hair from salons. Rosemary and nettle give body and strand strength to hair.

Lactic Acid. Found in blood and muscle tissue. Also in sour milk, beer, sauerkraut, pickles, and other food products made by bacterial fermentation. Used in skin fresheners, as a preservative, in the formation of plasticizers, etc. Alternative: plant milk sugars, synthetics.

Lactose. Milk sugar from milk of mammals. In eye lotions, foods, tablets, cosmetics, baked goods, medicines. Alternatives: plant milk sugars.

Laneth. (See Lanolin.)

Lanogene. (See Lanolin.)

Lanolin. Lanolin Acids. Wool Fat. Wool Wax. A product of the oil glands of sheep, extracted from their wool. Used as an emollient in many skin care products and cosmetics and in medicines. Derivatives: Aliphatic Alcohols, Cholesterin, Isopropyl Lanolate, Laneth, Lanogene, Lanolin Alcohols, Lanosterols, Sterols, Triterpene Alcohols. Alternatives: plant and vegetable oils.

Lanolin Alcohol. (See Lanolin.)

Lanosterols. (See Lanolin.)

Lard. Fat from hog abdomens. In shaving creams, soaps, cosmetics. In baked goods, French fries, refried beans, and many other foods. Alternatives: pure vegetable fats or oils.

L-Cysteine Hydrochloride. A flour additive often extracted from duck feathers. Found in commercial cereals and baking mixes.

Leather. Suede. Calfskin. Sheepskin. Alligator Skin. Other Types of Skin. Subsidizes the meat industry. Used to make wallets, handbags, furniture and car upholstery, shoes, etc. Alternatives: cotton, canvas, nylon, vinyl, ultrasuede, pleather, other synthetics.

Lecithin. Choline Bitartrate. Waxy substance in nervous tissue of all living organisms. But frequently obtained for commercial purposes from eggs and soybeans. Also from nerve tissue, blood, milk, corn. Choline bitartrate, the basic constituent of lecithin, is in many animal and plant tissues and prepared synthetically. Lecithin can be in eye creams, lipsticks, liquid powders, hand creams, lotions, soaps, shampoos, other cosmetics, and some medicines. Alternatives: soybean lecithin, synthetics.

Linoleic Acid. An essential fatty acid. Used in cosmetics, vitamins.

Alternatives: (See alternatives to Fatty Acids.)

Lipase. Enzyme from the stomachs and tongue glands of calves, kids, and lambs. Used in digestive aids as it helps the body break down fats. Also commonly found in cheese and dairy products. Alternatives: vegetable enzymes, castor beans.

Lipids. (See Lipoids.)

Lipoids. Lipids. Fat and fat-like substances that are found in animals and plants. Alternatives: vegetable oils.

Marine Oil. From fish or marine mammals (including porpoises). Used in soap-making. Used as a shortening (especially in some margarines), as a lubricant, and in paint. Alternatives: vegetable oils.

Methionine. Essential amino acid found in various proteins (usually from egg albumen and casein). Used as a texturizer and for freshness in potato chips. Alternatives: synthetics.

Milk Protein. Hydrolyzed milk protein. From the milk of cows. In cosmetics, shampoos, moisturizers, conditioners, etc. Alternatives: soy protein, other plant proteins.

Mink Oil. From minks. In cosmetics, creams, etc. Alternatives: vegetable oils and emollients such as avocado oil, almond oil, and jojoba oil.

Monoglycerides. Glycerides. (See Glycerin.) From animal fat. In margarines, cake mixes, candies, foods, etc. In cosmetics. Alternative: vegetable glycerides.

Musk (Oil). Dried secretion painfully obtained from musk deer, beaver, muskrat, civet cat, and otter genitals. In perfumes and in food flavorings. Alternatives: labdanum oil (which comes from various rockrose shrubs) and other plants with a musky scent.

Myristal Ether Sulfate. (See Myristic Acid.)

Myristic Acid. Organic acid in most animal and vegetable fats. In butter acids. Used in shampoos, creams, cosmetics. In food flavorings.

Derivatives: Isopropyl Myristate, Myristal Ether Sulfate, Myristyls, Oleyl Myristate. Alternatives: nut butters, oil of lovage, coconut oil, extract from seed kernels of nutmeg, etc.

Myristyls. (See Myristic Acid.)

"Natural Sources." Can mean animal or vegetable sources. Most often in the health food industry, especially in the cosmetics area, it means animal sources, such as animal elastin, glands, fat, protein, and oil. Alternatives: plant sources.

Nucleic Acids. In the nucleus of all living cells. Used in cosmetics, shampoos, conditioners, etc. Also in vitamins, supplements. Alternatives: plant sources.

Ocenol. (See Oleyl Alcohol.)

Octyl Dodecanol. Mixture of solid waxy alcohols. Primarily from stearyl alcohol. (See Stearyl Alcohol.)

Oleic Acid. Obtained from various animal and vegetable fats and oils. Usually obtained commercially from inedible tallow. (See Tallow.) In foods, soft soap, bar soap, permanent wave solutions, creams, nail polish, lipsticks, many other skin preparations. Derivatives: Oleyl Oleate, Oleyl Stearate. Alternatives: coconut oil. (See alternatives to Animal Fats and Oils.)

Oils. (See alternatives to Animal Fats and Oils.)

Oleths. (See Oleyl Alcohol.)

Oleyl Alcohol. Ocenol. Found in fish oils. Used in the manufacture of detergents, as a plasticizer for softening fabrics, and as a carrier for medications. Derivatives: Oleths, Oleyl Arachidate, Oleyl Imidazoline.

Oleyl Arachidate. (See Oleyl Alcohol.)

Oleyl Imidazoline. (See Oleyl Alcohol.)

Oleyl Myristate. (See Myristic Acid.)

Oleyl Oleate. (See Oleic Acid.)

Oleyl Stearate. (See Oleic Acid.)

Palmitamide. (See Palmitic Acid.)

Palmitamine. (See Palmitic Acid.)

Palmitate. (See Palmitic Acid.)

Palmitic Acid. From fats, oils (see Fatty Acids). Mixed with stearic acid. Found in many animal fats and plant oils. In shampoos, shaving soaps, creams. Derivatives: Palmitate, Palmitamine, Palmitamide. Alternatives: palm oil, vegetable sources.

Panthenol. Dexpanthenol. Vitamin B-Complex Factor. Provitamin B-5. Can come from animal or plant sources or synthetics. In shampoos, supplements, emollients, etc. In foods. Derivative: Panthenyl. Alternatives: synthetics, plants.

Panthenyl. (See Panthenol.)

Pepsin. In hogs' stomachs. A clotting agent. In some cheeses and vitamins. Same uses and alternatives as Rennet.

Placenta. Placenta Polypeptides Protein. Afterbirth. Animal placenta is widely used in skin creams, shampoos, masks, etc.Alternatives: kelp. (See alternatives to Animal Fats and Oils.)

Polyglycerol. (See Glycerin.)

Polysorbates. Derivatives of fatty acids. In cosmetics, foods.

Pristane. Obtained from the liver oil of sharks and from whale ambergris. (See Squalene, Ambergris.) Used as a lubricant and anti-corrosive agent. In cosmetics. Alternatives: plant oils, synthetics.

Progesterone. A steroid hormone used in anti-wrinkle face creams. Can have adverse systemic effects. Alternatives: synthetics.

Propolis. Tree sap gathered by bees and used as a sealant in beehives. In toothpaste, shampoo, deodorant, supplements, etc. Alternatives: tree sap, synthetics.

Provitamin A. (See Carotene.)

Provitamin B-5. (See Panthenol.)

Provitamin D-2. (See Vitamin D.)

Rennet. Rennin. Enzyme from calves' stomachs. Used in cheese-making, rennet custard (junket), and in many coagulated dairy products. Alternatives: microbial coagulating agents, bacteria culture, lemon juice, or vegetable rennet.

Rennin. (See Rennet.)

Resinous Glaze. (See Shellac.)
Ribonucleic Acid. (See RNA.)
RNA. Ribonucleic Acid. RNA is in all living cells. Used in many protein shampoos and cosmetics.
Royal Jelly.
Sable Brushes. From the fur of sables (weasel-like mammals). Used to make eye makeup, lipstick, and artists' brushes. Alternatives: synthetic fibers.
Sea Turtle Oil. (See Turtle Oil.)
Shark Liver Oil. Used in lubricating creams and lotions. Derivatives: Squalane, Squalene. Alternatives: vegetable oils.
Sheepskin. (See Leather.)
Shellac. Resinous Glaze. Resinous excretion of certain insects. Used as a candy glaze, in hair lacquer, and on jewelry. Alternatives: plant waxes.
Silk. Silk Powder.
Snails. In some cosmetics (crushed).
Sodium Caseinate. (See Casein.)
Sodium Steroyl Lactylate. (See Lactic Acid.)
Sodium Tallowate. (See Tallow.)
Spermaceti. Cetyl Palmitate. Sperm Oil. Waxy oil derived from the sperm whale's head or from dolphins. In many margarines. In skin creams, ointments, shampoos, candles, etc. Used in the leather industry. May become rancid and cause irritations. Alternatives: synthetic spermaceti, jojoba oil, and other vegetable emollients.
Sponge (Luna and Sea). A plant-like animal. Lives in the sea. Becoming scarce. Alternatives: synthetic sponges, loofahs (plants used as sponges).
Squalane. (See Shark Liver Oil.)
Squalene. Oil from shark livers, etc. In cosmetics, moisturizers, hair dyes, surface-active agents. Alternatives: vegetable emollients such as olive oil, wheat germ oil, rice bran oil, etc.
Stearamide. (See Stearic Acid.)
Stearamine. (See Stearic Acid.)
Stearamine Oxide. (See Stearyl Alcohol.)

Stearates. (See Stearic Acid.)
Stearic Acid. Fat from cows and sheep and from dogs and cats euthanized in animal shelters, etc. Most often refers to a fatty substance taken from the stomachs of pigs. Can be harsh, irritating. Used in cosmetics, soaps, lubricants, candles, hairspray, conditioners, deodorants, creams, chewing gum, food flavoring. Derivatives: Stearamide, Stearamine, Stearates, Stearic Hydrazide, Stearone, Stearoxytrimethylsilane, Stearoyl Lactylic Acid, Stearyl Betaine, Stearyl Imidazoline. Alternatives: Stearic acid can be found in many vegetable fats, coconut.
Stearic Hydrazide. (See Stearic Acid.)
Stearone. (See Stearic Acid.)
Stearoxytrimethylsilane. (See Stearic Acid.)
Stearoyl Lactylic Acid. (See Stearic Acid.)
Stearyl Acetate. (See Stearyl Alcohol.)
Stearyl Alcohol. Sterols. A mixture of solid alcohols. Can be prepared from sperm whale oil. In medicines, creams, rinses, shampoos, etc. Derivatives: Stearamine Oxide, Stearyl Acetate, Stearyl Caprylate, Stearyl Citrate, Stearyldimethyl Amine, Stearyl Glycyrrhetinate, Stearyl Heptanoate, Stearyl Octanoate, Stearyl Stearate. Alternatives: plant sources, vegetable stearic acid.
Stearyl Betaine. (See Stearic Acid.)
Stearyl Caprylate. (See Stearyl Alcohol.)
Stearyl Citrate. (See Stearyl Alcohol.)
Stearyldimethyl Amine. (See Stearyl Alcohol.)
Stearyl Glycyrrhetinate. (See Stearyl Alcohol.)
Stearyl Heptanoate. (See Stearyl Alcohol.)
Stearyl Imidazoline. (See Stearic Acid.)
Stearyl Octanoate. (See Stearyl Alcohol.)
Stearyl Stearate. (See Stearyl Alcohol.)
Steroids. Sterols. From various animal glands or from plant tissues. Steroids

include sterols. Sterols are alcohol from animals or plants (e.g., cholesterol). Used in hormone preparation. In creams, lotions, hair conditioners, fragrances, etc. Alternatives: plant tissues, synthetics.

Sterols. (See Stearyl Alcohol and Steroids.)

Suede. (See Leather.)

Tallow. Tallow Fatty Alcohol. Stearic Acid. Rendered beef fat. May cause eczema and blackheads. In wax paper, crayons, margarines, paints, rubber, lubricants, etc. In candles, soaps, lipsticks, shaving creams, other cosmetics. Chemicals (e.g., PCB) can be in animal tallow. Derivatives: Sodium Tallowate, Tallow Acid, Tallow Amide, Tallow Amine, Talloweth-6, Tallow Glycerides, Tallow Imidazoline. Alternatives: vegetable tallow, Japan tallow, paraffin and/or ceresin. Paraffin is usually from petroleum, wood, coal, or shale oil.

Tallow Acid. (See Tallow.)

Tallow Amide. (See Tallow.)

Tallow Amine. (See Tallow.)

Talloweth-6. (See Tallow.)

Tallow Glycerides. (See Tallow.)

Tallow Imidazoline. (See Tallow.)

Triterpene Alcohols. (See Lanolin.)

Turtle Oil. Sea Turtle Oil. From the muscles and genitals of giant sea turtles. In soap, skin creams, nail creams, other cosmetics. Alternatives: vegetable emollients (see alternatives to Animal Fats and Oils).

Tyrosine. Amino acid hydrolyzed from casein. Used in cosmetics and creams. Derivative: Glucose Tyrosinase.

Urea. Carbamide. Excreted from urine and other bodily fluids. In deodorants, ammoniated dentifrices, mouthwashes, hair colorings, hand creams, lotions, shampoos, etc. Used to "brown" baked goods, such as pretzels. Derivatives: Imidazolidinyl Urea, Uric Acid. Alternatives: synthetics.

Uric Acid. (See Urea.)

Vitamin A. Can come from fish liver oil (e.g., shark liver oil), egg yolk, butter, lemongrass, wheat germ oil, carotene in carrots, and synthetics. It is an aliphatic alcohol. In cosmetics, creams, perfumes, hair dyes, etc. In vitamins, supplements. Alternatives: carrots, other vegetables, synthetics.

Vitamin B-Complex Factor. (See Panthenol.)

Vitamin B Factor. (See Biotin.)

Vitamin B-12. Usually animal source. Alternatives: some vegetarian B-12-fortified yeasts and analogs available. Some nutritionists caution that fortified foods or supplements are essential.

Vitamin D. Ergocalciferol. Vitamin D-2. Ergosterol. Provitamin D-2. Calciferol. Vitamin D-3. Vitamin D can come from fish liver oil, milk, egg yolk, etc. Vitamin D-2 can come from animal fats or plant sterols. Vitamin D-3 is always from an animal source. All the D vitamins can be in creams, lotions, other cosmetics, vitamin tablets, etc. Alternatives: plant and mineral sources, synthetics, completely vegetarian vitamins, exposure of skin to sunshine. Many other vitamins can come from animal sources. Examples: choline, biotin, inositol, riboflavin, etc.

Vitamin H. (See Biotin.)

Wax. Glossy, hard substance that is soft when hot. From animals and plants. In lipsticks, depilatories, hair straighteners. Alternatives: vegetable waxes.

Whey. A serum from milk. Usually in cakes, cookies, candies, and breads. In cheese-making. Alternatives: soybean whey.

Wool.

Wool Fat. (See Lanolin.)

Wool Wax. (See Lanolin.)

AUTHOR BIOGRAPHIES

AFYA IBOMU is a Certified Holistic Health Counselor, Author, Freelance Journalist, Entrepreneur, Crochet Artist and Nutritionist. Afya is currently the CEO of her holistic lifestyle company, Nattral Unlimited, LLC and holds a bachelor's degree in nutrition. She is also the managing editor of her online magazine *Nattral Magazine*. Afya recently released her book *Vegan Soulfood Guide to the Galaxy* and continues to teach cooking classes and health workshops around the country.

AIYA ABRIHET is a former radio host and motivational speaker. A raw vegan diet cured her of severe asthma and allergies and brought about a near full recovery in her son who was diagnosed with autism. She is an herbalist-in-training, holistic mentor and vegan chef, pursuing her masters of science in herbal medicine.

C'BS ALIFE ALLAH started his journey into natural living growing up as an asthmatic child. A simple change in diet allowed him to become a state champion and letterman in Track and Field during high school. Since that time, he has been on a journey towards pure vegetarianism, sunlight, raw food and non-processed goodies. He is an opponent of dietary racism, environmental racism, ignorance and sloppy living. He is a full time advocate of Original people "taking it back to the basics" in terms of their health and seeing how they can fit what worked in the past into the present.

C. WISE "TAWA" HAAKIM ALLAH attended the Academy of Massage Therapy and Rising Spirit Institute of Natural Health. He is a Certified Reflexologist, Meditation Guide, Yoga Instructor, Raw/Live food advocate, and trained Chi Master. He specializes in systematic ways to assist people in the transition to Holistic Living.

CY has been a raw food practitioner and advocate for the past five years and vegan for the last ten. She is a firm believer in holistic health and has modeled and taught health practices locally and internationally. She has a connection with Latin American and Caribbean health issues and sees achieving radiant health as the most universal and radical goal that anyone can strive for, and a great infusion for any form of activism. She lives in Brooklyn, NY.

DENIZ LOPEZ is an artist, poet, and activist who has worked for over 6 years to bring the message of revolution and inner strength into community consciousness. She has helped organize events in the Houston area, dealing with the abolition of the death penalty, an end to police brutality, empowerment of women, migrant rights, Black/Brown unity, and indigenous pride. Once adopting the ancient Mexica way of life known as Mexicayotl, Deniz began to explore the parallels between mental and physical health and through learning her own body, has begun to teach others the process of learning theirs.

DR. NANCY J. WILLIAMS is a Holistic Detox Expert and the Visionary/CEO of First Fruit Natural Healing Home, an oasis sitting on 5 beautiful acres, located just 20 minutes from downtown Atlanta, Georgia. Founded on a mission to help others to heal body, mind and soul, a place to experience relaxation, positive atmosphere and therapeutic treatments. Dr. Nancy is also an accomplished author with an e-book series called *Detoxing Into A New You*.

DR. SCOTT WHITAKER is a board certified naturopathic doctor with over 20 years of experience in herbology, iridology, homeopathy, natural healing and detoxification. Over the years, Dr. Whitaker has traveled throughout the world learning and applying the healing sciences of China, Asia Minor, North Africa, and Southeast Asia to correct the maladies of our modern time. He is a sought-after lecturer that can be heard nationwide uncovering the myths associated with holistic medicine. He is also the co-author of the best-selling *Medisin*.

EARTH EM'MAYA JEWEL is the founder of Tendaheadz Holistic Livity, a seedling health counseling company that advocates healthy, wholesome lifestyles. They are based out of Mississippi where she shares her wealth of information within her own community. She is currently working toward building her practice into a nonprofit organization.

EBONI JOY is an award winning poet and freelance writer, and since 1999 has used her independent Zine, *The 14th Degree and Beyond Magazine*, to raise awareness about holistic health care, vegetarianism, environmentalism, and political issues affecting the African Diaspora. She has helped organize numerous "Feed The People" outings, Poets 4 Political Prisoners, Happily Natural Day Atlanta, and Black August Weekend.

GENIALLY GREEN EARTH (Queen Jade Osorio) is a timeless sistah who has experienced the very best and worst New York City has to offer. Through self-directed and professional study she has obtained a wealth of information concerning proper nutrition and holistic health. She is a certified instructor of the Living Foods Lifestyle and currently a student of Traditional Chinese Medicine. In her free time, Genially enjoys traveling, discovering new ways to refine self, and working on her home garden.

KING DIVINE ALLAH (David Williams) graduated from Bethune Cookman University in 2009 with a B.S. in Physical Education. He currently works as a Youth Director in Deland, Florida.

LETITIA SALAZAR MONK lives in Denver, Colorado. She is a practicing Herbalist and Massage Therapist with focused training in women's health including labor support. Her background and experience are rooted in the cultural tradition of Curanderismo. Letitia is an active grower and organizer for the Eastside Growers Collective of Northeast Denver and Delany Farm.

MENTAL SUN is a producer, director, rapper, graphics and clothing designer, vegan chef and the mastermind behind VeganHood TV and Art of Facts Clothing Company. Vegan for over half of his life, Mental Sun touches lives through educational and entertaining episodes of VeganHood TV, where he shows members of the Black community firsthand that you don't have to be rich to live and eat well.

QUEEN CIVILIZED ZAG has been in the Nation of Gods and Earths for over 10 years. She is a staff member and writer for *The 14th Degree and Beyond*, a magazine for Original women. She is also a songwriter and author working on her first novel, *Welcome to Me.*

QUEEN RIGHTEOUSLY REFINED (Tovah J. Hicks) is a 32-year-old mother of three daughters. She embraced healthy living when she acquired knowledge of self as a member of the Nation of Islam between the years of 2003-2005, ultimately becoming a member of the Nation of Gods and Earths in 2007. QRR is a Gary, Indiana native and now currently resides in the Twin Cities area of Minnesota, where she works to educate and improve the community around her.

SCIHONOR DEVOTION is a certified Childbirth Educator, a certified Labor Doula, certified Postpartum Doula and a Homebirth Midwife Assistant. She has been vegan since 2004 and Vegetarian since 1998. SciHonor has been a staff member and writer for the *14th Degree and Beyond* magazine for over a decade and is currently working on her upcoming parenting book entitled, *Even Without the Village.* She is also a homeschooling mother of her two children in Connecticut.

SEIDAH WILLIAMS is a Holistic Health Consultant and Iridologist. She is also CoFounder/President of The People's Lunch Counter, a nonprofit serving the needs of the poor in Dallas, Texas.

SINCERE JUSTICE ALLAH grew up in a traditional Chinese household that practiced the eastern Five Element theory of health, including diet and lifestyle choices. At 17, he challenged himself to practice a vegetarian lifestyle for a year. Since then, he has observed a holistic, plant-based diet for 6 years, practices meditation and has developed a recent interest in martial arts.

THE 14TH DEGREE AND BEYOND is a publication dedicated to furthering and nurturing the strength of Original women and children through education. 14th Degree and Beyond, Inc. is also involved in sponsoring, facilitating, and educating through classes and events throughout the community.

ZAFIRAH AQUEOUS EQUALITY is a graduate of York College who is pursuing a career in nursing. She has been a vegetarian for 7 years and is raising vegetarian children. She is passionate about disseminating information about disease and health care.

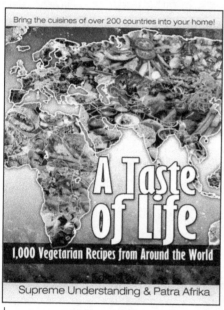

INDEX

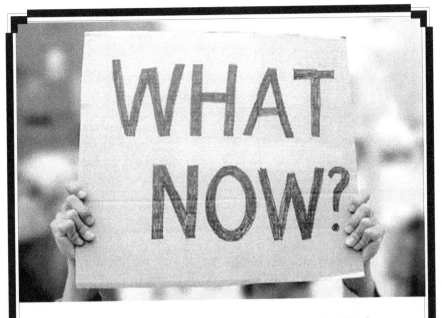

What should you do now that you're done reading?
Here are some suggestions:

- [ ] Complete any activities mentioned in this book, especially the discussions. See any of the films mentioned, but with others.
- [ ] Tell somebody about this book and what you've learned. Invite them to come read it. Don't let them steal the book.
- [ ] As another option, let them steal the book. It might help them.
- [ ] Mentor some young people or teach a class using this book as a handbook or reference.
- [ ] Talk about this book online, but don't stay on the Net forever.
- [ ] Join an organization or group that discusses concepts like the ones in this book and get into those discussions.
- [ ] Leave this book away somewhere it will be picked up and read.
- [ ] Identify the people in your community who could use a copy of this book. If they're people would want to buy a book like this, let em read a few pages and see if they can afford to buy a copy.

- [ ] If they're people who don't normally buy books – but you know that givin em a copy could change their life – give em a copy and tell em to come see you when they're ready for another one. This is why you can order copies at wholesale rates at our site.

We hope this helps you keep the knowledge contagious.

ALSO FROM OUR COMPANY

How to Hustle and Win, Part 1: A Survival Guide for the Ghetto

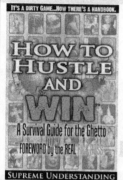

By Supreme Understanding
Foreword by the Real Rick Ross

This is the book that started it all. Now an international bestseller, this book has revolutionized the way people think of "urban literature." It offers a street-based analysis of social problems, plus practical solutions that anyone can put to use.

CLASS	PAGES	RETAIL	RELEASE
I-1	336	$14.95	Jun. 2008

ISBN: 978-0-9816170-0-8

How to Hustle and Win, Part 2: Rap, Race, and Revolution

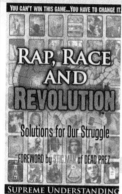

By Supreme Understanding
Foreword by Stic.man of Dead Prez

Seen here in its original green cover, the controversial follow-up to *How to Hustle and Win* digs even deeper into the problems we face, and how we can solve them. Part One focused on personal change, and Part Two explores the bigger picture of changing the entire hood.

CLASS	PAGES	RETAIL	RELEASE
I-1	384	$14.95	Apr. 2009

ISBN: 978-0-9816170-9-1

Knowledge of Self: A Collection of Wisdom on the Science of Everything in Life

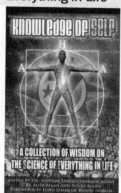

Edited by Supreme Understanding, C'BS Alife Allah, and Sunez Allah, Foreword by Lord Jamar of Brand Nubian

Who are the Five Percent? Why are they here? In this book, over 50 Five Percenters from around the world speak for themselves, providing a comprehensive introduction to the esoteric teachings of the Nation of Gods and Earths.

CLASS	PAGES	RETAIL	RELEASE
I-2	256	$14.95	Jul. 2009

ISBN: 978-0-9816170-2-2

The Hood Health Handbook, Volume One (Physical Health)

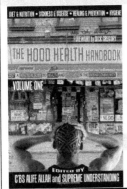

Edited by Supreme Understanding and C'BS Alife Allah, Foreword by Dick Gregory

Want to know why Black and brown people are so sick? This book covers the many "unnatural causes" behind our poor health, and offers hundreds of affordable and easy-to-implement solutions.

CLASS	PAGES	RETAIL	RELEASE
PH-1	480	$19.95	Nov. 2010

ISBN: 978-1-935721-32-1

The Hood Health Handbook, Volume Two (Mental Health)

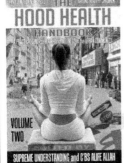

Edited by Supreme Understanding and C'BS Alife Allah

This volume covers mental health, how to keep a healthy home, raising healthy children, environmental issues, and dozens of other issues, all from the same down-to-earth perspective as Volume One.

CLASS	PAGES	RETAIL	RELEASE
MH-1	480_	$19.95	Nov. 2010

ISBN: 978-1-935721-33-8

A Taste of Life: 1,000 Vegetarian Recipes from Around the World

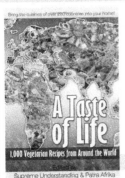

Edited by Supreme Understanding and Patra Afrika

This cookbook makes it easy to become vegetarian. In addition to over 1,000 recipes from everywhere you can think of, plus over 100 drink and smoothie recipes, this book also teaches how to transition your diet, what to shop for, how to cook, as well as a guide to nutrients and vitamins.

CLASS	PAGES	RETAIL	RELEASE
W-1	400	$19.95	Jun. 2011

ISBN: 978-1-935721-10-9

La Brega: Como Sobrevivir En El Barrio

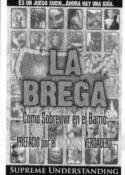

By Supreme Understanding

Thanks to strong demand coming from Spanish-speaking countries, we translated our groundbreaking How to Hustle and Win into Spanish, and added new content specific to Latin America. Because this book's language is easy to follow, it can also be used to brush up on your Spanish.

CLASS	PAGES	RETAIL	RELEASE
O-1	336	$14.95	Jul. 2009

ISBN: 978-0981617-08-4

Locked Up but Not Locked Down: A Guide to Surviving the American Prison System

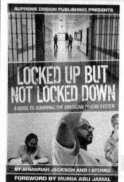

By Ahmariah Jackson and IAtomic Allah
Foreword by Mumia Abu Jamal

This book covers what it's like on the inside, how to make the most of your time, what to do once you're out, and how to stay out. Features contributions from over 50 insiders, covering city jails, state and federal prisons, women's prisons, juvenile detention, and international prisons.

CLASS	PAGES	RETAIL	RELEASE
J-1	288	$14.95	Jul. 2012

ISBN: 978-1935721-00-0

The Science of Self: Man, God, and the Mathematical Language of Nature

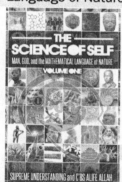

By Supreme Understanding and C'BS Alife Allah

How did the universe begin? Is there a pattern to everything that happens? What's the meaning of life? What does science tell us about the depths of our SELF? Who and what is God? This may be one of the deepest books you can read.

CLASS	PAGES	RETAIL	RELEASE
I-4	360	$19.95	Jun. 2012

ISBN: 978-1935721-67-3

The Science of Self: Man, God, and the Mathematical Language of Nature (Hardcover Edition)

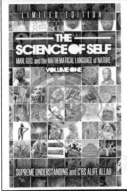

By Supreme Understanding

A beautiful hardcover edition of the bestselling work, *The Science of Self*. Under the full-color dust jacket is an embossed clothbound hard cover. Autographed and numbered as part of a special limited edition series, this book also includes the 16 full-color inserts found in the paperback edition.

CLASS	PAGES	RETAIL	RELEASE
I-4	360	$34.95	Jun. 2012

Only available direct from publisher.

365 Days of Real Black History Calendar (2012 Edition)

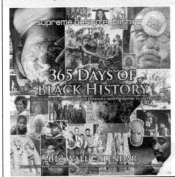

By Supreme Understanding and Robert Bailey

A calendar that'll never be out-dated! Over 365 important facts and quotes covering little-known, but important, moments in Black history. Written in brief chunks and easy language for all audiences.

CLASS	PGS	PRICE	RELEASE
I-2	26	$2.95	2011

Only available direct from publisher.

365 Days of Real Black History Calendar (2013 Edition)

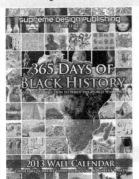

By Supreme Understanding

Our 2013 calendar and planner was also designed to be timeless, as it's a beautifully-designed companion to *When the World was Black*. You'll find dozens of striking full-color images that help tell the stories of global Black history.

CLASS	PAGES	PRICE	RELEASE
I-2	26	$4.95	2012

Only available direct from publisher.

When the World was Black, Part One: Prehistoric Cultures

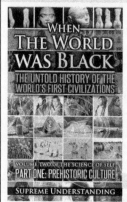

By Supreme Understanding
Foreword by Runoko Rashid

When does Black history begin? Certainly not with slavery. In two volumes, historian Supreme Understanding explores over 200,000 years of Black history from every corner of the globe. Part One covers the first Black communities to settle the world, establishing its first cultures and traditions. Their stories are remarkable.

CLASS	PAGES	RETAIL	RELEASE
I-3	400	$19.95	Feb. 2013

ISBN: 978-1-935721-04-8

When the World Was Black, Part Two: Ancient Civilizations

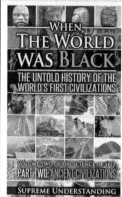

By Supreme Understanding

Part Two covers the ancient Black civilizations that gave birth to the modern world. Black people built the first urban civilizations in Africa, Asia, Europe, and the Americas. And every claim in these books is thoroughly documented with reputable sources. Do you want to know the story of your ancestors? You should. We study the past to see what the future will bring.

CLASS	PAGES	RETAIL	RELEASE
I-3	400	$19.95	Feb. 2013

ISBN: 978-1-935721-05-5

When the World was Black, Parts One and Two (Hardcover)

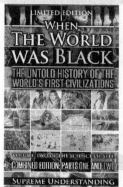

By Supreme Understanding

An incredible limited edition that combines Part One and Part Two into a single book, cased in an embossed clothbound hardcover and dust jacket. Autographed and numbered, this collector's item also includes both sets of full-color inserts.

CLASS	PAGES	RETAIL	RELEASE
I-3	800	$19.95	Dec. 2013

Only available direct from publisher.

Black Rebellion: Eyewitness Accounts of Major Slave Revolts

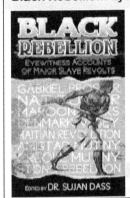

Edited by Dr. Sujan Dass

Who will tell the stories of those who refused to be slaves? What about those who fought so effectively that they forced their slavers to give up? Black Rebellion is a collection of historical "eyewitness" accounts of dozens of major revolts and uprisings, from the U.S. to the Caribbean, as well as a history of slavery and revolt.

CLASS	PAGES	RETAIL	RELEASE
P-3	272	$14.95	May 2010

ISBN: 978-0-981617-04-6

The Heroic Slave

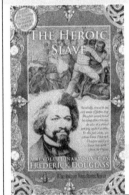

By Frederick Douglass

Most people don't know that Douglass wrote a novel...or that, in this short novel, he promoted the idea of violent revolt. By this time in his life, the renowned abolitionist was seeing things differently. This important piece of history comes with *David Walker's Appeal*, all in one book.

CLASS	PAGES	RETAIL	RELEASE
P-3	160	$14.95	Apr. 2011

ISBN: 978-1-935721-27-7

David Walker's Appeal

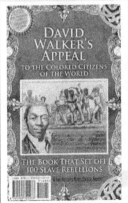

By David Walker

This is one of the most important, and radical, works ever published against slavery. Rather than call for an end by peaceful means, Walker called for outright revolution. His calls may have led to over 100 revolts, including those described in *Black Rebellion*. This important piece of history comes with Douglass' *The Heroic Slave*, which it may have helped inspire.

CLASS	PAGES	RETAIL	RELEASE
P-3	160	$14.95	Apr. 2011

ISBN: 978-1-935721-27-7

Darkwater: Voices from Within the Veil, Annotated Edition

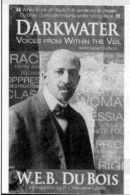

By W.E.B. Du Bois

This book makes Du Bois' previous work, like *Souls of Black Folk*, seem tame by comparison. *Darkwater* is revolutionary, uncompromising, and unconventional in both its content and style, addressing the plight of Black women, the rise of a Black Messiah, a critical analysis of white folks, and the need for outright revolution.

CLASS	PAGES	RETAIL	RELEASE
I-4	240	$14.95	Jun. 2011

ISBN: 978-0-981617-07-7

The African Abroad: The Black Man's Evolution in Western Civilization, Volume One

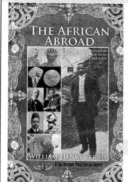

By William Henry Ferris

Who would think a book written in 1911 could cover so much? Ferris, chairman of the UNIA, speaks up for the Black man's role in Western civilization. He discusses a wealth of history, as well as some revolutionary Black theology, exploring the idea of man as God and God as man.

CLASS	PAGES	RETAIL	RELEASE
I-5	570	$29.95	Oct. 2012

ISBN: 978-1935721-66-6

The African Abroad: Volume Two

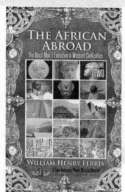

By William Henry Ferris

The second volume of Ferris' epic covers important Black biographies of great leaders, ancient and modern. He tells the stories of forty "Black Immortals." He also identifies the African origins of many of the world's civilizations, including ancient Egypt, Akkad, Sumer, India, and Europe.

CLASS	PAGES	RETAIL	RELEASE
I-5	330	$19.95	Oct. 2012

ISBN: 978-1-935721-69-7

From Poverty to Power: The Realization of Prosperity and Peace

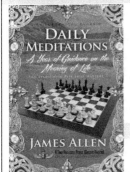

By James Allen

Want to transform your life? James Allen, the author of the classic *As a Man Thinketh,* explores how we can turn struggle and adversity into power and prosperity. This inspirational text teaches readers about their innate strength and the immense power of the conscious mind.

CLASS	PAGES	RETAIL	RELEASE
I-3	144	$14.95	May 2010

ISBN: 978-0-981617-05-3

Daily Meditations: A Year of Guidance on the Meaning of Life

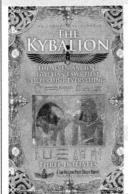

By James Allen

Need a guidebook to a productive and healthy year? This is it. James Allen delivers another great work in this book, this time offering 365 days of inspiration and guidance on life's greatest challenges. This book includes sections for daily notes.

CLASS	PAGES	RETAIL	RELEASE
C-3	208	$14.95	Apr. 2013

ISBN: 978-1-935721-08-6

The Kybalion: The Seven Ancient Egyptian Laws _

By the Three Initiates

Thousands of years ago, the ancients figured out a set of principles that govern the universe. In *The Kybalion*, these laws are explored and explained. This edition includes research into the authorship of the book, and where the laws came from.

CLASS	PAGES	RETAIL	RELEASE
C-4	130	$14.95	Oct. 2012

ISBN: 978-1-935721-25-3

Real Life is No Fairy Tale (w/ Companion CD)

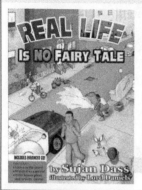

By Sujan Dass and Lord Williams

Looking for a children's book that teaches about struggle? Written for school age children, this full-color hardcover book is composed entirely in rhyme, and the images are as real as they get. Includes a CD with an audio book, animated video, review questions, and printable worksheets and activities.

CLASS	PGS	RETAIL	RELEASE
CD-4	36+	$16.95	Jun. 2010

ISBN: 978-0-9816170-2-2

Aesop's Fables: 101 Classic Tales and Timeless Lessons

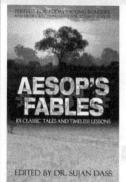

Edited by Dr. Sujan Dass

What's better to teach our children than life lessons? This easy-to-read collection of classic tales told by an African storyteller uses animals to teach valuable moral lessons. This edition includes dozens of black-and-white images to accompany the timeless fables. Color them in!

CLASS	PAGES	RETAIL	RELEASE
CD-3	112	$14.95	Feb. 2013

ISBN: 978-1-935721-07-9

Heritage Playing Cards (w/ Companion Booklet)

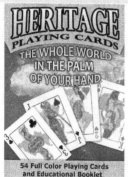

Designed by Sujan Dass

No more European royalty! This beautiful deck of playing cards features 54 full-color characters from around the world and a 16-page educational booklet on international card games and the ethnic backgrounds of the people on the cards.

CLASS	PGS	RETAIL	RELEASE
CD-2	16+	$6.95	May 2010

UPC: 05105-38587

Black God: An Introduction to the World's Religions and their Black Gods

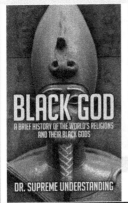

By Supreme Understanding

Have you ever heard that Christ was Black? What about the Buddha? They weren't alone. This book explores the many Black gods of the ancient world, from Africa to Europe, Asia, and Australia, all the way to the Americas. Who were they? Why were they worshipped? And what does this mean for us today?

CLASS	PAGES	RETAIL	RELEASE
C-3	200	$19.95	Jan. 2014

ISBN: 978-1-935721-12-3

Black People Invented Everything

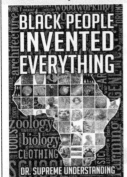

By Supreme Understanding

In *The Science of Self* we began exploring the origins of everything that modern civilization depends on today. In this book, we get into specifics, showing how Black people invented everything from agriculture to zoology, with dozens of pictures and references to prove it!

CLASS	PAGES	RETAIL	RELEASE
I-3	180	$14.95	Feb. 2014

NOT YET PUBLISHED

The Yogi Science of Breath: A Complete Manual of the Ancient Philosophy of the East

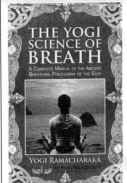

By Yogi Ramacharaka

A classic text on the science of breathing, one of the most ignored, yet important, aspects of our physical and emotional health. This book has been used by both martial arts experts and legendary jazz musicians. This edition explores the "secret science" of breath, and where its mysterious author learned such teachings.

CLASS	PAGES	RETAIL	RELEASE
PH-4	112	$14.95	Apr. 2012

ISBN: 978-1-935721-34-5

How to Get Our Books

To better serve our readers, we've streamlined the way we handle book orders. Here are some of the ways you can find our books.

In Stores

You can find our books in just about any Black bookstore or independent bookseller. If you don't find our titles on the shelves, just request them by name and publisher. Most bookstores can order our titles directly from us (via our site) or from the distributors listed below. We also provide a listing of retailers who carry our books at www.bestblackbooks.com

Online (Wholesale)

Now, you can visit our sites (like www.supremeunderstanding.com or www.bestblackbooks.com) to order wholesale quantities direct from us, the publisher. From our site, we ship heavily discounted case quantities to distributors, wholesalers, retailers, and local independent resellers (like yourself – just try it!). The discounts are so deep, you can afford to GIVE books away if you're not into making money.

Online (Retail)

If you're interested in single "retail" copies, you can now find them online at Amazon.com, or you can order them via mail order by contacting one of the mail order distributors listed below. You can also find many of our titles as eBooks in the Amazon Kindle, Nook, or Apple iBooks systems. You may also find full-length videobook or audiobook files available, but nothing beats the pass-around potential of a real book!

By Mail Order

Please contact any of the following Black-owned distributors to order our books! For others, visit our site.

Afrikan World Books
2217 Pennsylvania Ave.
Baltimore, MD 21217
(410) 383-2006

Lushena Books
607 Country Club Dr
Bensenville, IL 60106
(800) 785-1545

Special Needs X-Press
3128 Villa Ave
Bronx, NY 10468
(718) 220-3786